METHODS IN MOLECULAR BIOLOGY

Series Editor
John M. Walker
School of Life and Medical Sciences
University of Hertfordshire
Hatfield, Hertfordshire, UK

For further volumes:
http://www.springer.com/series/7651

For over 35 years, biological scientists have come to rely on the research protocols and methodologies in the critically acclaimed *Methods in Molecular Biology* series. The series was the first to introduce the step-by-step protocols approach that has become the standard in all biomedical protocol publishing. Each protocol is provided in readily-reproducible step-by-step fashion, opening with an introductory overview, a list of the materials and reagents needed to complete the experiment, and followed by a detailed procedure that is supported with a helpful notes section offering tips and tricks of the trade as well as troubleshooting advice. These hallmark features were introduced by series editor Dr. John Walker and constitute the key ingredient in each and every volume of the *Methods in Molecular Biology* series. Tested and trusted, comprehensive and reliable, all protocols from the series are indexed in PubMed.

Esophageal Squamous Cell Carcinoma

Methods and Protocols

Edited by

Alfred K. Lam

Cancer Molecular Pathology, School of Medicine, Griffith University, Gold Coast, Queensland, Australia

Humana Press

Editor
Alfred K. Lam
Cancer Molecular Pathology
School of Medicine
Griffith University
Gold Coast, Queensland, Australia

ISSN 1064-3745 ISSN 1940-6029 (electronic)
Methods in Molecular Biology
ISBN 978-1-0716-0376-5 ISBN 978-1-0716-0377-2 (eBook)
https://doi.org/10.1007/978-1-0716-0377-2

This Humana imprint is published by the registered company Springer Science+Business Media, LLC, part of Springer Nature.
The registered company address is: 1 New York Plaza, New York, NY 10004, U.S.A.

Preface

Oesophageal cancer, especially the squamous cell carcinoma type, is one of the most commonly occurring cancer worldwide. The aim of the book is to provide the current management and research protocols of oesophageal squamous cell carcinoma with the objective to identify the materials available for molecular biological research. Also, different research protocols are provided to improve the understanding of pathogenesis as well as improvement of the care of patients with oesophageal squamous cell carcinoma. Target audience of the book could include diverse groups of medical science students, medical students, academics, researchers and multidisciplinary team in management of oesophageal squamous cell carcinoma such as pathologists, gastroenterologists, gastrointestinal surgeons and oncologists.

Chapter 1 introduces the characteristics and the potential of improvement of management of patients with oesophageal squamous cell carcinoma. This chapter guides the readers to explore the other chapters of the book. Chapters 2–6 illustrate the clinical and pathological diagnostic information of oesophageal squamous cell carcinoma which comprises histopathology, staging, macroscopic examination, endoscopic diagnosis biopsy and resection. Chapters 7–10 identify the resources for translational research for oesophageal squamous cell carcinoma—including frozen sectioning, biobanking, whole section imaging and tissue microarray. Chapters 11 and 12 introduce the animal models for studying of the cancer. Chapters 13–21 highlights the different research approaches in studying oesophageal squamous cell carcinoma including detection of cancer stem cells, in vitro assays, liquid biopsy for cancer DNA and circulating tumour cells, genomic analysis, miRNAs and proteins (mass spectrometry, Western blotting and immunohistochemistry). Finally, it is important to aware of the current treatment protocols of oesophageal squamous cell carcinoma including radiotherapy, systemic therapy, surgical as well as anaesthetic management as presented in Chapters 22–26.

By using this book, the readers will understand the most updated information of different aspects of the processes, cost and resources available for research and management of patients with oesophageal squamous cell carcinoma. Increasing awareness and promoting research in this area will certainly translate to improving the management of oesophageal squamous cell carcinoma of high prevalence.

I thank all the authors for their invaluable contributions.

Gold Coast, Queensland, Australia *Alfred K. Lam*

Contents

Contributors

EVA Y. F. CHAN • *Department of Anaesthesiology, University of Hong Kong, Queen Mary Hospital, Pok Fu Lam, Hong Kong*
WENDY W. L. CHAN • *Department of Clinical Oncology, LKS Faculty of Medicine, The University of Hong Kong, Pok Fu Lam, Hong Kong; Clinical Oncology Centre, The University of Hong Kong-Shenzhen Hospital, Shenzhen, China*
SATOSHI FUJII • *Division of Pathology, Exploratory Oncology Research & Clinical Trial Center, National Cancer Center, Kashiwa, Chiba, Japan*
VINOD GOPALAN • *Cancer Molecular Pathology, School of Medicine, Griffith University, Gold Coast, Queensland, Australia*
FAYSAL BIN HAMID • *Cancer Molecular Pathology, School of Medicine, Griffith University, Gold Coast, Queensland, Australia*
DANNY K. Y. IP • *Department of Anaesthesiology, University of Hong Kong, Queen Mary Hospital, Pok Fu Lam, Hong Kong*
JOSEPH C. Y. IP • *Department of Clinical Oncology, Li Ka Shing Faculty of Medicine, The University of Hong Kong, Pokfulam, Hong Kong; Vium Inc., San Mateo, CA, USA*
MICHAEL G. IRWIN • *Department of Anaesthesiology, University of Hong Kong, Queen Mary Hospital, Pok Fu Lam, Hong Kong*
FARHADUL ISLAM • *Cancer Molecular Pathology, School of Medicine, Griffith University, Gold Coast, Queensland, Australia; Department of Biochemistry and Molecular Biology, University of Rajshahi, Rajshahi, Bangladesh*
KAIS KASEM • *Clinical Pathology Department, Melbourne Medical School, University of Melbourne, Melbourne, VIC, Australia*
JOSEPHINE M. Y. KO • *Department of Clinical Oncology, Li Ka Shing Faculty of Medicine, The University of Hong Kong, Pokfulam, Hong Kong; Vium Inc., San Mateo, CA, USA*
DORA L. W. KWONG • *Department of Clinical Oncology, LKS Faculty of Medicine, The University of Hong Kong, Pok Fu Lam, Hong Kong; Clinical Oncology Centre, The University of Hong Kong-Shenzhen Hospital, Shenzhen, China*
ALFRED K. LAM • *Cancer Molecular Pathology, School of Medicine, Griffith University, Gold Coast, Queensland, Australia*
KA ON LAM • *Department of Clinical Oncology, LKS Faculty of Medicine, The University of Hong Kong, Pok Fu Lam, Hong Kong; Clinical Oncology Centre, The University of Hong Kong-Shenzhen Hospital, Shenzhen, China*
LOUIS H. S. LAU • *Division of Gastroenterology and Hepatology, Department of Medicine and Therapeutics, Faculty of Medicine, The Chinese University of Hong Kong, Hong Kong, SAR, China*
SIMON LAW • *Division of Esophageal and Upper Gastrointestinal Surgery, Department of Surgery, The University of Hong Kong, Hong Kong, China*
MELISSA LEUNG • *Cancer Molecular Pathology of School of Medicine, Griffith University, Gold Coast, Queensland, Australia*
DAVID K. LOR • *Department of Biomedical Engineering, National Taiwan University, Taipei City, Taiwan*
MARIA L. LUNG • *Department of Clinical Oncology, Li Ka Shing Faculty of Medicine, The University of Hong Kong, Pokfulam, Hong Kong*

Neven Maksemous • *Genomics Research Centre, Institute of Health and Biomedical Innovation, School of Biomedical Sciences, Queensland University of Technology, Brisbane, Queensland, Australia*
María Carmen Fernández Moreno • *Division of Esophageal and Upper Gastrointestinal Surgery, Department of Surgery, The University of Hong Kong, Hong Kong, China*
Suja Pillai • *School of Biomedical Science, Faculty of Medicine, University of Queensland, Brisbane, Queensland, Australia*
Robert A. Smith • *Genomics Research Centre, Institute of Health and Biomedical Innovation, Queensland University of Technology, Kelvin Grove, Queensland, Australia*
Tsz Him So • *Department of Clinical Oncology, LKS Faculty of Medicine, The University of Hong Kong, Pok Fu Lam, Hong Kong; Clinical Oncology Centre, The University of Hong Kong-Shenzhen Hospital, Shenzhen, China*
Johnny C. Tang • *Kamford Health and Genetics Centre, Central, Hong Kong*
Lihua Tao • *Department of Clinical Oncology, Li Ka Shing Faculty of Medicine, The University of Hong Kong, Pokfulam, Hong Kong*
Sunny H. Wong • *Division of Gastroenterology and Hepatology, Department of Medicine and Therapeutics, Faculty of Medicine, The Chinese University of Hong Kong, Hong Kong, SAR, China*
Peter I. C. Wu • *Department of Gastroenterology and Hepatology, St George Hospital, University of New South Wales, Sydney, NSW, Australia*
Hon-Chi Yip • *Division of Upper Gastrointestinal and Metabolic Surgery, Department of Surgery, Faculty of Medicine, The Chinese University of Hong Kong, Hong Kong, SAR, China*
Valen Z. Yu • *Department of Clinical Oncology, Li Ka Shing Faculty of Medicine, The University of Hong Kong, Pokfulam, Hong Kong*
Ru Zhang • *Division of Gastroenterology and Hepatology, Department of Medicine and Therapeutics, Faculty of Medicine, The Chinese University of Hong Kong, Hong Kong, SAR, China; Division of Gastroenterology, Department of Medicine, Shenzhen People's Hospital, Shenzhen, China*

Chapter 1

Introduction: Esophageal Squamous Cell Carcinoma—Current Status and Future Advances

Alfred K. Lam

Abstract

Esophageal squamous cell carcinoma is the most common histological subtype of esophageal cancer. The carcinoma is more common in high-incidence areas such as in Central and Southeast Asia, Eastern and Southern Africa, South America, etc. Common risk factors associated with the cancer are tobacco smoking and excessive alcohol consumption. Dietary factors, genetic factors, microorganisms, and some other environmental factors may contribute to the etiopathogenesis of the disease. Despite the global incidence of esophageal squamous cell carcinoma decreases slightly in the recent years, esophageal squamous cell carcinoma is still a major cause of cancer-related morbidity and mortality worldwide. Further improvement of the outcomes of the patients with the disease could be achieved by early diagnosis, collaborative efforts of multidisciplinary clinical and research teams, use of standardized protocol for pathological reporting and staging of the disease, proper use of cancer tissue, as well as improvement in clinical, pathological, therapeutic, and research approaches to the cancer.

Key words Esophageal, Squamous cell carcinoma, Epidemiology, Incidence, Metastases, ICCR

1 Global Burden of Esophageal Squamous Cell Carcinoma

Esophageal cancer comprises mainly squamous cell carcinoma and adenocarcinoma. Globally, the cancer ranked ninth for cancer incidence in 2013 [1]. In general, esophageal squamous cell carcinoma (ESCC) is predominately found in regions of high incidence whereas adenocarcinoma in areas of low incidence. In addition, the age-standardized incidence rates of the cancer are higher in developing countries [1]. The high cancer incidence areas are in Central and Southeast Asia, Eastern and Southern Africa along the Indian Ocean coast (Malawi, Kenya, South Africa, etc.), as well as Central and South America (Brazil, Uruguay, etc.) [2]. In these regions, Asia is the region of highest incidence of esophageal cancer, with highest incidence in China, Iran, Korea, and Japan. China alone accounts for approximately half of the world's esophageal cancer incidence. In all these high-incidence areas, the histology

Alfred K. Lam (ed.), *Esophageal Squamous Cell Carcinoma: Methods and Protocols*, Methods in Molecular Biology, vol. 2129, https://doi.org/10.1007/978-1-0716-0377-2_1,

of esophageal cancer noted is almost exclusively squamous cell carcinoma.

Globally, squamous cell carcinoma accounted for approximately 90% of esophageal cancer [3]. In the recent years, as opposed to esophageal adenocarcinoma, the esophageal squamous cell carcinoma shows a trend of decrease in incidence almost globally [4, 5]. The decrease could be related to the decrease prevalence of risk factors such as cigarette smoking.

2 Risk Factors

In esophageal adenocarcinoma, the roles and pathogenesis of esophagogastric reflux is well established [6]. In contrast, the risk factors for esophageal squamous cell carcinoma are less well defined [7–10]. The carcinoma is most often detected in the patients with lower social economic status in both developed and undeveloped countries which point to the possibility of environmental risk effects.

Overall, smoking and consumption of alcohol alone or in combination are the factors most strongly related to esophageal squamous cell carcinoma. Betel nut and chowing tobacco also increase the risk of ESCC in Asian populations [11]. However, smoking and alcohol consumption are common to many cancers. They could not completely explain the occurrence of the cancer especially in high-incidence regions. There are other dietary factors including high intake of pickled vegetables and low intake of fresh fruit and vegetables which may contribute to the etiology of ESCC. In addition, high temperature on the esophageal mucosa (thermal injury), such as taking hot food, tea, and beverages, may potentiate the effects of other etiological factors. Exposure to polycyclic aromatic hydrocarbons (from opium, indoor air pollution, food, milky tea, and other sources) has also been associated with high risk of ESCC [12].

Poor oral health (including tooth loss), change in microtome populations, and human papilloma virus [13–16] are etiological factors for ESCC requiring further research. Other environmental factors for ESCC include the type of drinking water and radiation exposure [17]. In addition, hormone factors are postulated to be related to the high male predominance for the cancer. Furthermore, obesity is a weak protective factor for ESCC.

The high incidence of the carcinoma in Asian populations suggests some roles of genetic predisposition of ESCC. In addition, genetic disorders such as tylosis (characterized by hyperkeratosis of the palms of the hands and soles of the feet as well as hyperkeratosis in the esophagus) [18] and Fanconi anemia (an inherited bone marrow failure with impaired response to DNA damage) [19] are associated with high risk of development of esophageal squamous cell carcinoma. Furthermore, some candidate genes discovered by genomic studies of families with predisposition of ESCC were shown to be important in the etiology of this subgroup of patients with ESCC [20].

3 Predisposing Lesions

Some rare esophageal pathologies including achalasia (esophageal motility disorder) [21] and Plummer-Vinson syndrome with esophageal membrane [22] are associated with increased risk of having ESCC. More commonly, squamous carcinoma in the head and neck is associated with an increased risk of squamous carcinoma of the esophagus [23]. This is related to the field effect of carcinogen(s) in the squamous mucosa of the anatomical region. In addition, squamous dysplasia shares the same etiological factor as squamous cell carcinoma. The presence of squamous dysplasia in the esophagus is associated with progression to squamous cell carcinoma [24, 25].

4 Clinicopathological Features

Many of the patients with esophageal squamous cell carcinoma presented in the late adult life mainly in the seventh decade of life [5, 26, 27]. There is a male preponderance with average male-to-female ratio of 2.5 to 1 [2]. Patients with esophageal squamous cell carcinoma often present symptoms related to difficulty in swallowing as well as weight loss. The diagnosis of the esophageal squamous cell carcinoma is by endoscopic biopsy of esophageal lesion with pathological examination (*see* Chapter 5). Radiological examinations are needed for pretreatment clinical staging of the disease to decide the management of the patient. Endoscopic ultrasound (EUS) uses an endoscope with a probe, which releases sound waves that can help to study if the squamous cell carcinoma has spread into the esophageal wall or lymph nodes.

The cancer is most often seen in the mid third of the esophagus [26, 27]. Approximately half of the squamous cell carcinoma is moderately differentiated, and most of the cases presented at stage III (*see* Chapter 3). Treatment options include systemic therapy, radiotherapy, and surgery (Chapters 22–25).

5 Prognosis

Esophageal cancer is the sixth most common cause of cancer death worldwide. The prognosis for patients with esophageal squamous cell carcinoma has improved recently [4]. However, the prognosis of the patients with cancer remains poor. The 5-year survival rate of patients with esophageal squamous cell carcinoma is approximately 20% [28]. At autopsy, distant metastases occur in approximately half of the patients with esophageal squamous cell carcinoma [29]. Common sites of metastases include the lung, liver, and bone [30]. Metastatic esophageal squamous cell carcinomas are noted in autopsy series of adrenal gland [31], heart [32], and spleen [33].

Improvement of survival of patients with ESCC can theoretically be via detection of early cancer by screening. Screening of esophageal squamous cell carcinoma by endoscopic examination could be useful in people from high-incidence areas and patients with history of head and neck squamous cell carcinoma [34]. In other regions, studies are being performed to investigate non-endoscopic methods (e.g., liquid biopsy, circulating tumor cells; *see* Chapters 15 and 16) for detecting esophageal squamous carcinoma [34].

6 Future Perspectives

Esophageal squamous cell carcinoma continues to be an important health issues despite the global decrease in incidence and mortality. There are ways to further decrease the social and economic burdens of the disease in the future. The improved accuracy of registration of the disease and advanced knowledge of the risk factors of the disease will allow the public health measures to decrease the incidence of the disease. The detection of early cancer in the high-risk regions may allow the disease to be treated early with improved survival rates of patients with cancer.

There is an urgent need for an understanding of the collaborative efforts and achievements made in the multidisciplinary team (clinical, pathological, molecular biology, and translational research) in the management of ESCC. The advancements include the development of standardized protocol for pathological reporting and staging of the disease (*see* Chapter 3). One important milestone for standardization of pathology reporting is based on an international effort of specialists including pathologists, surgeons, and oncologists working on the International Collaboration on Cancer Reporting (ICCR). ICCR is a project which issues datasets and guidelines for international standardization of cancer reporting including esophageal cancer (http://www.iccr-cancer.org/). This will provide the framework for evidence-based and personalized approach to predict prognosis of patients with ESCC and response to various new therapeutic interventions.

Molecular studies are increasingly being used in research in ESCC. Features of ideal molecular tests include high sensitivity, high specificity, technically simple, cheap to perform, as well as fast turnaround time. It is important that the tests could be performed on formalin-fixed paraffin-embedded tissues as the tissues are most commonly available for diagnosis and research from patients with ESCC. In addition, mouse models as well as biobanking of frozen tissue and blood samples are important resources for research on the cancer.

The improved clinical, pathological, therapeutic, and research approaches in the field of management of esophageal squamous cell carcinoma will allow for improved outcomes of patients with this cancer.

References

1. Global Burden of Disease Cancer Collaboration, Fitzmaurice C, Dicker D, Pain A, Hamavid H, Moradi-Lakeh M et al (2015) The global burden of cancer 2013. JAMA Oncol 1:505–527
2. Malhotra GK, Yanala U, Ravipati A, Follet M, Vijayakumar M, Are C (2017) Global trends in esophageal cancer. J Surg Oncol 115:564–579
3. Wang SM, Abnet CC, Qiao YL (2019) What have we learned from Linxian esophageal cancer etiological studies? Thorac Cancer 10:1036–1042
4. Shin A, Won YJ, Jung HK, Kong HJ, Jung KW, Oh CM, Choe S, Lee J (2018) Trends in incidence and survival of esophageal cancer in Korea: analysis of the Korea Central Cancer Registry Database. J Gastroenterol Hepatol 33:1961–1968
5. Wang QL, Xie SH, Wahlin K, Lagergren J (2018) Global time trends in the incidence of esophageal squamous cell carcinoma. Clin Epidemiol 10:717–728
6. Lam AK (2018) Introduction: esophageal adenocarcinoma: updates of current status. Methods Mol Biol 1756:1–6
7. Xie SH, Lagergren J (2018) Risk factors for oesophageal cancer. Best Pract Res Clin Gastroenterol 36-37:3–8
8. Abnet CC, Arnold M, Wei WQ (2018) Epidemiology of esophageal squamous cell carcinoma. Gastroenterology 154:360–373
9. Sheikh M, Poustchi H, Pourshams A, Etemadi A, Islami F, Khoshnia M, Gharavi A, Hashemian M, Roshandel G, Khademi H, Zahedi M, Abedi-Ardekani B, Boffetta P, Kamangar F, Dawsey SM, Pharaoh PD, Abnet CC, Day NE, Brennan P, Malekzadeh R (2019) Individual and combined effects of environmental risk factors for esophageal cancer based on results from the Golestan cohort study. Gastroenterology 156:1416–1427
10. Castro C, Peleteiro B, Lunet N (2018) Modifiable factors and esophageal cancer: a systematic review of published meta-analyses. J Gastroenterol 53:37–51
11. Akhtar S (2013) Areca nut chewing and esophageal squamous-cell carcinoma risk in Asians: a meta-analysis of case-control studies. Cancer Causes Control 24:257–265
12. Mwachiro MM, Parker RK, Pritchett NR, Lando JO, Ranketi S, Murphy G, Chepkwony R, Burgert SL, Abnet CC, Topazian MD, Dawsey SM, White RE (2019) Investigating tea temperature and content as risk factors for esophageal cancer in an endemic region of Western Kenya: Validation of a questionnaire and analysis of polycyclic aromatic hydrocarbon content. Cancer Epidemiol 60:60–66
13. Hošnjak L, Poljak M (2018) A systematic literature review of studies reporting human papillomavirus (HPV) prevalence in esophageal carcinoma over 36 years (1982-2017). Acta Dermatovenerol Alp Pannonica Adriat 27:127–136
14. He D, Zhang DK, Lam KY, Ma L, Ngan HY, Liu SS, Tsao SW (1997) Prevalence of HPV infection in esophageal squamous cell carcinoma in Chinese patients and its relationship to the p53 gene mutation. Int J Cancer 72:959–964
15. Lam KY, He D, Ma L, Zhang D, Ngan HY, Wan TS, Tsao SW (1997) Presence of human papillomavirus in esophageal squamous cell carcinomas of Hong Kong Chinese and its relationship with p53 gene mutation. Hum Pathol 28:657–663
16. Lam AK (2000) Molecular biology of esophageal squamous cell carcinoma. Crit Rev Oncol Hematol 33:71–90
17. Talagala IA, Nawarathne M, Arambepola C (2018) Novel risk factors for primary

prevention of oesophageal carcinoma: a case-control study from Sri Lanka. BMC Cancer 18:1135

18. Ellis A, Risk JM, Maruthappu T, Kelsell DP (2015) Tylosis with oesophageal cancer: diagnosis, management and molecular mechanisms. Orphanet J Rare Dis 10:126
19. Itskoviz D, Tamary H, Krasnov T, Yacobovich J, Sahar N, Zevit N, Shamir R, Ben-Bassat O, Leibovici Wiseman Y, Dickman R, Ringel Y, Dotan I, Goldberg Y, Morgenstern S, Levi Z (2019) Endoscopic findings and esophageal cancer incidence among Fanconi Anemia patients participating in an endoscopic surveillance program. Dig Liver Dis 51:242–246
20. Donner I, Katainen R, Tanskanen T, Kaasinen E, Aavikko M, Ovaska K, Artama M, Pukkala E, Aaltonen LA (2017) Candidate susceptibility variants for esophageal squamous cell carcinoma. Genes Chromosomes Cancer 56:453–459
21. Ponds FA, Moonen A, Smout AJPM, Rohof WOA, Tack J, van Gool S, Bisschops R, Bredenoord AJ, Boeckxstaens GE (2018) Screening for dysplasia with Lugol chromoendoscopy in longstanding idiopathic achalasia. Am J Gastroenteol 113:855–862
22. Nasa M, Patil G, Sharma Z, Puri R (2017) Plummer-Vinson syndrome with simultaneous mid-esophageal growth. J Assoc Physicians India 65:96–97
23. Priante AV, Castilho EC, Kowalski LP (2011) Second primary tumors in patients with head and neck cancer. Curr Oncol 13:132–137
24. Dawsey SM, Lewin KJ, Wang GQ, Liu FS, Nieberg RK, Yu Y, Li JY, Blot WJ, Li B, Taylor PR (1994) Squamous esophageal histology and subsequent risk of squamous cell carcinoma of the esophagus. A prospective follow-up study from Linxian, China. Cancer 74:1686–1692
25. Wang GQ, Abnet CC, Shen Q, Lewin KJ, Sun XD, Roth MJ, Qiao YL, Mark SD, Dong ZW, Taylor PR, Dawsey SM (2005) Histological precursors of oesophageal squamous cell carcinoma: results from a 13 year prospective follow up study in a high risk population. Gut 54:187–192
26. Lam KY, Law S, Tin L, Tung PH, Wong J (1999) The clinicopathological significance of p21 and p53 expression in esophageal squamous cell carcinoma: an analysis of 153 patients. Am J Gastroenterol 94:2060–2068
27. Lam KY, Ma L (1997) Pathology of esophageal cancers: local experience and current insights. Chin Med J 110:459–464
28. Lagergren J, Smyth E, Cunningham D, Lagergren P (2017) Oesophageal cancer. Lancet 390:2383–2396
29. Lam KY, Law S, Wong J (2003) Low prevalence of incidentally discovered and early stage esophageal cancers in a 30-year autopsy study. Dis Esophagus 16:1–3
30. Wu SG, Zhang WW, Sun JY, Li FY, Lin Q, He ZY (2018) Patterns of distant metastasis between histological types in esophageal cancer. Front Oncol 8:302
31. Lam KY, Lo CY (2002) Metastatic tumours of the adrenal glands: a 30-year experience in a teaching hospital. Clin Endocrinol 56:95–101
32. Lam KY, Dickens P, Chan AC, Tumors of the heart (1993) A 20-year experience with a review of 12,485 consecutive autopsies. Arch Pathol Lab Med 117:1027–1031
33. Lam KY, Tang V (2000) Metastatic tumors to the spleen: a 25-year clinicopathologic study. Arch Pathol Lab Med 124:526–530
34. Codipilly DC, Qin Y, Dawsey SM, Kisiel J, Topazian M, Ahlquist D, Iyer PG (2018) Screening for esophageal squamous cell carcinoma: recent advances. Gastrointest Endosc 88:413–426

Chapter 2

Histopathological Assessment for Esophageal Squamous Cell Carcinoma

Alfred K. Lam

Abstract

Histological assessment of esophageal squamous malignancies is crucial for management of patients with the cancer as well as working in research on the cancer. The squamous malignancies in the esophagus comprise squamous dysplasia and squamous cell carcinoma. Current classification of squamous dysplasia in the esophagus is to divide it into low grade and high grade. Most of the esophageal squamous cell carcinomas are of conventional type and divided into well, moderately, and poorly differentiated. The variants of esophageal squamous cell carcinoma include basaloid squamous carcinoma, spindle cell carcinoma, and verrucous carcinoma. Preoperative chemoradiation is used commonly in the treatment of esophageal squamous cell carcinoma and induces changes in morphology. Tumor regression grading systems based on the percentage of the remaining carcinoma cells are used to assess the response to the neoadjuvant therapy in the cancer. Additional histological parameters including lymphovascular invasion, perineural invasion, clearance of resection margins, and carcinoma in the nodal and distant metastatic sites provide essential information for the management of the patient with the cancer.

Key words Esophagus, Squamous dysplasia, Squamous cell carcinoma, Basaloid squamous carcinoma, Spindle cell carcinoma, Grade, Neoadjuvant therapy, Pathology

1 Introduction

Squamous cell carcinoma is most common histological type of esophageal cancer in areas with high prevalence of esophageal carcinoma [1]. In these areas, squamous cell carcinoma accounts approximately 90% of esophageal cancer in surgical series and more than 95% esophageal cancer in autopsy series [1, 2]

Histopathological examination of esophageal squamous carcinoma is essential to determine the pathological staging of the cancer and hence the management of the patients with the cancer [3]. It is also important to aware of the different characteristics of the squamous malignancy in the esophagus before planning research. Esophageal squamous carcinoma could present with multiple lesions because of the rich lymphatics in the wall of the

Alfred K. Lam (ed.), *Esophageal Squamous Cell Carcinoma: Methods and Protocols*, Methods in Molecular Biology, vol. 2129, https://doi.org/10.1007/978-1-0716-0377-2_2, © Springer Science+Business Media, LLC, part of Springer Nature 2020

esophagus as well as the field effect of smoking [4]. The carcinoma often invades extensively locally, and the tumor becomes inoperable.

More importantly, neoadjuvant therapies (medical therapies – most commonly chemotherapy and radiotherapy given before operation) before surgery were being employed to down stage the locally advanced cancer [5]. The treatment could make the carcinoma shrunken and easier to be operated. These treatments have altered the histological features of the carcinoma seen at the surgically removed specimen. In addition, clinical complete response may occur, there could be no residual carcinoma in the resected specimen, or there may be no additional surgery done [5]. In this case, the initial endoscopic biopsy is an important source of tissue for assessment of the pathological and molecular profiles of the cancer. For early squamous malignancies, endoscopic resection is done for esophageal squamous cell carcinoma (*see* Chapter 5). The material obtained from this procedure for histological examination is also limited in volume.

2 Materials

1. Clinical information of the resected or biopsied esophageal squamous cell carcinoma.

   These could include the information of the histological examination of the biopsy result(s), radiological examination result(s), etc.
2. Macroscopic information of the specimen (*see* Chapter 4).
3. Hematoxylin and eosin-stained sections after sampling and processing of specimen.
4. Light microscope.

3 Methods

1. Determine the types of squamous malignancy.

   Squamous malignancy in the esophagus shows keratinocyte-type cells with intercellular bridges and/or keratinization. It could be pre-invasive or invasive. Squamous dysplasia is unequivocal neoplastic alteration of squamous epithelium without invasion of basement membrane. Squamous cell carcinoma of the esophagus is squamous malignancy with invasion of basement membrane (*see* **Note 1**).

2. Determine the grade of squamous dysplasia.

   The severity of the cytological atypia and the level of involvement of the cytological atypia in the esophageal epithelium determine the grade of squamous dysplasia in the esophagus (*see* **Note 2**).

3. Determine the grade of squamous cell carcinoma.

   Grading of the squamous cell carcinoma is based on degree of resemblance to squamous epithelium. The common system used is a three-tier system (grade 1 [well differentiated], grade 2 [moderately differentiated], and grade 3 [poorly differentiated]) (*see* **Note 3**).

4. Determine the histological variant of squamous cell carcinoma.

   The histological variants are basaloid squamous carcinoma, spindle cell carcinoma, and verrucous carcinoma (*see* **Note 4**).

5. Determine the response to the neoadjuvant therapy in esophageal squamous cell carcinoma (*see* **Note 5**).
6. Identify the presence of lymphovascular invasion and perineural invasion by esophageal squamous cell carcinoma (*see* **Note 6**).
7. Record the distance of carcinoma from the proximal, distal, and circumferential margins.
8. Document the number of lymph nodes involved by squamous cell carcinoma.
9. Document the presence of squamous cell carcinoma in metastatic site biopsies if received for examination.

4 Notes

1. Squamous dysplasia is uncommon and often found adjacent to the squamous carcinoma. It may be difficult to determine the presence or absence of invasion in endoscopic biopsy (due to the small size). In this instance, correlations with radiological and clinical information are essential to make a proper judgment.
2. The current World Health Organization Classification of Tumors favors a two-tier (low-grade and high-grade) system for grading of esophageal squamous dysplasia [6]. Low-grade esophageal squamous dysplasia has mild cytological atypia and limits to the lower half of the squamous epithelium of the esophagus (Fig. 1). In contrast, high-grade esophageal squamous dysplasia shows more than half of the squamous epithelium involved by cytological dysplasia or in the presence of severe cytological dysplasia (regardless of extent of epithelial involvement) (Fig. 2). High-grade dysplasia in the esophagus

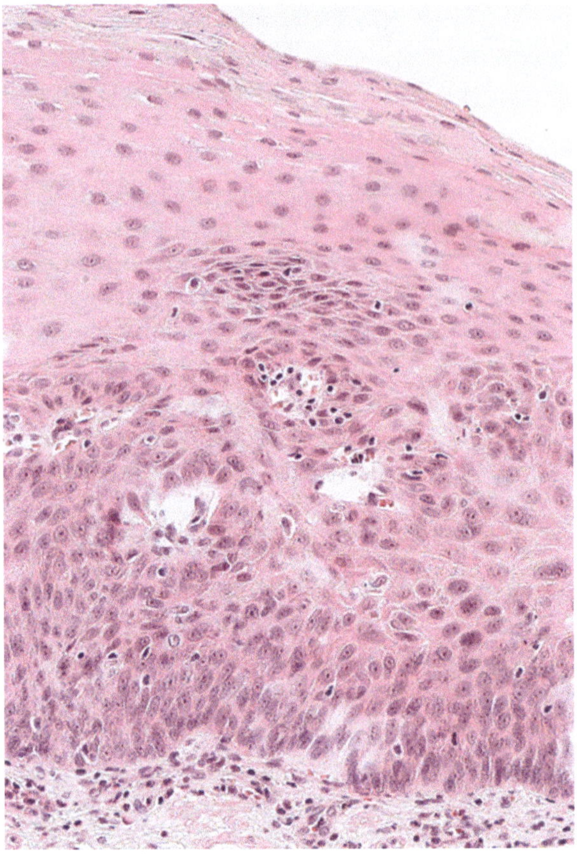

Fig. 1 Low-grade dysplasia: the squamous epithelium shows mild cytological atypia and limits to the lower half (hematoxylin and eosin ×20)

includes carcinoma in situ (dysplasia involves the full thickness of the squamous epithelium).

3. The three grades of squamous cell carcinoma depend on cytological features including cytological atypia, mitotic activity, and extent of keratinization (Figs. 3 and 4). The grading depends on the resemblance of the carcinoma to normal squamous epithelium. Poorly differentiated squamous carcinoma (grade 3) shows basaloid cells, high mitotic activities, and minimal/focal keratinization (Fig. 5). Well-differentiated (grade 1) squamous cell carcinoma (grade 1) has prominent keratinization with pearl formation and a minor component of non-keratinizing basal-like cells, tumor cells arranged in sheets, and mitotic counts that are low. Moderately differentiated (grade 2) squamous cell carcinoma has features between well-differentiated squamous cell carcinoma and poorly differentiated squamous cell carcinoma. It shows variable histological features ranging from parakeratotic to poorly keratinizing lesions, and pearl formation is generally absent.

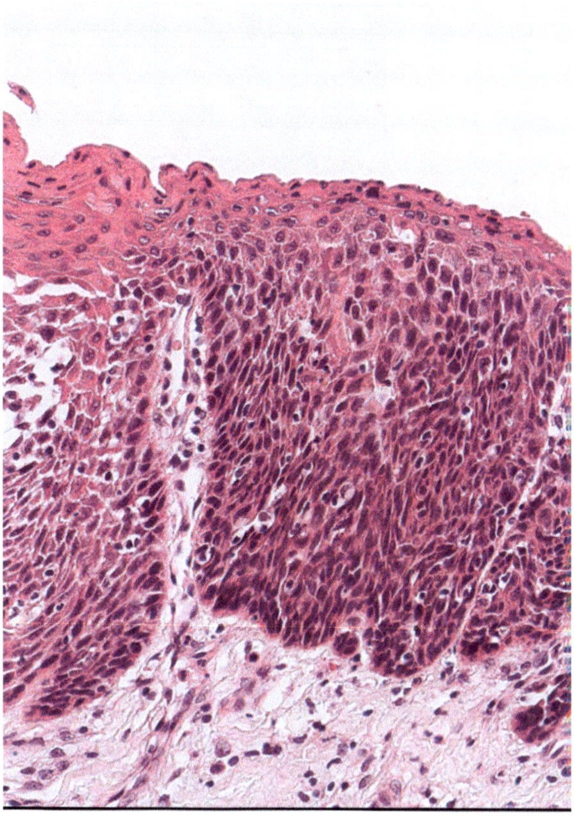

Fig. 2 High-grade dysplasia: the squamous epithelium shows high cytological atypia and extends to more than lower half (hematoxylin and eosin ×20)

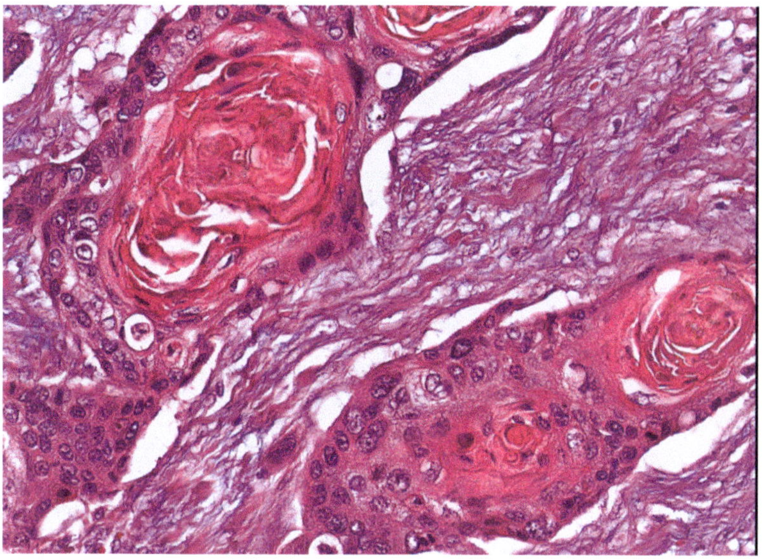

Fig. 3 Well differentiated squamous cell carcinoma. Note the prominent keratinization (hematoxylin and eosin ×20)

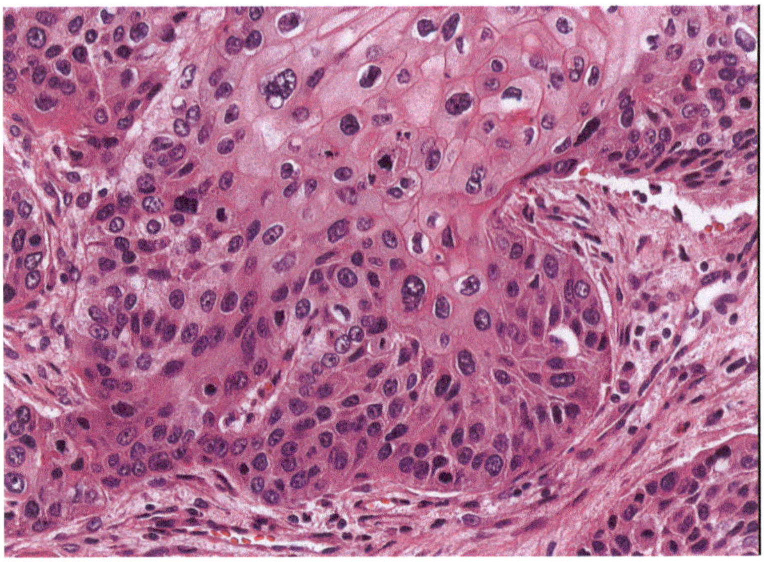

Fig. 4 Moderately differentiated squamous cell carcinoma. Note the presence of mild nuclear atypia and presence of mitotic activities (hematoxylin and eosin $\times 20$)

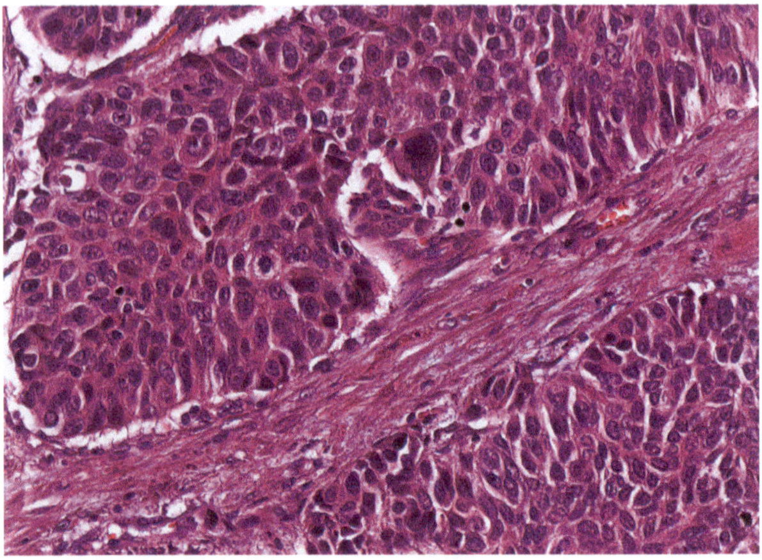

Fig. 5 Poorly differentiated squamous cell carcinoma. Note the presence of basaloid cells, high mitotic activities, and prominent nuclear atypia (hematoxylin and eosin $\times 20$)

4. The histological variants of squamous cell carcinoma are basaloid squamous carcinoma, spindle cell carcinoma and verrucous carcinoma with details as follows:
   (a) Basaloid squamous cell carcinoma.

Basaloid squamous cell carcinoma is a common variant of squamous cell carcinoma other than conventional squamous cell carcinoma. Despite this, the carcinoma accounts for only 4–5% of primary esophageal cancer in large series [7, 8]. Patients with basaloid squamous carcinoma often have shorter overall survival than conventional squamous cell carcinoma, but the difference is often not significant [7–9].

The carcinoma comprises a major component of basaloid tumor cells (resemble basal cells in squamous epithelium) in lobules, nests, or cribriform patterns with peripheral palisading as well as a distinctive component of squamous tumor cells. There is abrupt transition between the basaloid component and squamous component, which is a key differential feature from poorly differentiated squamous cell carcinoma. Frequent mitosis, single-cell necrosis, and comedonecrosis (necrosis in the center of the tumor nests) occur in basaloid squamous carcinoma (Fig. 6). In addition, this variant shows hyalinization both within and outside tumor nests, and the hyaline material is the same as that in the basement membrane. Stroma may also be myxoid and with variable pseudo-glandular spaces resembling adenoid cystic carcinoma [10].

(b) Spindle cell (squamous) carcinoma.

Spindle cell (squamous) carcinoma, also known as sarcomatoid carcinoma or carcinosarcoma, comprises

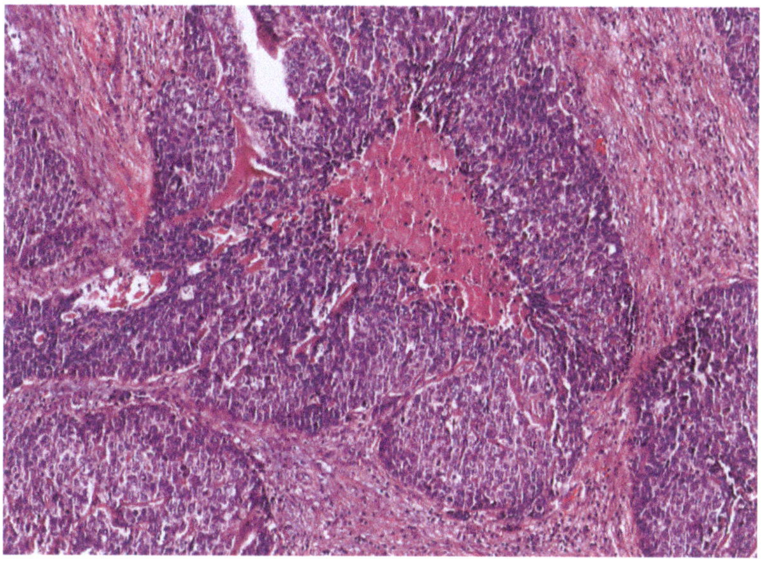

Fig. 6 Basaloid squamous carcinoma. Note the basaloid-looking tumor cells with central necrosis (hematoxylin and eosin ×10)

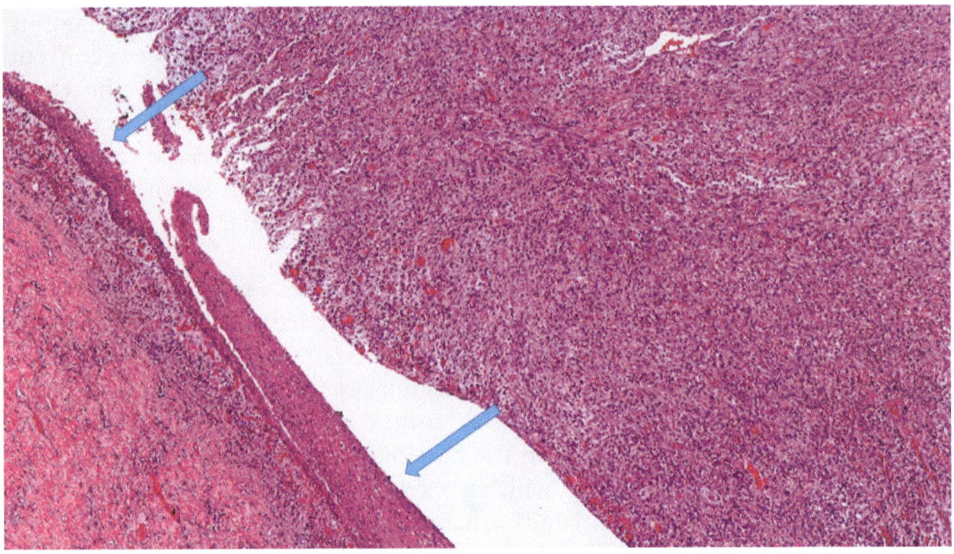

Fig. 7 Spindle cell carcinoma. Note the epithelium shows dysplasia (arrows) (hematoxylin and eosin ×5)

approximately 2% of primary esophageal cancer [1, 11]. Double spindle cell carcinoma could occur in the esophagus [12]. The short-term survival of the patients with spindle cell carcinoma is slightly better than conventional squamous cell carcinoma because of its exophytic growth rather than deep invasion. However, the long-term survival of these patients is like those with conventional esophageal squamous cell carcinoma [13].

The carcinoma often has intraluminal/polypoid growth pattern because of the spindle cell component. Microscopically, the carcinoma has a biphasic pattern of neoplastic squamous epithelium and spindle cells that resemble sarcoma. The squamous component may present as high-grade dysplasia in the squamous epithelium and be missed in initial histological examination (Fig. 7). The neoplastic spindle cell component typically is undifferentiated and arranged in fascicular or storiform pattern (Fig. 8). Rarely, bizarre giant cells with osseous, cartilaginous, or skeletal muscle differentiation occur [11]. As sarcoma or stromal tumor is very uncommon in the esophagus, presence of spindle cell malignancy should alter the pathologist to consider the spindle cell (squamous) carcinoma as more likely diagnosis.

(c) Verrucous (squamous) carcinoma.

Verrucous (squamous) carcinoma of the esophagus is a rare variant with only a few series reported [14]. The carcinoma could represent a malignant counterpart of squamous papilloma of the esophagus. Human

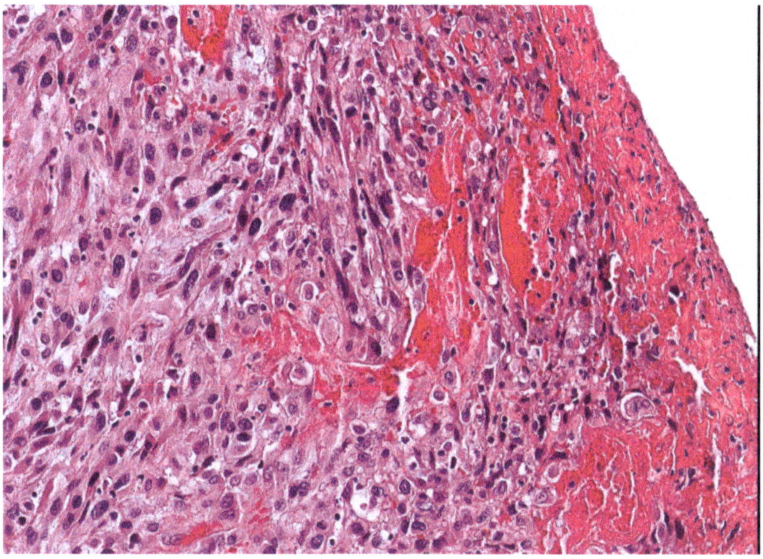

Fig. 8 Spindle cell carcinoma. Higher magnification shows the spindle tumor cells with surface ulceration and lacking epithelium which makes the correct diagnosis difficult (hematoxylin and eosin ×15)

papillomavirus (such as types 11 and 51) could occur in the verrucous carcinoma [15, 16]. Nevertheless, most of the cases were not associated with human papillomavirus infection [17].

The carcinoma is an extremely well-differentiated type of squamous carcinoma with minimal cytological atypia and mitotic activities. The architecture of the carcinoma is characterized by papillary projections at the surface and broad bullous pushing base. Keratinization occurs abruptly without an intervening granular cell layer with cup-like collections of keratins. Verrucous carcinoma is often of T1 stage and rarely has lymph node or distant metastases. Prognosis of the patients with verrucous carcinoma is often good [14].

(d) Other carcinomas.

Adenosquamous carcinoma and mucoepidermoid carcinoma are carcinomas with both squamous carcinoma and mucin-secreting neoplastic component [6, 18, 19]. In the current World Health Organization (WHO) classification, they are separate entities from squamous cell carcinoma or adenocarcinoma [6].

5. Tumor regression grade is an independent predicator of overall survival of patient with esophageal squamous cell carcinoma having neoadjuvant therapy [20, 21]. In the literature, many studies used percentage of tumor cells remaining in the

resection specimen as the grading system [20–22]. Other systems may use the relative proportion of the tumor cells and stromal cells in a tumor for grading of the response to neoadjuvant therapy. None of these systems show better performance than others in assessment of grading of tumor regression. In the current version of WHO classification, the two most common systems used are listed out for reference to be used in both esophageal squamous cell carcinoma and adenocarcinoma [23, 24]. One is based on percentage of tumor cells (Becker) and one based on relative amount of tumor cells as compared to the stromal cells (Mandard).

If endoscopic biopsy is being used to assess the response of the tumor to chemoradiation, the biopsy should be obtained from deep portion of the lesion in the esophagus when possible. In addition, pathologist should pay attention to the changes related to neoadjuvant therapy in the assessment. The carcinoma may appear small or even totally disappear. Histological examination may reveal morphological changes in the carcinoma cytoplasm (vacuolation, oncocytic changes, and neuroendocrine changes) and nuclei (Fig. 9). Reactive atypia in non-cancer tissue (fibroblasts, glands, and endothelium) could mimic changes in malignancy. In addition, keratin may be present even if no viable tumor cells are noted (Fig. 10). Degenerative and reparative changes such as fibrosis, calcification, necrosis, inflammation, and cholesterol clefts may occur.

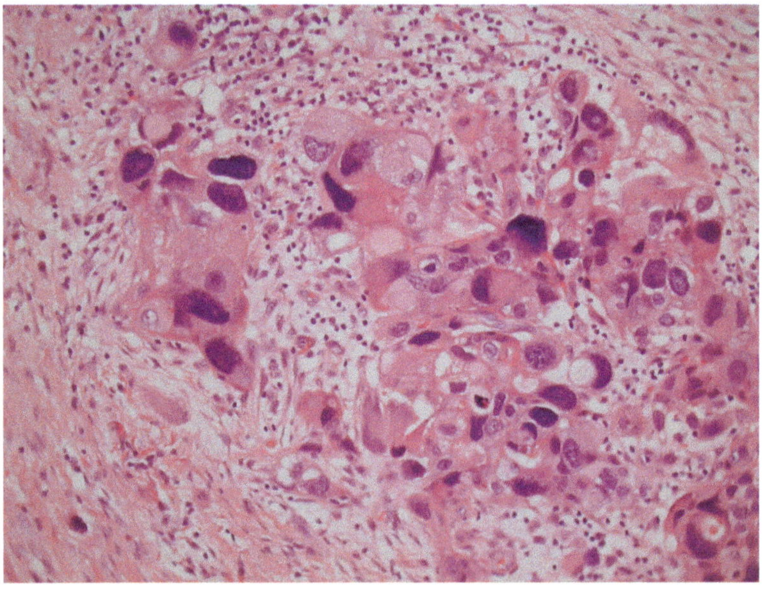

Fig. 9 Squamous cell carcinoma post-chemoradiation. Note the changes in the cytoplasm (vacuolation and foamy) and nuclei (hyperchromatic and irregular) (hematoxylin and eosin ×20)

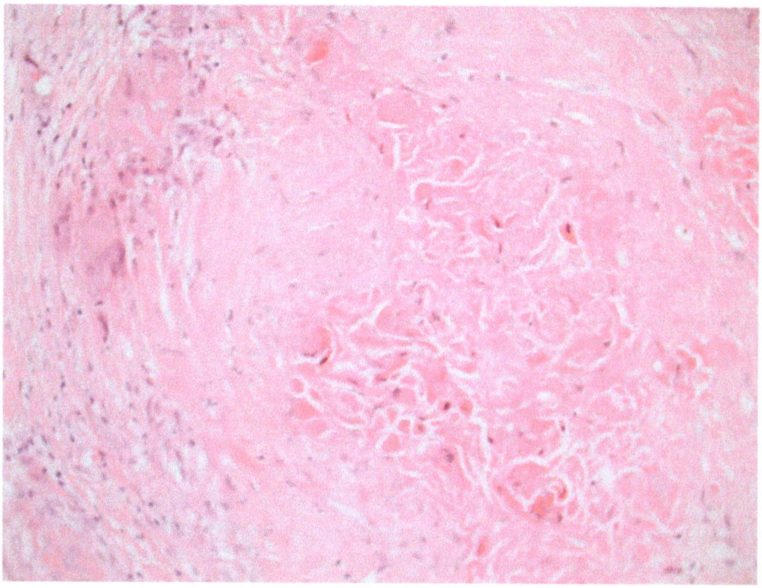

Fig. 10 Degenerative changes in tumor stroma showing the giant cells, fibrosis, and keratin of pre-existing squamous cell carcinoma (hematoxylin and eosin ×20)

6. In patients treated with neoadjuvant therapy followed by esophagectomy, histological parameters such as lymphovascular permeation and perineural invasion have important prognostic impacts and may identify patients at high risk of recurrence [25].

References

1. Lam KY, Ma L (1997) Pathology of esophageal cancers: local experience and current insights. Chin Med J 110:459–464
2. Lam KY, Law S, Wong J (2013) Low prevalence of incidentally discovered and early-stage esophageal cancers in a 30-year autopsy study. Dis Esophagus 16:1–3
3. Rice TW, Kelsen D, Blackstone E, Ishwaran H, Patil DT, Bass AJ, Erasmus JJ, Gerdes H, Hofstetter WL (2016) Esophagus and esophagogastric junction. In: Amin MB, Edge S, Greene F, Byrd DR, Brookland RK, Washington MK, Gershenwald JE, Compton CC, Hess KR, Sullivan DC, Jessup JM, Brierley JD, Gaspar LE, Schilsky RL, Balch CM, Winchester DP, Asare EA, Madera M, Gress DM, Meyer LR (eds) Chapter 16: AJCC cancer staging manual, 8th edn. Springer, Berlin, pp 185–202
4. Lam KY, Ma LT, Wong J (1996) Measurement of extent of spread of oesophageal squamous carcinoma by serial sectioning. J Clin Pathol 49:124–129
5. Wang J, Qin J, Jing S, Liu Q, Cheng Y, Wang Y, Cao F (2018) Clinical complete response after chemoradiotherapy for carcinoma of thoracic esophagus: is esophagectomy always necessary? A systematic review and meta-analysis. Thorac Cancer 9:1638–1647
6. Lam AK, Ochiai A, Odze RD (2019) Tumours of the oesophagus: introduction. In: Odze RD, Lam AK, Ochiai A, Washington MK (eds) Chapter 2: WHO classification of tumours, 5th edn, pp 28–29
7. Li TJ, Zhang YX, Wen J, Cowan DF, Hart J, Xiao SY (2004) Basaloid squamous cell carcinoma of the esophagus with or without adenoid cystic features. Arch Pathol Lab Med 128:1124–1130
8. Lam KY, Law S, Luk JM, Wong J (2001) Oesophageal basaloid squamous cell carcinoma: a unique clinicopathological entity with

telomerase activity as a prognostic indicator. J Pathol 195:435–442
9. Salami A, Abbas AE, Petrov R, Jhala N, Bakhos CT (2018) Comparative analysis of clinical, treatment, and survival characteristics of basaloid and squamous cell carcinoma of the esophagus. J Am Coll Surg 226:1086–1092
10. Lam AK (2019) Oesophageal adenoid cystic carcinoma. In: Odze RD, Lam AK, Ochiai A, Washington MK (eds) Chapter 2: WHO classification of tumours, 5th edn, pp 44–45
11. Raza MA, Mazzara PF (2011) Sarcomatoid carcinoma of esophagus. Arch Pathol Lab Med 135:945–948
12. Lam KY, Law SY, Loke SL, Fok M, Ma LT (1996) Double sarcomatoid carcinomas of the oesophagus. Pathol Res Pract 192:604–609
13. Iyomasa S, Kato H, Tachimori Y, Watanabe H, Yamaguchi H, Itabashi M (1990) Carcinosarcoma of the esophagus: a twenty-case study. Jpn J Clin Oncol 20:99–106
14. Behrens A, Stolte M, Pech O, May A, Ell C (2014) Verrucous oesophageal carcinoma: single case report and case series including 15 patients—issues for consideration of therapeutic strategies. Viszeralmedizin 30:346–352
15. Vieira CL, Lopes JC, Velosa J (2013) A case of esophageal squamous cell carcinoma with positive HPV 11. Gastroenterol Hepatol 36:311–315
16. Tonna J, Palefsky JM, Rabban J, Campos GM, Theodore P, Ladabaum U (2010) Esophageal verrucous carcinoma arising from hyperkeratotic plaques associated with human papilloma virus type 51. Dis Esophagus 23:E17–E20
17. Cappellesso R, Coati I, Barzon L, Peta E, Masi G, Scarpa M, Lanza C, Michelotto M, Ruol A, Cesaro S, Castoro C, Palù G, Nuovo GJ, Fassan M, Rugge M (2019) Human papillomavirus infection is not involved in esophageal verrucous carcinoma. Hum Pathol 85:50–57
18. Lam AK (2018) Histopathological assessment for esophageal adenocarcinoma. Methods Mol Biol 1756:67–76
19. Lam KY, Dickens P, Loke SL, Fok M, Ma L, Wong J (1994) Squamous cell carcinoma of the oesophagus with mucin-secreting component (muco-epidermoid carcinoma and adenosquamous carcinoma): a clinicopathologic study and a review of literature. Eur J Surg Oncol 20:25–31
20. Tong DK, Law S, Kwong DL, Chan KW, Lam AK, Wong KH (2010) Histological regression of squamous esophageal carcinoma assessed by percentage of residual viable cells after neoadjuvant chemoradiation is an important prognostic factor. Ann Surg Oncol 17:2184–2192
21. Chao YK, Chang CB, Chuang WY, Wen YW, Chang HK, Tseng CK, Yeh CJ, Liu YH (2015) Correlation between tumor regression grade and clinicopathological parameters in patients with squamous cell carcinoma of the esophagus who received neoadjuvant chemoradiotherapy. Medicine (Baltimore) 94:e1407
22. Fujishima F, Taniyama Y, Nakamura Y, Okamoto H, Ozawa Y, Ito K, Ishida H, Konno-Kumagai T, Kasajima A, Taniuchi S, Watanabe M, Kamei T, Sasano H (2018) Residual carcinoma cells after chemoradiotherapy for esophageal squamous cell carcinoma patients: striving toward appropriate judgment of biopsy. Dis Esophagus 31:1–6
23. Lam AK, Kumarasinghe MP (2019) Adenocarcinoma of the oesophagus and oesophagogastric junction NOS. In: Odze RD, Lam AK, Ochiai A, Washington MK (eds) Chapter 2: WHO classification of tumours, 5th edn, pp 38–43
24. Brown IS, Fujii S, Kawachi H, Lam AK, Saito T (2019) Oesophageal squamous cell carcinoma NOS. In: Odze RD, Lam AK, Ochiai A, Washington MK (eds) Chapter 2: WHO classification of tumours, 5th edn, pp 48–53
25. Lagarde SM, Phillips AW, Navidi M, Disep B, Immanuel A, Griffin SM (2015) The presence of lymphovascular and perineural infiltration after neoadjuvant therapy and oesophagectomy identifies patients at high risk for recurrence. Br J Cancer 113:1427–1433

Chapter 3

Application of Pathological Staging in Esophageal Squamous Cell Carcinoma

Alfred K. Lam

Abstract

Pathological staging is the most important factor that determines the prognosis and management of patients with esophageal squamous cell carcinoma. The method for the pathological staging in esophageal squamous cell carcinoma involves assessment of standard parameters—extent of tumor (T), lymph node status (N), presence of distant metastasis (M), as well as grade (G) and anatomical location of the carcinoma. In addition, other relevant factors, such as use of neoadjuvant therapy, could affect the pathological staging of esophageal squamous cell carcinoma.

Key words Esophageal, Squamous carcinoma, Staging, Pathology, Neoadjuvant therapy

1 Introduction

Cancer staging is the most important factor in predicting prognosis and formulating management in patients with esophageal squamous cell carcinoma. It is a measurement of the extent of the cancer in a patient with esophageal squamous cell carcinoma. For many years, pathological staging of esophageal cancers depends on anatomical factors—tumor extent (T), lymph node status (N), and occurrence of distant metastases (M) [1]. However, there are drawbacks in this old approach. These may include (1) some predictive factors known to affect the prognosis of the patient missed out; (2) lack of awareness of the biology of the cancer that has been altered by therapy; and (3) the survival data being based on the relative small number of patients.

For esophageal cancer, there are major modifications starting in the seventh edition of AJCC published in 2009 (adopted in 2010) [2]. In the seventh edition of AJCC Staging Manual, for the first time, histological type accounted for the staging of esophageal cancer. The difference in survival between adenocarcinoma and squamous cell carcinoma of the esophagus could reflect better in two separate stage groupings. In addition, the stage grouping

Alfred K. Lam (ed.), *Esophageal Squamous Cell Carcinoma: Methods and Protocols*, Methods in Molecular Biology, vol. 2129, https://doi.org/10.1007/978-1-0716-0377-2_3,

adopted two new parameters—the grade of the carcinoma and the location of the carcinoma in the esophagus. Of great importance is the survival information being constructed from worldwide data—the Worldwide Esophageal Cancer Collaboration (WECC) [3]. WECC was inaugurated in 2006 at the initiative of Drs. Thomas W. Rice and Eugene H. Blackstone in United States. They collected data from 13 institutions, over 5 countries and 3 continents (Asia, Europe, and North America), summarizing 4627 patients with esophageal cancers underwent esophagectomy with no induction or adjuvant therapy to develop a staging system for the seven edition of AJCC.

Cancer staging of the esophageal squamous cell carcinoma is now based on the eighth edition of Staging Manual published in 2016 by the American Joint Committee on Cancer (AJCC) [4]. The manual commenced its application globally for management of cancers in 2018. The eighth edition of AJCC increases the cover of the WECC data [5]. The populations being recruited included patients who received neoadjuvant treatment as a large portion of patients with esophageal cancer received neoadjuvant treatment. In addition, invitation to submit data to WECC extends to 6 continents and over 79 institutions. Of these, 33 institutions submitted their data by September 30, 2014, and 22,654 patients with esophageal cancers collected. The stage grouping is much refined because of the more robust and reliable random forest-based machine learning analysis of large amount of data. This chapter will highlight the principle and changes in the most recent pathological staging information concerning esophageal squamous cell carcinoma.

2 Materials

1. Have the surgical specimens dissected and with the hematoxylin and eosin-stained slides reviewed by pathologists collected (*see* Chapter 4).
2. The pathological report of these patients.
3. Clinical information obtained by clinical records (electronic medical records) as well as from multidisciplinary team meeting for management of cancer.
4. Eighth edition of the American Joint Committee on Cancer (AJCC) Staging Manual.

3 Methods

1. Select the section for the type of staging specific for the status of the patients in the eighth edition of the AJCC Staging Manual (*see* **Note 1**).
2. Determine the extent of involvement of the squamous cell carcinoma in the esophagus and the adjacent structures (T stage). T stage of the tumors can be classified as T0, Tis, T1 (T1a and T1b), T2, T3, and T4 (T4a and T4b) (*see* **Note 2**).
3. Count the number of regional lymph nodes involved by the squamous cell carcinoma, and assign the cancer to subgroups N0, N1, N2, and N3 (*see* **Note 3**).
4. Determine whether there are distant metastases, and group the cancer into Mo or M1 (*see* **Note 4**).
5. Determine the grade of esophageal squamous cell carcinoma (*see* **Note 5**),
6. Define the anatomical location of esophageal squamous cell carcinoma (*see* **Note 6**).
7. Refer to the table in the eighth edition of the AJCC Staging Manual (based on the T, N, M, and G) and location in order get an overall staging prognostic group.

   The staging prognostic groups broadly divide the esophageal squamous cell carcinoma into four stage groups: I, II, III, and IV (*see* **Note 7**).
8. Additional factors recommended for clinical care include tumor length, lymphovascular invasion, histoviability (tumor regression grading system), clearance of surgical margin, and extranodal extension of carcinoma.

4 Notes

1. This is the first time that there are three prognostic stage groups for esophageal squamous cell carcinoma. The first one is clinical staging (cTMN) based on clinical, radiological, and endoscopic findings before operation. This allows planning of treatment of patients with esophageal squamous cell carcinoma. The resolution of the imaging techniques will limit the accuracy of the staging. Histological examination of lymph node is recommended if there is suspicion of lymph node metastases.

   The second group (pathological stage group) is for patients after surgery or endoscopic mucosal resection (pTNM). The patients in this group do not have any preoperative neoadjuvant therapy (administration of therapeutic agents such as chemoradiation before a main treatment).

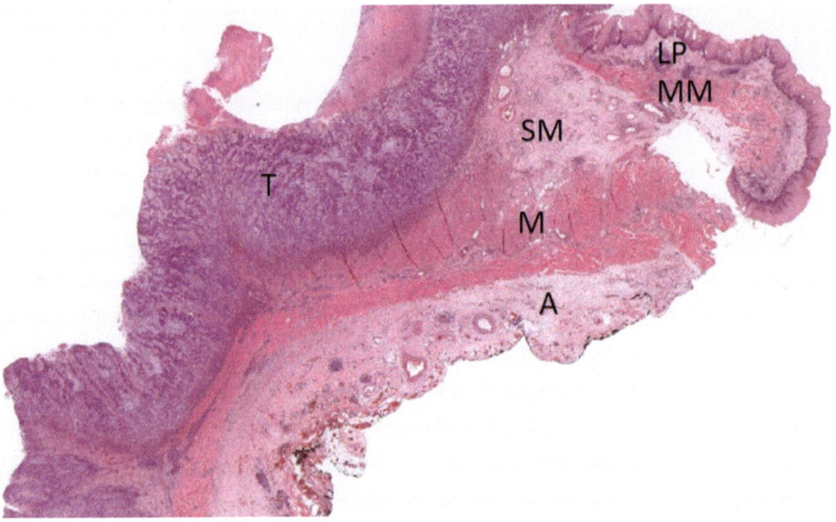

Fig. 1 The different layers of the esophagus with the squamous cell carcinoma (T) in the muscularis propria (M) of the esophagus; *LP* lamina propria, *MM* muscularis propria, *SM* submucosa, *A* adventitia (hematoxylin and eosin ×0.5)

The third group (neoadjuvant pathological stage group (ypTNM)) is for patients after receiving neoadjuvant therapy.

2. T stage measures the local extent of the carcinoma in the wall of the esophagus and the adjacent tissue (Fig. 1). T0 is no residual malignancy detected (after neoadjuvant therapy). Tis means high-grade squamous dysplasia of the esophagus (*see* Chapter 2). Starting from eighth edition of the AJCC Staging Manual, T1 includes T1a and T1b to provide improve subgrouping of stage I carcinoma. T1a carcinoma is intramucosal squamous cell carcinoma in which the carcinoma invades lamina propria or muscularis mucosae. T1b carcinoma is submucosal squamous carcinoma in which the carcinoma invades submucosa (Fig. 2). T2 carcinoma is squamous cell carcinoma that invades muscularis propria (Fig. 3). T3 carcinoma is squamous cell carcinoma reaching the adventitia (Fig. 4). T4 carcinoma is squamous carcinoma that invades structure adjacent to the esophagus. The documentation of T4 carcinoma needs clinical or radiological findings. Ongoing from the seventh edition, T4 had two subgroups: T4a and T4b. T4a is generally resectable tumor invading the pleura, pericardium, azygos vein, or diaphragm or peritoneum. It is worth noting that in the eighth version of AJCC, T4a carcinoma includes carcinoma with direct invasion of peritoneum. T4b carcinoma is unresectable carcinoma that invades the other structures such as the aorta, vertebral body, trachea, etc.

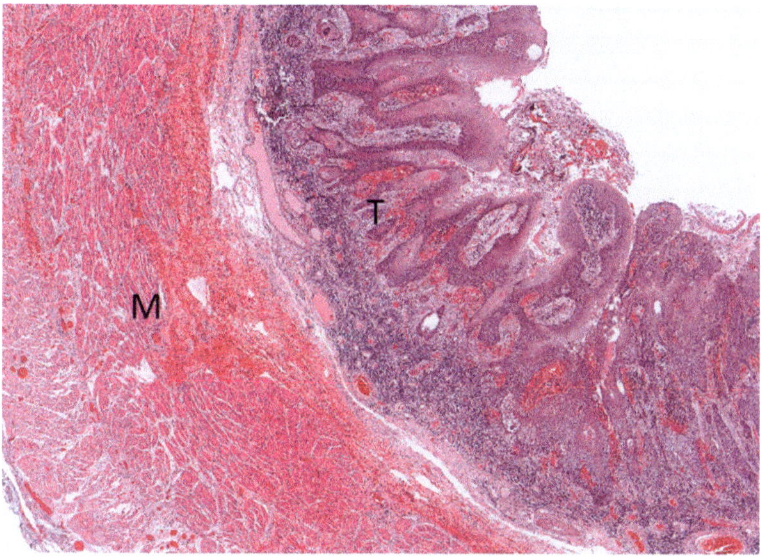

Fig. 2 Stage T1: esophageal squamous cell carcinoma (T) involves the submucosa of the esophagus; *M* muscularis propria (hematoxylin and eosin ×1.5)

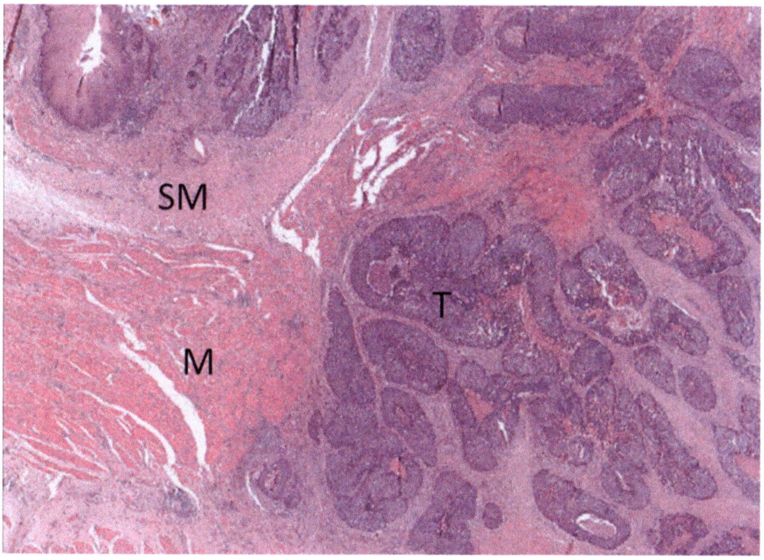

Fig. 3 Stage T2: esophageal squamous cell carcinoma (T) involves the muscularis propria (M) of the esophagus; *SM* submucosa (hematoxylin and eosin ×1)

3. The regional lymph nodes to search for metastases are adventitia or peri-esophageal lymph nodes from the upper esophageal sphincter to the coeliac artery, which includes supraclavicular cervical nodes to coeliac lymph nodes (Fig. 5). N0 stage means absence of regional lymph nodes metastases; N1 stage means one to two lymph nodes are positive for metastatic squamous

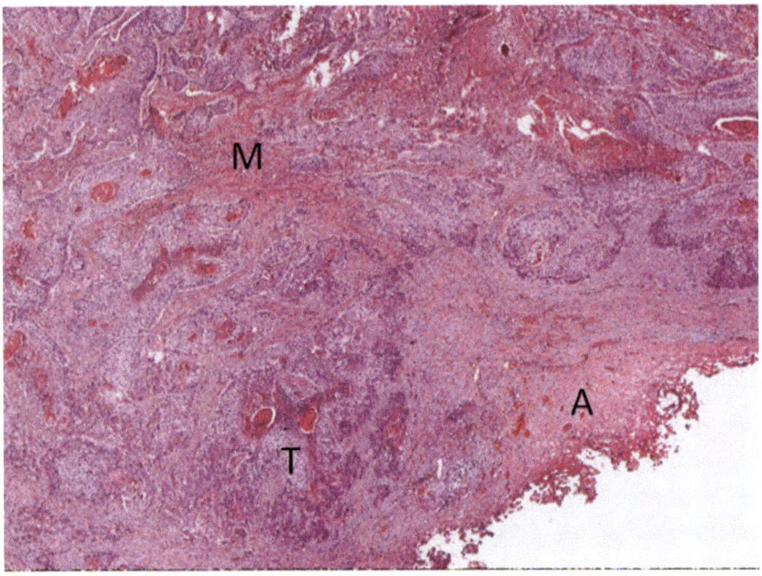

Fig. 4 Stage T3: esophageal squamous cell carcinoma (T) involves the adventitia (A) of the esophagus (hematoxylin and eosin ×1.5)

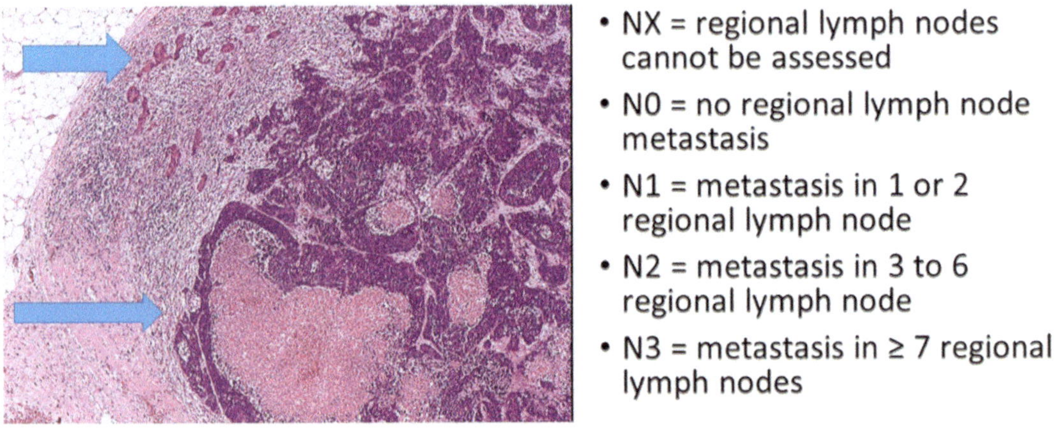

Fig. 5 The definition of regional lymph node (N) stage in AJCC. The right side of the figure reveals a peri-esophageal lymph node infiltrated by esophageal squamous cell carcinoma (arrows). The left side showing the different N stages as classified by the number of lymph nodes with metastases

cell carcinoma; N2 stage refers to three to six lymph nodes that are positive for metastatic squamous cell carcinoma, and N3 stage refers to seven or more lymph nodes involved by metastatic squamous cell carcinoma.

It is important to sample as many regional lymph nodes as possible in pathological examination for accurate N staging of patients with esophageal squamous cell carcinoma. In addition, the number of lymph node required for accurate staging depends on the grade and T stage of the cancer [6–9]. Rizk and colleagues proposed that in T1 stage carcinoma, approximately 10 lymph nodes must be sampled; in T2 stage carcinoma, 20 lymph nodes; and for T3 stage or T4 stage carcinomas, 30 lymph nodes or more [6]. Other studies have suggested sampling of 12 to 23 nodes [7, 8]. As the highest N classification (N3) is seven or more lymph nodes, theoretically, it would not be acceptable to sample less than seven lymph nodes in each patient with esophageal squamous cell carcinoma.

4. Radiological examination as well as observation plus or minus biopsy examination during the operation could determine the presence or absence of distant metastases in patients with esophageal squamous cell carcinoma. The absence of distant metastasis is M0. Squamous cell carcinoma with separate focus/foci of carcinoma in distant organ(s) is being defined as M1. M1 stage also includes non-regional lymph nodes involved by squamous cell carcinoma.

5. In esophageal squamous cell carcinoma, the grade of the tumor is a new criterion in addition to the TNM staging starting in the seventh edition of the Staging Manual. It is a parameter only useful in the pTNM stage group (not in other ypTNM or cTNM).

   In the current Staging Manual, the grades of squamous carcinoma include grade 1 (G1, well differentiated), grade 2 (G2, moderately differentiated), grade 3 (G3, poorly differentiated), and grade X (GX, differentiation cannot be assessed). "Undifferentiated" grade does not exist. Additional test (s) should be performed to uncover the grade of the carcinoma [10]. Otherwise, "undifferentiated" mentioned in the last edition is categorized as G3 squamous cell carcinoma.

   The grade (differentiation) of squamous cell carcinoma is important in the subgrouping of the early pTNM stages (stage I or II) for squamous cell carcinoma—carcinoma without lymph node or distant metastasis.

6. The esophagus starts below the hypopharynx. Clinically, the determination of location of the esophageal cancer is by endoscopic measurements from the incisors. The esophagus starts at approximately 15 cm from the incisors at around the upper esophageal sphincter [11]. The upper esophagus is from cervical esophagus to lower border of azygos vein (approximately 25 cm from the incisors) (Fig. 6). It comprises of two portions, the cervical esophagus which extends to the sternal notch (approximately 20 cm from incisors), and the upper thoracic esophagus (below the sternal notch). The middle esophagus starts from lower border of azygos vein to lower border of

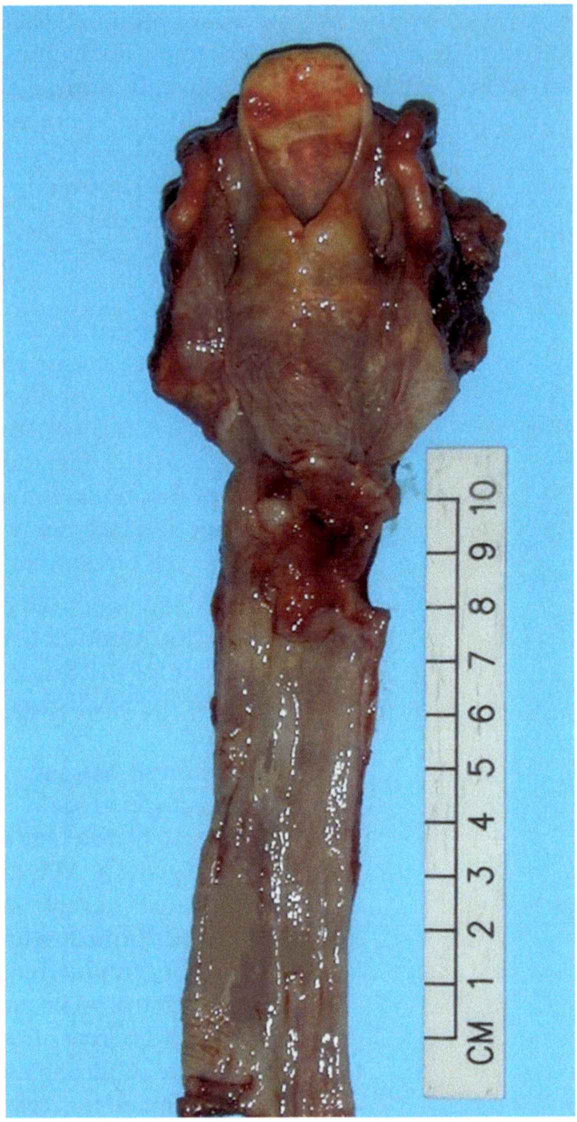

Fig. 6 Squamous cell carcinoma in the upper esophagus

inferior pulmonary vein (approximately 30 cm from the incisors) (Fig. 7). The lower esophagus is from the lower border of inferior pulmonary vein. The lower extent of an esophageal cancer is a controversial concept. The location of the carcinoma is the position of the epicenter of the tumor in the esophagus (Fig. 8). A carcinoma of the epicenter within 2 cm of the esophagogastric junction is an esophageal cancer. Nevertheless, squamous cell carcinoma of the stomach is extremely rare; presence of squamous cell carcinoma in the region around esophagogastric junction is practically a carcinoma from the esophagus.

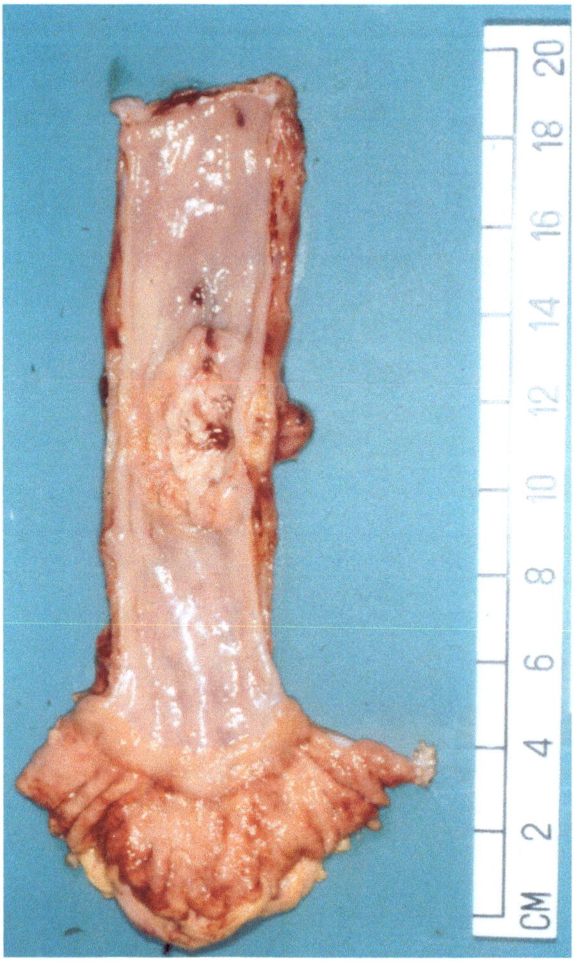

Fig. 7 Squamous cell carcinoma in the middle esophagus

It is a parameter of limit use in the pTNM stage group (not in other ypTNM or cTNM). For T3N0M0 grade 2–3/X squamous cell carcinomas, if they occur in lower esophagus, they are stage IIA, whereas those in upper/middle are stage IIB carcinomas.

7. For post-neoadjuvant pathological (yp) staging, the criteria for determining the staging of esophageal squamous cell carcinoma and adenocarcinoma are identical. The survival of patients with post-neoadjuvant pathological (yp) staging is less distinctive between different stage groups. In addition, these patients have poorer survival for early stage groups when compared with corresponding group for patients without neoadjuvant therapy.

   Table 1 summarizes the changes in pathological stage grouping from the seventh edition to eighth edition of AJCC Staging Manual. When compared to previous grouping, the

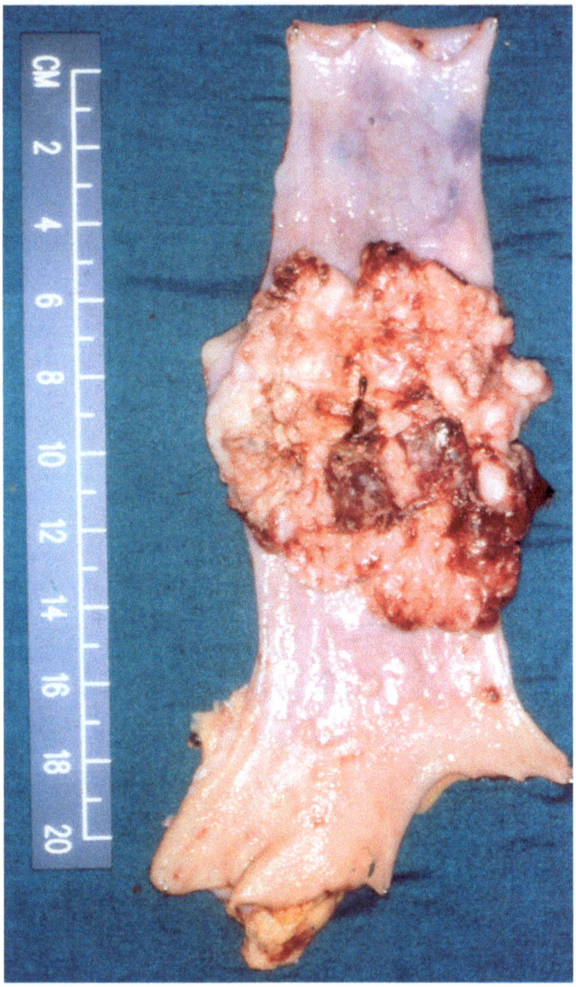

Fig. 8 Squamous cell carcinoma in the lower esophagus

advanced-stage squamous cell carcinomas show changes in subgroupings that are of prognostic significance. Stage III cancers comprise stage IIIA and stage IIIB cancers (in contrast to stage IIIA, stage IIIB, and stage IIIC in the seventh edition), and stage IV cancers are divided into stage IVA and stage IVB cancers (in contrast to a single category of stage IV).

In the eighth edition of the AJCC Staging Manual, presence of deep invasive squamous cell carcinoma (T3 stage) is an important criterion. Carcinomas with T3N0M0 classify the carcinomas into stage II (either A or B depending on grade and location), whereas in the seventh edition, carcinomas having T3N0M0 status could be either of stage IB or stage II. Furthermore, in the eighth edition of stage grouping, M1 carcinomas (with distant metastases) are stage IVB. Many of

Table 1
Comparisons between stage groupings for esophageal squamous cell carcinoma in the seventh and eighth edition of AJCC Squamous cell carcinoma stage groupings (without having neoadjuvant therapy)

Seventh edition						Eighth edition (pTNM)					
Stage	**T**	**N**	**M**	**G**	**Location**	**Stage**	**T**	**N**	**M**	**G**	**Location**
0	Tis	N0	M0	G1/X	Any	0	Tis	N0	M0	NA	Any
IA	T1	N0	M0	G1/X	Any	IA	T1a	N0	M0	G1/X	Any
IB	T1	N0	M0	G2–3	Any	IB	T1a	N0	M0	G2–3	Any
							T1b	N0	M0	G1–3/X	Any
	T2	N0	M0	G1/X	Lower/X		T2	N0	M0	G1	Any
	T3	N0	M0	G1/X	Lower/X	IIA	T3	N0	M0	Any	Lower
IIA	T2	N0	M0	G1	Upper/middle						
	T2	N0	M0	G2–3	Lower/X		T2	N0	M0	G2–3/X	Any
	T3	N0	M0	G1	Upper/middle		T3	N0	M0	G1	Upper/middle
	T3	N0	M0	G2–3	Lower/X						
IIB	T2	N0	M0	G2–3	Upper/middle						
	T3	N0	M0	G2–3	Upper/middle	IIB	T3	N0	M0	G2–3/X	Upper/middle
	T1	N1	M0	Any	Any		T1	N1	M0	Any	Any
	T2	N1	M0	Any	Any	IIIA	T2	N1	M0	Any	Any
IIIA	T1	N2	M0	Any	Any		T1	N2	M0	Any	Any
	T2	N2	M0	Any	Any	IIIB	T2	N2	M0	Any	Any
	T3	N1	M0	Any	Any		T3	N1	M0	Any	Any
	T4a	N0	M0	Any	Any		T4a	N0	M0	Any	Any
IIIB	T3	N2	M0	Any	Any		T3	N2	M0	Any	Any
IIIC	T4a	N1	M0	Any	Any		T4a	N1	M0	Any	Any
	T4a	N2	M0	Any	Any	IVA	T4a	N2	M0	Any	Any
	T4b	Any N	M0	Any	Any		T4b	Any N	M0	Any	Any
	Any T	N3	M0	Any	Any		Any T	N3	M0	Any	Any
IV	Any T	Any N	M1	Any	Any	IVB	Any T	Any N	M1	Any	Any

Table 2
Comparisons of the staging in esophageal squamous cell carcinoma in patients with and without neoadjuvant therapy

ypTNM (post-neoadjuvant therapy)				pTNM (pathological)					
Stage	T	N	M	Stage	T	N	M	G	Location
				0	Tis	N0	M0	NA	Any
I	T0	N0	M0						
	T1	N0	M0	IA	T1a	N0	M0	G1/X	Any
				IB	T1a	N0	M0	G2–3	Any
					T1b	N0	M0	G1–3/X	Any
	T2	N0	M0		T2	N0	M0	G1	Any
II	T3	N0	M0	IIA	T2	N0	M0	G2–3/X	Any
					T3	N0	M0	Any	Lower
					T3	N0	M0	G1	Upper/middle
				IIB	T3	N0	M0	G2–3/X	Upper/middle
IIIA	T0	N1	M0						
	T1	N1	M0		T1	N1	M0	Any	Any
	T2	N1	M0	IIIA	T2	N1	M0	Any	Any
IIIB	T0	N2	M0						
	T1	N2	M0		T1	N2	M0	Any	Any
	T2	N2	M0	IIIB	T2	N2	M0	Any	Any
	T3	N1	M0		T3	N1	M0	Any	Any
	T4a	N0	M0		T4a	N0	M0	Any	Any
	T3	N2	M0		T3	N2	M0	Any	Any
IVA	T4a	N1	M0		T4a	N1	M0	Any	Any
	T4a	N2	M0	IVA	T4a	N2	M0	Any	Any
	T4b	Any N	M0		T4b	Any N	M0	Any	Any
	Any T	N3	M0		Any T	N3	M0	Any	Any
IV	Any T	Any N	M1	IVB	Any T	Any N	M1	Any	Any

the advanced-stage carcinomas labeled as stage IIIC in the seventh edition of stage grouping (with T4b, N3, or T4aN2) now belong to stage IVA even if they have no distant metastasis (M0).

Table 2 shows the difference between the staging in esophageal squamous cell carcinoma with (yTNM) and without (pTNM) preoperative neoadjuvant therapy. For post-neoadjuvant therapy (yp) TNM group, grade and location of squamous cell carcinoma are not parameters for staging. In addition, stage I and stage II do not have prognostic staging subgroups (in contrast to having stage IA, stage IB, stage IIA, and stage IIB in pTNM grouping). Furthermore, N1 M0 (with low number of lymph node metastasis and without distant metastasis) esophageal squamous cell carcinoma in ypTNM group indicates a stage III carcinoma (it is stage IIB in pTNM grouping).

References

1. Lam AK (2018) Application of pathological staging in esophageal adenocarcinoma. Methods Mol Biol 1756:93–103
2. (2010) Esophagus and Esophagogastric junction. In: Chapter 10: AJCC cancer staging manual, 7th. edn, Part 3. Springer, New York, pp p103–p155
3. Rice TW, Blackstone EH, Rusch VW (2010) 7th edition of the AJCC cancer staging manual: esophagus and esophagogastric junction. Ann Surg Oncol 17:1721–1724
4. Rice TW, Kelsen D, Blackstone E, Ishwaran H, Patil DT, Bass AJ, Erasmus JJ, Gerdes H, Hofstetter WL (2016) Esophagus and Esophagogastric junction. In: Amin MB, Edge S, Greene F, Byrd DR, Brookland RK, Washington MK, Gershenwald JE, Compton CC, Hess KR, Sullivan DC, Jessup JM, Brierley JD, Gaspar LE, Schilsky RL, Balch CM, Winchester DP, Asare EA, Madera M, Gress DM, Meyer LR (eds) Chapter 16: AJCC cancer staging manual, 8th edn. Springer, New York, pp 185–202
5. D'Journo XB (2018) Clinical implication of the innovations of the 8(th) edition of the TNM classification for esophageal and esophago-gastric cancer. J Thorac Dis 10: S2671–S2681
6. Rizk NP, Ishwaran H, Rice TW, Chen LQ, Schipper PH, Kesler KA, Law S, Lerut TE, Reed CE, Salo JA, Scott WJ, Hofstetter WL, Watson TJ, Allen MS, Rusch VW, Blackstone EH (2010) Optimum lymphadenectomy for esophageal cancer. Ann Surg 251:46–50
7. Chen YJ, Schultheiss TE, Wong JY, Kernstine KH (2009) Impact of the number of resected and involved lymph nodes on esophageal cancer survival. J Surg Oncol 100:127–132
8. Peyre CG, Hagen JA, DeMeester SR, Altorki NK, Ancona E, Griffin SM, Hölscher A, Lerut T, Law S, Rice TW, Ruol A, van Lanschot JJ, Wong J, DeMeester TR (2008) The number of lymph nodes removed predicts survival in esophageal cancer: an international study on the impact of extent of surgical resection. Ann Surg 248:549–556
9. Rice TW, Ishwaran H, Hofstetter WL, Schipper PH, Kesler KA, Law S, Lerut EM, Denlinger CE, Salo JA, Scott WJ, Watson TJ, Allen MS, Chen LQ, Rusch VW Cerfolio RJ, Luketich JD, Duranceau A, Darling GE, Pera M, Apperson-Hansen C, Blackstone EH (2017) Esophageal cancer: associations with (pN+) lymph node metastases. Ann Surg 265:122–129
10. Brown IS, Fujii S, Kawachi H, Lam AK, Saito T Oesophageal squamous cell carcinoma NOS. In: Odze RD, Lam AK, Ochiai A, Washington MK (eds) Chapter 2: WHO classification of tumours, 5th edn, pp 48–53
11. Rice TW, Ishwaran H, Ferguson MK, Blackstone EH, Goldstraw P (2017) Cancer of the esophagus and esophagogastric junction: an eighth edition staging primer. J Thorac Oncol 12:36–42

Chapter 4

Macroscopic Examination of Surgical Specimen of Esophageal Squamous Cell Carcinoma

Alfred K. Lam

Abstract

Macroscopic examination of the surgical specimen of esophageal squamous cell carcinoma by pathologist is important for quality clinical management, research, as well as education purposes. The process includes dissection of the specimen, identification of the lesion, measurements, and taking appropriate samples for histopathological examination. The basic principle of the examination is to study the characteristics and extent of the cancer. In addition, examination of proximal resection margin and circumferential resection margin are important in the cancer. A standardized approach for macroscopic examination by professionals is needed for accurate diagnosis and to optimize the use of the surgical specimen with esophageal squamous cell carcinoma.

Key words Esophageal squamous cell carcinoma, Macroscopic, Cut up, Resection

1 Introduction

Macroscopic examination of the surgical specimen by pathologist is one, if not the most, important step for quality clinical management and research for patients with esophageal squamous cell carcinoma. The process includes dissection of the specimen, identification of the cancer, measurements, as well as taking appropriate samples (blocking) for histopathological examination. The information obtained provides histopathological parameters and pathological staging which are important for predicting prognosis and planning postoperative treatment of patients with esophageal squamous cell carcinoma (ESCC) (*see* Chapter 3). Macroscopic examination of the specimen with ESCC must be performed or supervised by a pathologist having knowledge of the anatomy, histopathology, and oncology relevant to the ESCC. Unprofessional handing of the specimen results in errors or inadequacy of information provided in the pathological reports which will endanger the life of patients with ESCC.

Alfred K. Lam (ed.), *Esophageal Squamous Cell Carcinoma: Methods and Protocols*, Methods in Molecular Biology, vol. 2129, https://doi.org/10.1007/978-1-0716-0377-2_4,

In this process of macroscopic examination, tissues could be triage to research purposes such as tissue biobanking for genomic researches, raising of cancer cell lines, xenografts in mice, etc. (*see* Chapters 8 and 11) [1–9]. It is worth noting that taking of these research samples is best supervised by a pathologist to ensure adequate tissue for pathological diagnosis and not to damage the specimen in a way to hinder the correct macroscopic and microscopic examination for proper pathology reporting.

The macroscopic specimen is an invaluable teaching resource. The process involves the use of pictures taken at macroscopic examination as well as the potting of the specimens in pathology museum. They could be used to teach undergraduate students in medicine, dentistry, and medical science for knowledges in the anatomy, histology, and pathology [10, 11]. The digital pictures taken from the specimen could be used in pathology lectures and as electronic resources in the internet. The pathology gross specimens could be used in pathology practical session [12]. The availability of digital pictures of the specimen allows the teaching of clinical pathology to medical personnel including to those in the remote rural sites [13]. For postgraduate level, these specimens are often used in the teaching and professional examination of medical specialists in training in surgery, pathology, oncology, and radiology. The pictures taken on the macroscopic examination could also be used for research presentations including poster and platform presentations, research papers, and book chapters. Proper dissection technique by pathologist to ensure the specimen could be reconstructed for potting in pathology museum is important for these teaching purposes.

In this chapter, the essential steps in macroscopic examination of esophageal squamous cell carcinoma are presented. The basic principle for macroscopic examination of esophageal squamous cell carcinoma is akin to esophageal adenocarcinoma [14]. In specimen with ESCC, it is important to examine the status of proximal resection margin and the possibility of multiple tumors. Because of rich networks of lymphatic in the esophagus as well as the field effect of carcinogenesis, ESCC often spread along the wall of the esophagus [15]. Synchronous carcinoma could occur in the esophagus [16]. Multiple squamous cell carcinoma occurs commonly in the esophagus and aerodigestive tract [17]. In addition, due to the anatomical limitations, resection could not extend as proximal as possible in patients with esophageal squamous cell carcinoma in upper portion of the esophagus. Thus, squamous dysplasia or carcinoma may occur in the proximal resection margin of the specimen which could lead to cancer recurrence. The margin should be sampled and examined in detail. On the other hand, Barrett esophagus and Barrette dysplasia are not associated with ESCC; less attention should be paid on these pathologies in surgical specimen from patients with ESCC.

2 Materials

1. Specimen obtained at surgery.
2. 10% formaldehyde (formalin) for fixation of specimen.
3. Personal protective equipment (disposable gloves, aprons, etc.).
4. Specimen request forms (paper or electronic copies).
5. Photographic facilities (digital camera or more complex pathology digital imaging system with digital camera and labelling options).
6. Photo printing papers and card papers.
7. Rulers and labels.
8. Recording equipment to document the findings at examination (digital recording, voice recognition software, etc.).
9. Ink (tissue marking dye).
10. Dissecting equipment (forceps, scissors, and surgical scalpels and disposable blades).
11. Pencil or digital labelling printer to label the cassette.
12. Tissue cassette.
13. Tissue processing machine.
14. Microtome.
15. Glass slides labelled with patient identifier.
16. Hematoxylin and eosin staining station/Autostainer.
17. Automatic glass cover slipper/coverslips and mounting medium.

3 Methods

1. Label the specimen with information for correct identification of the patient as well as supply of the correct clinical information. The clinical information may include clinical staging information, location of the cancer (from endoscopic biopsy examination—*see* Chapters 2 and 5), history of neoadjuvant therapy, and presence or history of other cancers.
2. Follow the protocol in your instituion in receiving the specimen after surgery (*see* **Note 1**).
3. Check the patient identity and clinical information on laboratory request form, or check from the electronic medical record which is of widespread use nowadays [18].

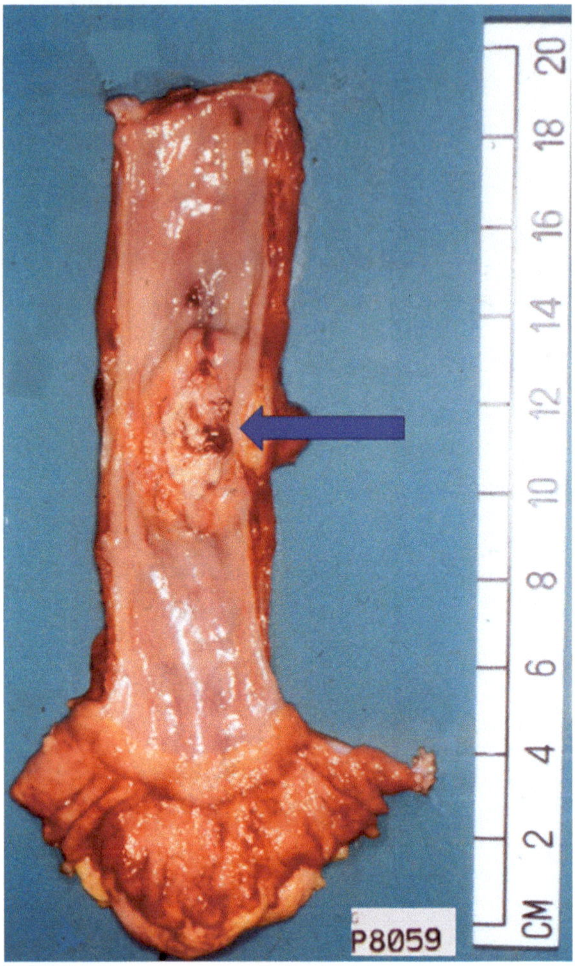

Fig. 1 The most common appearance of ESCC showing an ulcerative growth in the middle portion of the esophagus (arrow)

4. Open the specimen longitudinally in the esophagus, and open the stomach along the greater curve. Avoid transection of the tumor if possible.
5. Orientate the specimen on a piece of card paper with ruler (acts as a scale for photo), and label it (normally with histology number that can later identify the patient) (Fig. 1).
6. Take a picture of the specimen with the ESCC with either a digital camera or using photo station (*see* **Note 2**).
7. Set up the voice recording system to document the findings at examination and dissection of the specimen.
8. Recognize the type of specimen. For proximal ESCC, the specimen may include the upper aerodigestive tract (pharyngolaryngo-esophagectomy) (Fig. 2), whereas for

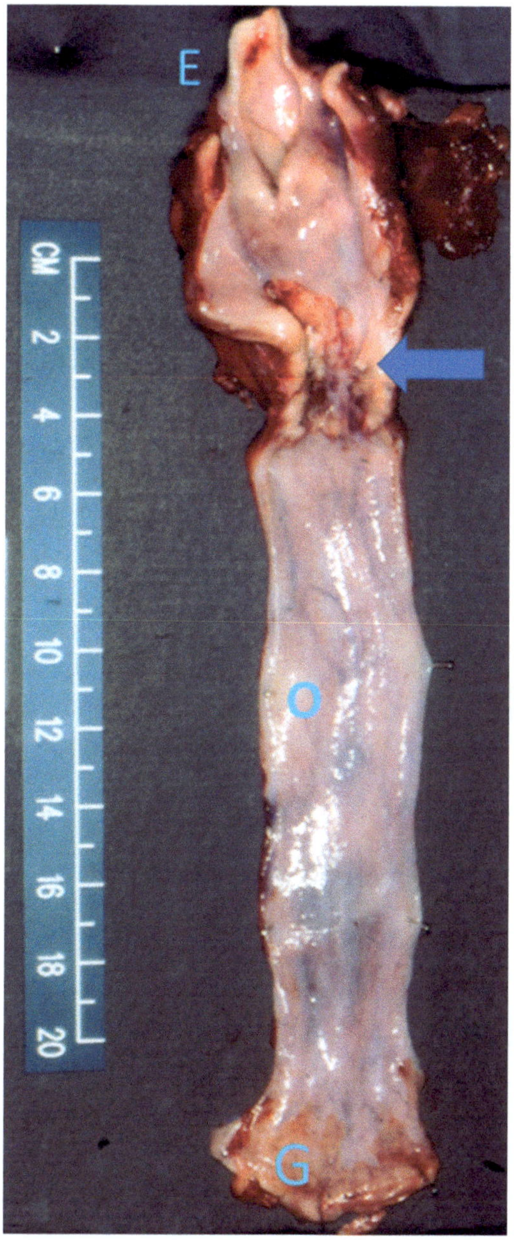

Fig. 2 The specimen with ESCC in the upper third of the esophagus (arrow). The specimen includes the epiglottis (E) in hypopharynx, esophagus (O), and stomach (G)

ESCC in another portion of the esophagus, the specimen could be esophagogastrectomy.

9. Make measurements of the specimen to get an overall dimension of the specimen. These include the longitudinal dimensions of the esophagus and the attached tissues (stomach and hypopharynx).

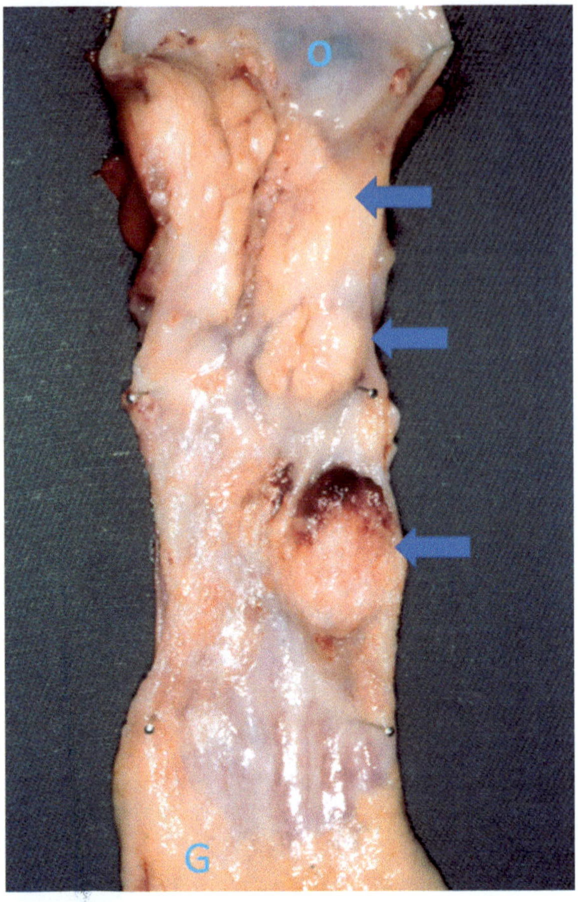

Fig. 3 The specimen shows a tumor with sclerotic growth in the upper part (arrow) together with two tumors distal to the main tumor (arrows). (O, esophagus; G, stomach)

10. Identify the tumor(s) and note the macroscopic appearance of the tumor.

    The macroscopic appearance is most commonly an ulcerative growth (Fig. 1). The appearance could be sclerotic, and occasionally, there may be satellite tumor nodules (Fig. 3). In patients with adjuvant chemotherapy, there may be no microscopically visible tumor or more commonly a linear fibrotic lesion (Fig. 4). Occasionally, there may be satellite tumor nodules.

11. Measure the size (maximum length of the tumor) of the tumor.

12. Measure the status of the longitudinal resection margins: these include distance from the proximal edge of tumor to proximal end of specimen and distance from the distal edge of the tumor to distal resection margin.

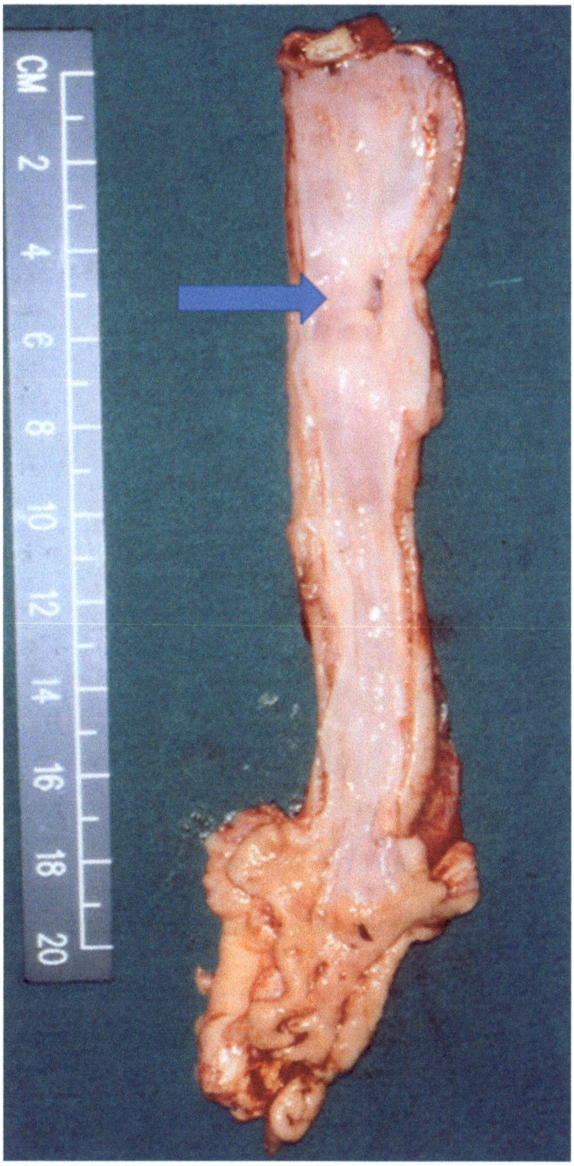

Fig. 4 The patient with confirmed ESCC was treated with adjuvant chemoradiation. The resected specimen shows no tumor growth but a tiny scar (arrow)

13. Measure the center of the tumor from the esophagogastric junction. This serves as a checkpoint for the anatomical location of the tumor to compare with the clinical information provided.
14. Note the involvement of adjacent structures (e.g., in pharyngolaryngo-esophagectomy, note any involvement of the larynx, any tumor on the adventitia, etc.).

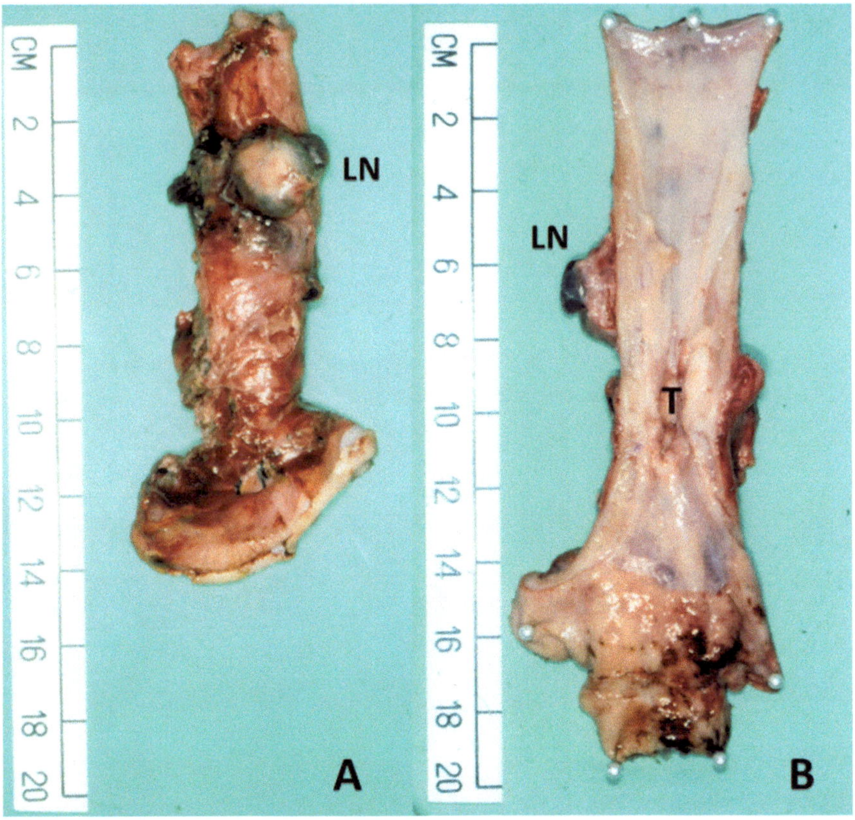

Fig. 5 (**a**) Before cutting open the specimen, there is an enlarged lymph node (LN) with cancer identified in the peri-esophageal tissue. (**b**) After the specimen being cut open, there is a sclerotic tumor (T) in the lower esophagus. The enlarged lymph node (LN) could also be seen

15. Note any enlarged lymph node(s) with cancer (can sample for biobanking if the specimen is received in fresh) (Fig. 5).
16. There may be some other specimens submitted by the surgeons as they may dissect other adjacent structures to confirm or exclude the presence of cancer invasion. They are helpful in staging (*see* Chapter 3).
17. Ink the circumferential esophageal margins (*see* **Note 3**) (Fig. 6).
18. Document the location of sampling of blocks for microscopic examination by either making drawing on the printed photo or using labelling on screen by software in pathology digital imaging system (Fig. 7).
19. Using dissecting equipment, sample (blocking) the proximal (esophageal resection margin) and distal (gastric resection margin) of the specimen. In pharyngolaryngo-esophagectomy specimen, the epiglottic and tracheal resection margins should also be sampled. Samples could be taken on the esophagogastric junction and unremarkable esophageal mucosa.

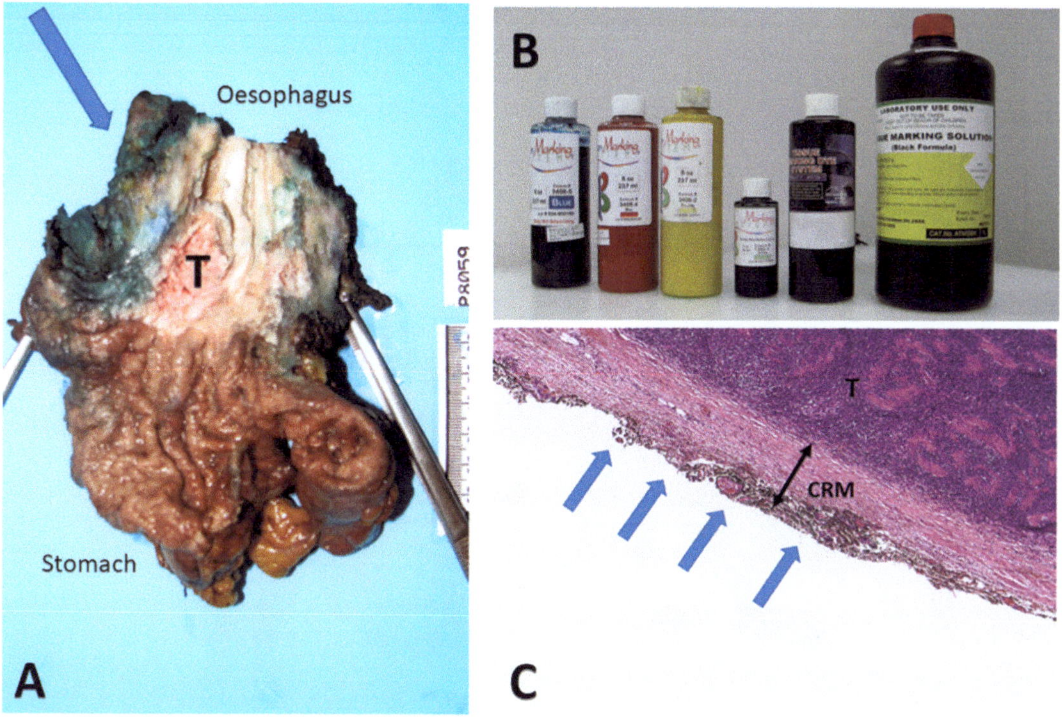

Fig. 6 (**a**) The circumferential margin of the specimen is inked by tissue marking dye (arrow): T = tumor. (**b**) Tissue dyes of different colors are used in histology to ink different resection margins. (**c**) On microscopic examination, the color will survive the processing and appears in the microscopic section to identify the margin (arrows). The distance (CRM) of the tumor (T) to the resection margin can thus be measured

20. Dissect the tumor (*see* **Note 4**).
21. There may be no visiable lesion in the esophagus after adjuvant chemoradiation. In this instance, embed the whole scar area, and sample areas proximal and distal to the scars to ensure microscopic clearance.
22. Sample the lymph nodes.

    Surgeons may submit the regional lymph nodes separately. Other than this, sample as much as possible the peri-esophageal soft tissue as many lymph nodes are in hidden in the tissue. If no obvious lymph nodes are identified macroscopically, all the peri-esophageal soft tissue could be sampled.
23. Embed the other tissues submitted for pathological examination separately by the surgeon(s).
24. The whole specimen is wrapped together to allow reconstruction and taking additional blocks if required.
25. The blocks are put in plastic cassettes (labelled with identifier number) in a container with formalin (Fig. 8).

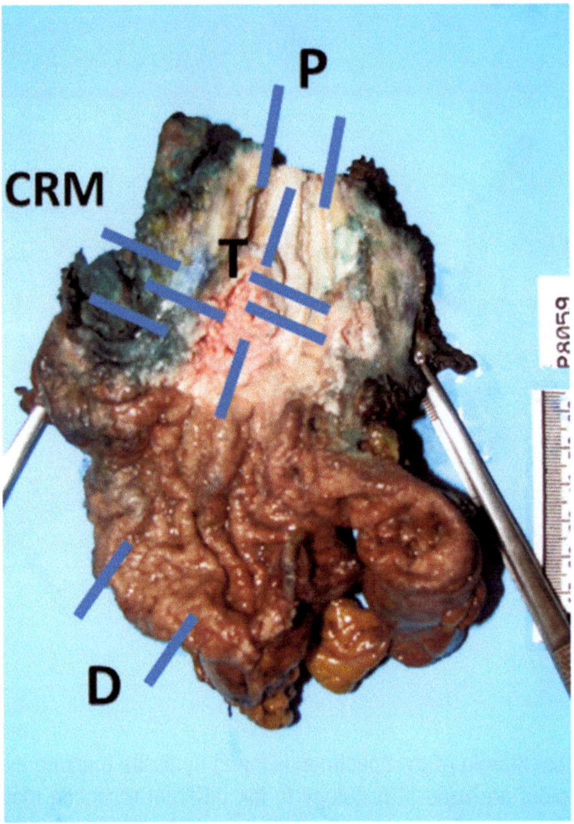

Fig. 7 Drawings (digital) on the picture of the specimen showing the areas where blocks have been taken from histological examination (blue lines). Blocks were taken from the proximal resection margin (P), distal resection margin (D), circumferential resection margin (CRM), esophagogastric junction (OG), and the tumor (T). It is better to take more blocks from the tumour. The CRM should be included in the block(s) sampled from the tumour

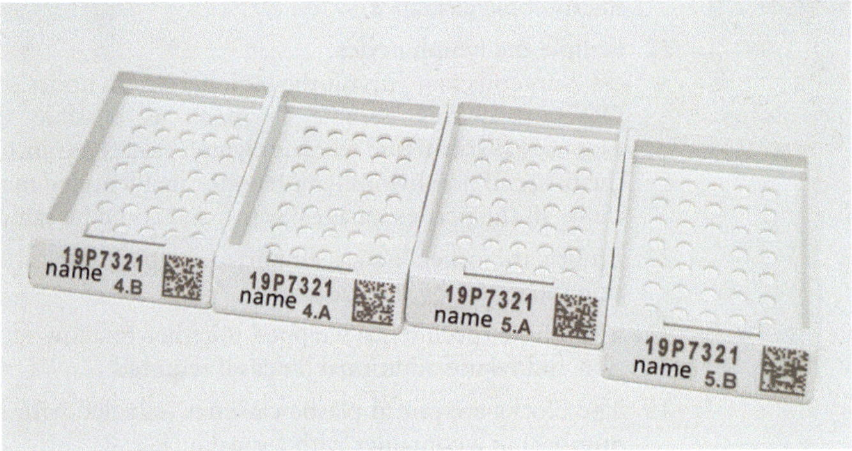

Fig. 8 Modern cassettes for the tissues have labellers printed with identifiers. Two identifiers are recommended to prevent errors. The first identifier is normally the pathology number/accession number (generated from the barcode attached to the specimen). The second could be the family name of the patient

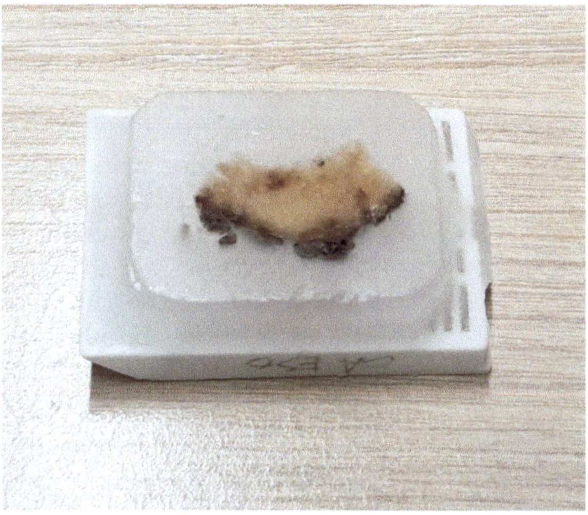

Fig. 9 Paraffin block made from the tissue in the cassette showing ESCC tissue embedded in wax. Sections of approximately 5 μm thick are cut from the block and stained with hematoxylin and eosin for microscopic examination

26. The plastic cassettes were put in tissue processing machine to make paraffin blocks (Fig. 9).
27. The paraffin blocks were cut by microtome into sections and mounted on glass slides (labelled with identifier number).
28. The sections were stained with hematoxylin and eosin.
29. Cover the stained sections with mounting medium and cover-slips either manually or by automatic glass cover slipper.
30. Examine all the sections under light microscope.

4 Notes

1. If tissues from ESCC are needed for biobanking, patient-derived xenograft, and frozen section diagnosis, the resection specimen with cancer will be received in fresh as soon as after operation (*see* Chapters 7, 8, and 11). For most patients, the specimen will need to be fixed in 10% formaldehyde immediately to prevent degradation of the tissues [19]. Poor or delayed fixation will produce low-quality morphology for histopathology assessment as well as affect the results of immunohistochemistry and genomic studies (*see* Chapter 8). For esophagectomy specimen, the specimen should be cut open for better penetration of fixative. The volume of fixatures should be enough to cover the whole specimen. On the other hand, the specimen preferably should not be fixed in formalin

for more than 1 day. Long fixation time will affect the validity of tests such as in detection of protein or RNA [20].

2. Good digital pictures are essential for documentation of the findings of extent of ESCC. The pictures are used to guide the pathologists for writing the histopathology report as wells as for teaching, assessment, and publication [21]. As the specimen is cut and dissembled in pathological examination, the digital pictures are the best documentation of the status of the cancer. The specimen should be opened, orientated, and cleaned before the photography. Proper lighting and background color as well as using right-sized scale and patient identifier should be employed [22].
3. Circumferential resection margin is an independent prognostic factor for survival in patients with resected ESCC [23]. In patients without lymph node metastasis, tumours with the circumferential margin more than 600 μm have better survivals than those with the margin closer to the tumour. Circumferential margin in this situation is the adventitia soft tissue that was resected with the esophagus. Unlike other portion of the gut, the esophagus does not have serosa lining for assessment. It is important to identify the landbank by tissue marking dye used in histopathology [24]. The dye should be able to survive processing in histopathology and could be seen microscopically in the resection margin, so the distance of cancer from the margin could be measured microscopically. The circumferential margin is important.
4. Dissection of the specimen is the most important step as it allows the study of biobanking and animal experiments (*see* Chapters 8 and 11). After collection of the tissue, additional blocks should be taken for histological examination. If the tumor is small (e.g., 4 cm or below), the whole tumor should be embedded. It the tumor is large, at least one block per centimeter of tumor should be sampled. The tumor blocks should include a block of the tumor to be cut to see the depth of involvement by the tumor in the esophagus. Sampling should be taken to study the relation between the tumor and the inked circumferential adventitia margin. The blocks taken should include the deepest extent of the tumor in the wall of the esophagus. The tumor should also be sampled with mucosa adjacent to the tumor. Squamous dysplasia is common in the area. Biobanking focusing on research requiring squamous dysplasia needs to obtain tissue in this area [25].

References

1. Dai W, Ko JMY, Choi SSA, Yu Z, Ning L, Zheng H, Gopalan V, Chan KT, Lee NP, Chan KW, Law SY, Lam AK, Lung ML (2017) Whole-exome sequencing reveals critical genes underlying metastasis in oesophageal squamous cell carcinoma. J Pathol 242:500–510
2. Haque MH, Gopalan V, Chan KW, Shiddiky MJ, Smith RA, Lam AK (2016) Identification of novel FAM134B (JK1) mutations in oesophageal squamous cell carcinoma. Sci Rep 6:29173
3. Wong ML, Tao Q, Fu L, Wong KY, Qiu GH, Law FB, Tin PC, Cheung WL, Lee PY, Tang JC, Tsao GS, Lam KY, Law S, Wong J, Srivastava G (2006) Aberrant promoter hypermethylation and silencing of the critical 3p21 tumour suppressor gene, RASSF1A, in Chinese oesophageal squamous cell carcinoma. Int J Oncol 28:767–773
4. Hu YC, Lam KY, Law S, Wong J, Srivastava G (2001) Profiling of differentially expressed cancer-related genes in esophageal squamous cell carcinoma (ESCC) using human cancer cDNA arrays: overexpression of oncogene MET correlates with tumor differentiation in ESCC. Clin Cancer Res 7:3519–3525
5. Hu YC, Lam KY, Law S, Wong J, Srivastava G (2001) Identification of differentially expressed genes in esophageal squamous cell carcinoma (ESCC) by cDNA expression array: overexpression of Fra-1, Neogenin, Id-1, and CDC25B genes in ESCC. Clin Cancer Res 7:2213–2221
6. Tang JC, Wan TS, Wong N, Pang E, Lam KY, Law SY, Chow LM, Ma ES, Chan LC, Wong J, Srivastava G (2001) Establishment and characterization of a new xenograft-derived human esophageal squamous cell carcinoma cell line SLMT-1 of Chinese origin. Cancer Genet Cytogenet 124:36–41
7. Hu Y, Lam KY, Wan TS, Fang W, Ma ES, Chan LC, Srivastava G (2000) Establishment and characterization of HKESC-1, a new cancer cell line from human esophageal squamous cell carcinoma. Cancer Genet Cytogenet 118:112–120
8. Hu YC, Lam KY, Law SY, Wan TS, Ma ES, Kwong YL, Chan LC, Wong J, Srivastava G (2002) Establishment, characterization, karyotyping, and comparative genomic hybridization analysis of HKESC-2 and HKESC-3: two newly established human esophageal squamous cell carcinoma cell lines. Cancer Genet Cytogenet 135:120–127
9. Ip JC, Ko JM, Yu VZ, Chan KW, Lam AK, Law S, Tong DK, Lung ML (2015) A versatile orthotopic nude mouse model for study of esophageal squamous cell carcinoma. Biomed Res Int 2015:910715
10. Gopalan V, Dissabandara L, Nirthanan S, Forwood MR, Lam AK (2016) Integrating gross pathology into teaching of undergraduate medical science students using human cadavers. Pathol Int 66:511–517
11. Ariana A, Amin M, Pakneshan S, Dolan-Evans-E, Lam AK (2016) Integration of traditional and e-learning methods to improve learning outcomes for dental students in histopathology. J Dent Educ 80:1140–1148
12. Gopalan V, Kasem K, Pillai S, Olveda D, Ariana A, Leung M, Lam AKY (2018) Evaluation of multidisciplinary strategies and traditional approaches in teaching pathology in medical students. Pathol Int 68:459–466
13. Lam AK, Veitch J, Hays R (2005) Resuscitating the teaching of anatomical pathology in undergraduate medical education: web-based innovative clinicopathological cases. Pathology 37:360–363
14. Kumarasinghe MP, Brown IS, Charlton A, De Boer B, Eckstein R, Epari K, Gill A. Lam A, Lauwers G, Raftopoulos S, Price T (2013) Tumours of the oesophagus and gastro-oesophageal junction structured reported protocol, 1st edition, Published on web by Royal College of Pathologists of Australasia. http://www.rcpa.edu.au//Library/Practising-Pathology/Structured-Pathology-Reporting-of-Cancer/Cancer-Protocols
15. Lam KY, Ma LT, Wong J (1996) Measurement of extent of spread of oesophageal squamous carcinoma by serial sectioning. J Clin Pathol 49:124–129
16. Lam KY, Law SY, Loke SL, Fok M, Ma LT (1996) Double sarcomatoid carcinomas of the oesophagus. Pathol Res Pract 192(6):604–609
17. Priante AV, Castilho EC, Kowalski LP (2011) Second primary tumors in patients with head and neck cancer. Curr Oncol Rep 13:132–137
18. Carter JT (2015) Electronic medical records and quality improvement. Neurosurg Clin N Am 26:245–251
19. Kim SW, Roh J, Park CS (2016) Immunohistochemistry for pathologists: protocols, pitfalls, and tips. J Pathol Transl Med 50:411–418
20. Evers DL, Fowler CB, Cunningham BR, Mason JT, O'Leary TJ (2011) The effect of formaldehyde fixation on RNA: optimization

of formaldehyde adduct removal. J Mol Diagn 13:282–288

21. Hays R, Veitch J, Lam A (2005) Teaching clinical pathology by flexible delivery in rural sites. Aust J Rural Health 13:232–235
22. Rampy BA, Glassy EF (2015) Pathology gross photography: the beginning of digital pathology. Surg Pathol Clin 8:195–211
23. Yang YS, Wang YC, Deng HY, Yuan Y, Wang ZQ, He D, Chen LQ (2018) Prognostic value of circumferential resection margin in T3N0M0 esophageal squamous cell carcinoma. Ann Transl Med 6:303
24. Williams AS, Hache KD (2014) Recognition and discrimination of tissue-marking dye color by surgical pathologists: recommendations to avoid errors in margin assessment. Am J Clin Pathol 142:355–361
25. Tang JC, Lam KY, Law S, Wong J, Srivastava G (2001) Detection of genetic alterations in esophageal squamous cell carcinomas and adjacent normal epithelia by comparative DNA fingerprinting using inter-simple sequence repeat PCR. Clin Cancer Res 7:1539–1545

Chapter 5

Endoscopic Diagnosis and Treatment of Esophageal Squamous Cell Carcinoma

Ru Zhang, Louis H. S. Lau, Peter I. C. Wu, Hon-Chi Yip, and Sunny H. Wong

Abstract

Esophageal squamous cell carcinoma (ESCC) is a deadly disease, partly because it is often diagnosed late in disease stage. An accurate early diagnosis by endoscopy could detect advanced carcinoma as well as curable dysplasia and early ESCC. This could save patients from incurable advanced malignancy. Important progress has been made in high-quality endoscopic diagnosis, including magnifying endoscopy, narrow-band imaging, and other image enhancement, as well as in techniques in endoscopic resection. These emerging techniques will aid the early diagnosis of ESCC that lead to higher chance of curing the cancer.

Key words Esophageal cancer, Squamous cell carcinoma, Esophagogastroduodenoscopy, Image-enhanced endoscopy, Endoscopic resection

1 Introduction

Esophageal cancer is a common cancer and represents a major global health burden. It is the eighth commonest cancer and sixth commonest cause of cancer death, with over 456,000 new cases and 400,000 deaths [1]. Whereas esophageal adenocarcinoma (EAC) is more common in developed countries, esophageal squamous cell carcinoma (ESCC) is prevalent in East Asia, East Africa, and South America and commonly affects the upper two-third of the esophagus. ESCC is an aggressive cancer with rapid growth and high lymph node metastasis rate [2, 3]. It is known to be frequently associated with synchronous or metachronous cancers, especially with primary head and neck squamous cell cancer. The main risk factors of ESCC include alcohol consumption and smoking [4]. The majority of patients with ESCC present with advanced disease with the 5-year survival rate of less than 20%; however, with early diagnosis, the survival of early staged cancers can be up to 80–90% especially when amenable to surgical or endoscopic therapies [2, 3]. Therefore, early detection strategies can significantly improve outcomes of patients with ESCC.

Alfred K. Lam (ed.), *Esophageal Squamous Cell Carcinoma: Methods and Protocols*, Methods in Molecular Biology, vol. 2129, https://doi.org/10.1007/978-1-0716-0377-2_5,

Endoscopy is regarded as the gold standard for the detection and diagnosis of esophageal cancer. ESCC can often be diagnosed with high-resolution white-light endoscopy, and its sensitivity can be further improved by image-enhanced endoscopy techniques such as narrowband imaging (NBI) or Lugol chromoendoscopy [5, 6]. The diagnosis of ESCC can be confirmed by targeted biopsies [7]. Endoscopic ultrasound (EUS) can often aid cancer staging in both tumor (T) and nodal (N) staging [8, 9]. Once the diagnosis has been made, endoscopic treatment can be used for epithelial dysplasia or early superficial mucosal carcinomas, using endoscopic resection techniques including endoscopic mucosal resection (EMR) or endoscopic submucosal dissection (ESD) [10–12]. In this chapter, we summarize the role of endoscopy in diagnosing and managing ESCC in clinical practice.

2 Materials

2.1 Diagnostic Endoscopy

1. Oral medications such as anti-foaming agent (e.g., dimethicone) and mucolytic agents (e.g., pronase, *N*-acetylcysteine).
2. Intravenous medications such as antispasmodic (e.g., butylscopolamine), sedative (e.g., midazolam), and analgesics (e.g., fentanyl).
3. High-definition gastroscope (preferably with optical magnification and NBI functions).
4. Biopsy forceps for possible need of tissue histology.
5. 1.2% Lugol's iodine solution and a plastic spray catheter for performing Lugol chromoendoscopy. To prepare the solution, mix 12 g of iodine and 24 g of potassium iodide in 1000 mL water.

2.2 Endoscopic Ultrasound (EUS)

1. Medications as in usual endoscopy (*see* Subheading 2.1).
2. Echoendoscope with ultrasound probes typically at frequencies of 7.5–12 MHz. High-frequency miniprobes (20 MHz) can be used for more detailed visualization of the esophageal wall.
3. Aspiration needle for EUS-guided fine needle aspiration (FNA).

2.3 Endoscopic Resection

1. Medications as in usual endoscopy (*see* Subheading 2.1). Note that higher doses of sedative and analgesia, monitored anesthesia care (MAC), or general anesthesia may be required if longer procedure is expected.
2. Argon plasma coagulation (APC) probe or snare/knife tip with soft coagulation for marking.

3. Endoscopic caps for cap-assisted endoscopic mucosal resection (EMR) or dedicated kits for ligation-EMR.
4. Injection catheter for submucosal injection.
5. For EMR requiring submucosal injection, prepare the injectate by mixing saline and diluted epinephrine (1:1).
6. A disposable polypectomy snare for the EMR procedure.
7. For endoscopic submucosal dissection (ESD), prepare the lifting agent (colloid solution, methylcellulose, or hyaluronic acid). Special dye such as indigo carmine can be added to the injectate.
8. Electrosurgical knives and forceps devices for the ESD procedure.

3 Methods

3.1 Diagnostic Endoscopy

The goal of the diagnostic endoscopy is to determine the presence and location of esophageal neoplasia, and/or to biopsy any suspicious lesions. Endoscopy can also provide information about the tumor size, extent, and presence of synchronous lesion. Advanced ESCC often manifest as a mass or a stricture (Fig. 1), whereas early neoplasms may be flat and subtle and therefore challenging to be detected (*see* **Note 1**). These early neoplasms can appear as well-demarcated areas with changes in color or brightness on white-light endoscopy (Fig. 2a), and their detection can be aided by image-enhanced endoscopy techniques [5], such as NBI [13] or Lugol chromoendoscopy [14, 15]. It is suggested that the use of sedation [16], antispasmodic agent [17, 18], and anti-foaming agent [19] can enhance the detection rate of superficial esophageal neoplasms. Endoscopic biopsies are recommended for suspected lesions (*see* **Note 2**). Lastly, EUS may be useful for selected cases for staging of the ESCC [8, 9].

3.1.1 White-Light Endoscopy

1. Patients should be fasted for at least 6 h before endoscopy.
2. Pre-medications such as antispasmodic (e.g., butylscopolamine) and anti-foaming (e.g., dimethicone) agents may be given 10 min prior to endoscopy.
3. Prepare patient to lie in left lateral position. Give intravenous sedation as required. Apply topical analgesia by administration of 10% lidocaine spray to the pharyngeal mucosa.
4. Prepare the endoscope and release the brakes for angulation controls. Pass the endoscope through the bite guard and over the tongue to reach the oropharynx. Advance gently past the epiglottis and cricoarytenoid cartilage, and pass posteriorly to reach the esophagus.

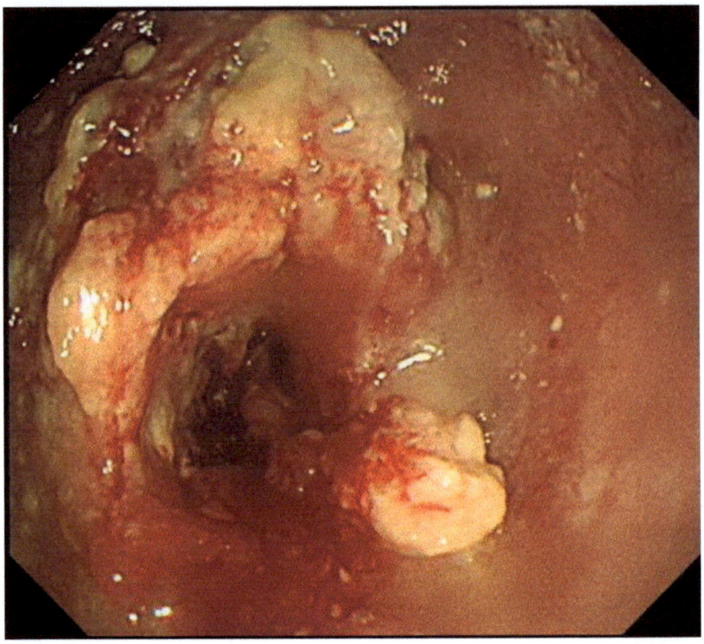

Fig. 1 Diagnosis of ESCC using endoscopy. A circumferential and necrotic tumor causing luminal stenosis is seen

5. Systematically examine the esophagus, stomach, and proximal duodenum.
6. For examination of the esophagus, visually inspect the organ from gastro-esophageal junction to the upper esophageal sphincter. Examine the mucosa for abnormalities that may appear as a tumor, nodule, stricture, plaque, erosion, ulcer, white patch, or focal erythema.
7. Upon detection of lesions, describe their size, site, extent, circumferential involvement, presence of obstruction, and distance into stomach or from the incisor teeth.

3.1.2 Narrowband Imaging (NBI) (Fig. 2b, c)

1. After white-light endoscopy, change the light filter to NBI mode using a control knob on the endoscope.
2. Examine the esophagus carefully again from the gastro-esophageal junction to the upper esophageal sphincter.
3. Look for well-demarcated brownish areas which may point to early neoplasia (*see* **Note 3**). Magnify and zoom in the area, to examine and classify the microvascular patterns (*see* **Notes 4–6**). Also describe the size, location, extent, and margin of the lesions.

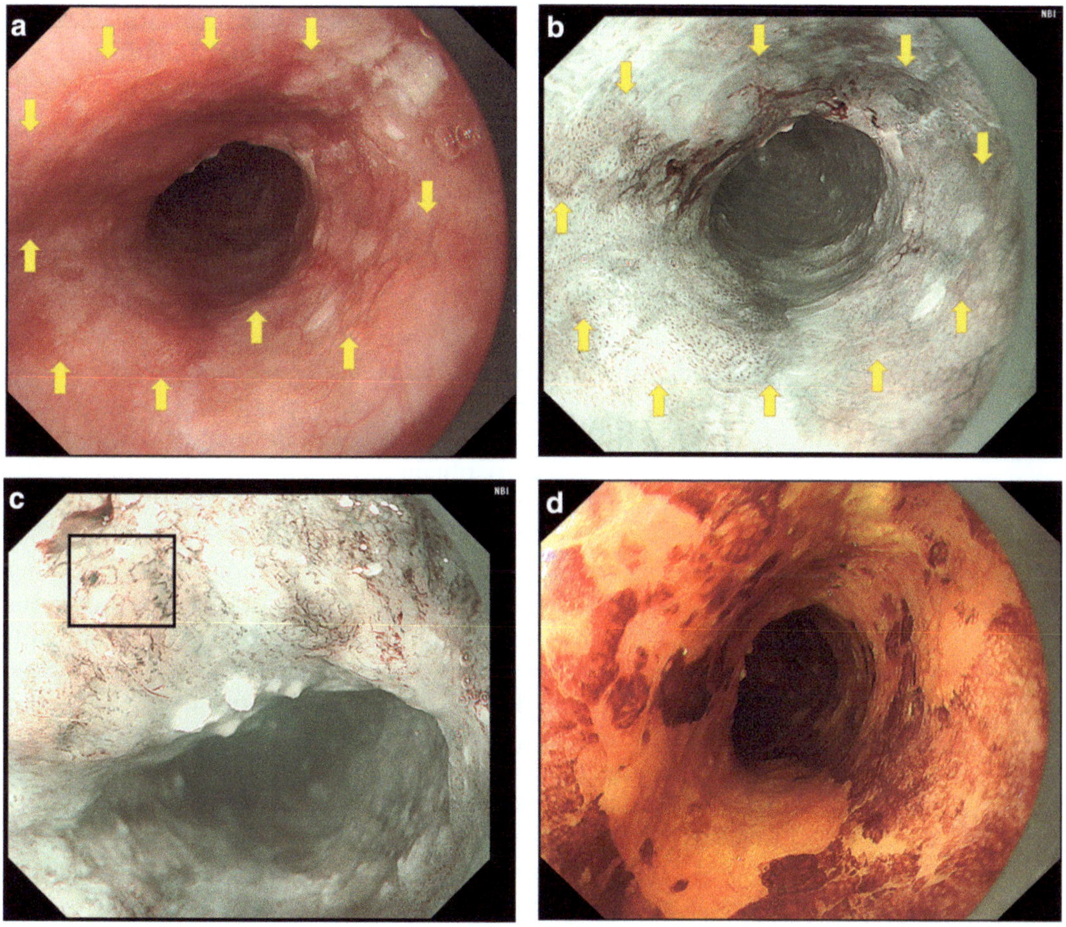

Fig. 2 Diagnosis of superficial ESCC using endoscopy. (**a**) White-light endoscopic image of superficial ESCC. A reddish flat lesion is seen. (**b**) Narrowband imaging identifies the same lesion as a well-demarcated brownish area. (**c**) Magnifying endoscopy with narrowband imaging showing dilated and irregular microvessels. Some avascular areas are visualized in the region marked by the square. (**d**) Lugol chromoendoscopy. After staining, neoplastic lesions are clearly seen as irregularly shaped Lugol-voiding lesions

3.1.3 Lugol Chromoendoscopy (Fig. 2d)

1. Spray the esophagus evenly with 20–30 mL of the Lugol solution from the gastro-esophageal junction to the upper esophageal sphincter, using a plastic spray catheter through the endoscopic channel.
2. Examine the esophagus for the staining (*see* **Notes 7** and **8**). Describe and photograph all unstained or overstained areas.
3. Look for suspicious unstained areas of Lugol-voiding lesions (LVLs). The size, location, extent, and margin of the LVL should be recorded.

3.1.4 Endoscopic Ultrasound (EUS)

1. The EUS procedure is an adjunct to standard endoscopy. The patient is prepared and sedated in the same manner for an endoscopy.

2. Insert the echoendoscope into the esophagus to obtain a robust image of the esophageal wall lining. Identify the five structured layers of the esophageal wall, including the superficial mucosa, deep mucosa, submucosa, muscularis propria, and adventitia.
3. Locate the esophageal neoplasia, and assess the T staging according to the depth of invasion (*see* **Note 9**). High-frequency catheter may permit more accurate determination of tumor invasive depth especially for small superficial cancers.
4. For selected cancers, EUS can be used to assess the N staging by identifying suspicious lymph nodes, which typically show up with an echo-poor pattern, round shape, smooth border, and a width >10 mm. EUS FNA can be performed by advancing an aspiration needle to obtain cytological confirmation of the malignant lymph nodes.

3.1.5 Endoscopic Resection

The management of ESCC depends on the tumor stage and other patient conditions including physical fitness and performance status [2, 3]. Early cancers may be suitable for endoscopic treatment, whereas locally advanced cancers are treated with chemotherapy, radiotherapy, surgical resection, or combinations of these. Due to difference in the cancer biology, ESCC generally infiltrates and invades through the epithelium earlier than esophageal adenocarcinoma [20]. As such, the therapeutic window for endoscopic resection is relatively narrow for ESCC. Generally, endoscopic resection for ESCC is limited to dysplasia and superficial mucosal cancers, whereas surgery is recommended for those with deep mucosal or submucosal invasion (*see* **Note 10**). Nevertheless, treatment may be individualized according to patient comorbidities and performance status, as well as expertise of individual centers. Endoscopic resection in carefully selected patients can achieve long-term cure [21–23]. Compared with esophagectomy that carries significant short-term mortality and morbidity [23, 24], endoscopic resection provides a chance for complete tumor resection, with reduced operative risks, adverse events, and length of hospital stay but equivalent oncological outcomes in selected cases (*see* **Notes 11** and **12**).

3.1.6 Endoscopic Mucosal Resection (EMR)

1. EMR can achieve complete resection especially for smaller mucosal lesions. Several techniques have been developed (*see* **Note 13**).
2. For cap-assisted EMR, first identify the target lesion, and mark the area for resection by placing cautery marks around the lesion, by APC or touching the mucosa with snare or knife tip with soft coagulation current.

3. Apply a submucosal injection with saline and diluted epinephrine to the base of lesion. Special dye such as methylene blue or indigo carmine can be added for better visualization and differentiation of layers.
4. The lesion is approached with the edge of the clear cap attached to endoscope. Suction should be applied, with the lesion and surrounding mucosa to be pulled inside the clear cap.
5. A snare is used to grasp and ligate the lesion with cutting current of electrocautery. Any superficial blood vessels would be cauterized simultaneously.
6. An alternative method of ligation-EMR can also be performed using a dedicated EMR kit with multiple small rubber bands.
7. For ligation-EMR, the lesion is first approached by suction. A pseudo-polyp will be formed and resected by standard polypectomy fashion using snare. Submucosal injection of saline is not necessary for this technique.
8. This technique can be applied repeatedly to remove larger lesions in a piecemeal manner, known as multi-band mucosectomy (MBM). It contains six modified band ligators to allow up to six resections at a time.

3.1.7 Endoscopic Submucosal Dissection (ESD) (Fig. 3)

1. ESD is characterized by three steps, namely, submucosal injection, circumferential mucosal incision, and submucosal dissection (*see* **Note 14**).
2. The perimeter of lesion is marked by cautery, again by APC or touching the mucosa with snare or knife tip with soft coagulation current (Fig. 3a).
3. Perform submucosal injection with a lifting agent (colloid solution, methylcellulose, or hyaluronic acid) and an injection needle catheter. A special dye, typically indigo carmine, can be used to help differentiation of tissue planes. Addition of diluted epinephrine can be considered.
4. Make a circular mucosal incision around the lesion using a specially designed electrosurgical knife (Fig. 3b) (*see* **Note 15**). Dissect through the submucosal layer beneath the lesion, using either cutting or high-voltage coagulation current.
5. A transparent hood should be attached distally to the endoscope for better visualization throughout the dissection (*see* **Note 16**). Hemostatic forceps can be used for pre-emptive coagulation of blood vessels or control of active bleeding during the dissection. Carbon dioxide insufflation is generally recommended throughout the procedure.
6. Carefully dissect out the neoplastic lesion en bloc (Fig. 3c). The mucosal defect can be closed by deploying repositionable clips consecutively from one end to another end.

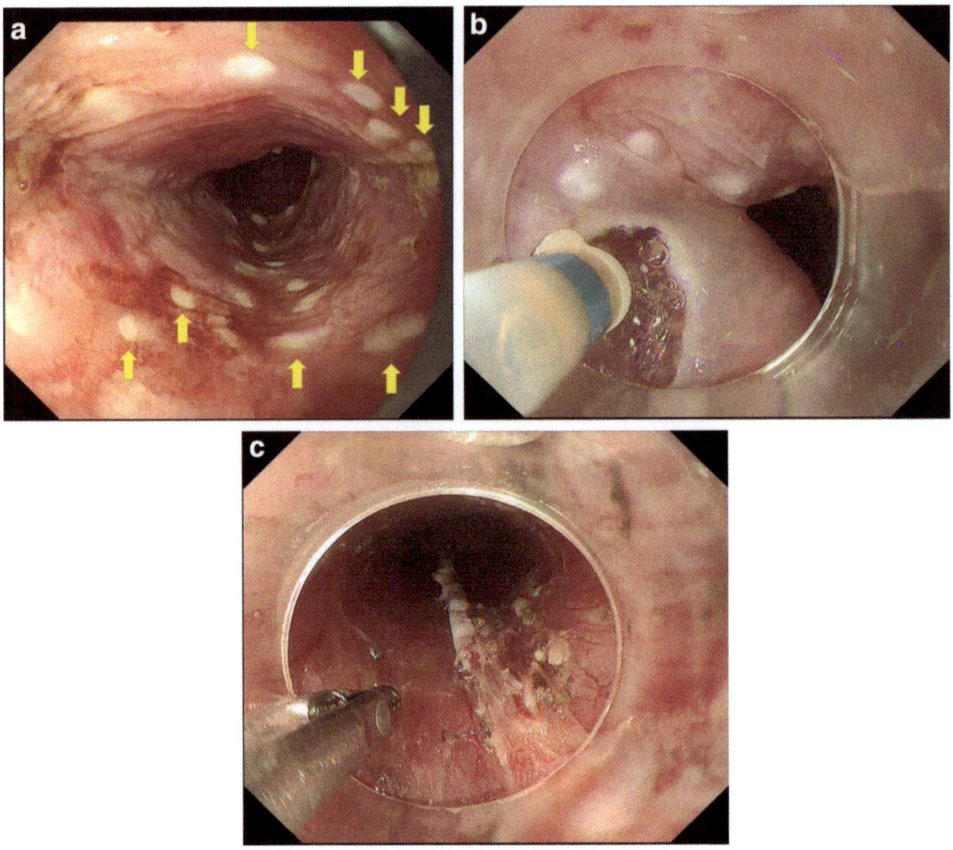

Fig. 3 Endoscopic resection of ESCC by endoscopic submucosal dissection. (**a**) Margins of the mucosal cancer marked by a snare tip with soft coagulation. (**b**) Mucosal incision with electrosurgical knife. (**c**) Near-circumferential dissection of the lesion, after which the lesion would be removed en bloc

4 Notes

1. Esophageal cancers may appear as a gross tumor but may also mimic a stricture or an ulcer especially with irregular shape or hemorrhagic base. Early neoplasms may be flat and subtle and may appear as color or brightness changes on white-light endoscopy or image-enhanced endoscopy.
2. Tissue diagnosis should be obtained by taking a biopsy. The lesions should be approached face on so that firm pressure can be applied with the widely opened cups on the forceps. Multiple biopsies should be taken from areas suspicious of malignancy, and necrotic areas are best to be avoided as they may produce non-diagnostic specimens.
3. NBI is a form of image enhancement that uses filters to limit light penetration at wavelengths of 415 (390–445) nm and 540 (530–550) nm. In these wavelengths, hemoglobin readily

absorbs light. Therefore, in sharp contrast to the background tissue, blood vessels on the mucosal surface are highlighted brown. NBI could thus be used to identify the microvascular architecture of the mucosa and delineate the margin of neoplasia as a brownish area [25, 26].

4. When such brownish areas are detected, further endoscopic magnification is employed to identify and classify the microvascular patterns. Based on the appearance of microvascular dilatation, meandering, irregular caliber, and form variation, the original intrapapillary capillary loop (IPCL) pattern classification was proposed by Inoue et al. [27]. The IPCL classification corresponded to five groups of histological grades (types I–V). This classification system was subsequently updated and simplified into three larger groups [28]: Group 1 (non-neoplastic), Group 2 (borderline), and Group 3 (cancer).
5. Apart from this classification, the Japan Esophageal Society (JES) has also developed a simplified magnifying endoscopic classification for estimating invasion depth of superficial ESCC [29]. Based on the morphology, microvessels are classified into type A or type B (B1, B2, and B3). It has been shown that the overall accuracy of type B microvessels in estimating tumor invasion depth was 90.5% [29].
6. A multicenter randomized controlled trial demonstrated that NBI detected more superficial ESCC than white-light endoscopy (97% vs. 55%, $p < 0.001$) [13]. NBI has been showed to have comparable sensitivity yet superior specificity compared with Lugol chromoendoscopy [30, 31]. Furthermore, apart from detecting and diagnosing neoplasia, the IPCL patterns have been shown to predict depth of tumor infiltration with an accuracy exceeding 80% [25, 32] and important information in selecting cancers amendable for endoscopic therapies.
7. Lugol chromoendoscopy is commonly used to screen or visualize neoplastic lesions. In Lugol chromoendoscopy, the combination of iodine with glycogen can give a brown-color change to enhance lesion detection. Normal squamous cell epithelium produces glycogen, whereas abnormal epithelium is depleted of glycogen [33]. Hence, unstained areas of LVLs may indicate precancerous neoplastic lesions. Lugol chromoendoscopy has been shown to enhance detection of superficial ESCC [14, 15], increasing the sensitivity for neoplastic lesions to over 90% [30, 31, 34].
8. Despite excellent sensitivity, low-grade neoplastic or non-neoplastic lesions (e.g., inflammation) may show up as under-stained areas in Lugol chromoendoscopy. Thus, it has been reported to have a suboptimal specificity [35, 36]. Furthermore, Lugol chromoendoscopy also has a disadvantage of

causing retrosternal discomfort [37] or even severe allergic reaction [38], esophagitis [39], or gastritis [40].

9. EUS may be useful for staging of the ESCC in selected cases [8, 9]. Conventional EUS probes can differentiate between T1 and T2 tumor and can detect locoregional lymph nodes [41, 42]. A meta-analysis has reported high sensitivity and specificity of EUS for the diagnosis of T1a (mucosal) lesion at 85% and 87%, respectively [43]. In addition, EUS enables sampling of suspicious lymph nodes to assess the N stage [44], for patients who are being considered for surgery after excluding distant metastases by computed tomography (CT) and/or positron emission tomography (PET) scan. EUS FNA may improve the accuracy of lymph node staging by providing cytological confirmation [45].

10. Generally, endoscopic resection for ESCC is limited to epithelial dysplasia and superficial mucosal cancer involving the epithelium (T1a-EP or m1) or the lamina propria layer (T1a-LP or m2) [12]. The risk of lymph node metastasis in such dysplasia and superficial mucosal cancer was estimated to be 0–5% but could rise to about 10% in mucosal cancers involving the muscularis mucosa (T1a-MM or m3) [46]. Infiltration into the submucosa is classified by its invasive depth, with sm1 representing infiltration into the superficial third, sm2 the middle third, and sm3 the deepest third. Once involving the submucosa (T1b), the risk of metastasis increased to 20% [46]. Endoscopic resection for tumors invading the muscularis mucosa (m3) or superficial submucosa (sm1) must be individualized, with benefits and risks carefully balanced in selected cases [46, 47].

11. Several studies have compared outcomes of ESD versus EMR in treating superficial ESCC. In previous studies in patients with high-grade dysplasia or intramucosal carcinoma, ESD allowed en bloc resection of large mucosal lesions [48, 49], at higher curative resection and lower local recurrence rates [50–52]. Therefore, ESD is recommended as the first option for treating early ESCC, although EMR may be considered for smaller lesions if en bloc resection can be ascertained [53].

12. Other endoscopic treatments such as radiofrequency ablation [54], cryotherapy [55], APC [56], and photodynamic therapy (PDT) [57] have been proposed and tested. Radiofrequency ablation probes deliver a specific waveform of energy, to vaporize the mucosal esophageal tissue with a depth of around 500 μm. While radiofrequency ablation has been used extensively to treat early neoplasia in Barrett's esophagus, it has been applied for intraepithelial neoplasia and early ESCC. Favorable complete response rates were observed up to 12 months after

therapy, with some cases developing strictures and requiring dilatation [58, 59]. Nevertheless, a UK registry showed 30% progression to invasive malignancy at 1 year [60], casting doubts on the accuracy in recognizing superficial mucosal lesions amendable to radiofrequency ablation during endoscopy [61].

13. EMR can achieve curative complete local resection, particularly for mucosal lesions less than 2 cm, of well-differentiated (grade 1) and with non-ulcerated surface. It is generally safe with a complication rate of perforation of less than 2% [62]. Reported en bloc resection rates ranged from 20% to 53%, whereas the local recurrence rates ranged from 10% to 26% [52, 63].
14. ESD involves dissecting the submucosa to remove a larger lesion. Compared to EMR, ESD is technically a more challenging technique, but it allows en bloc resection of neoplastic lesions of much larger sizes [64]. Reported outcomes of ESD for ESCC in more than 700 patients showed en bloc resection rates of 95.1% and histologically complete resection rates of 89.4% [65, 66]. Perforation, bleeding, mediastinal emphysema, and esophageal strictures requiring balloon dilatation have been reported [67, 68].
15. Different types of electrosurgical knives have been approved for ESD, including but not limited to ITKnife, ITKnife Nano, HookKnife, Triangle Tip Knife, DualKnife, FlexKnife, Hybrid-Knife, and FlushKnife. Some of them have pressurized water jet function, which enables delivery of submucosal injection without further needle puncture. Alternative forceps-like devices such as Clutch Cutter, SB Knife, and Endo-Dissector are also available to allow direct grasping and cutting of tissues [69].
16. Various traction methods have been introduced to improve the visualization during ESD procedures. Clip-with-line method using a hemostatic clip and dental floss has been described to allow safe and accurate dissection [70]. Pocket-creation method has also been investigated to counteract with the peristalsis and respiratory movement during procedure [71].

References

1. Ferlay J, Soerjomataram I, Dikshit R, Eser S, Mathers C, Rebelo M, Parkin DM, Forman D, Bray F (2015) Cancer incidence and mortality worldwide: sources, methods and major patterns in GLOBOCAN 2012. Int J Cancer 136(5):E359–E386. https://doi.org/10.1002/ijc.29210
2. Lagergren J, Smyth E, Cunningham D, Lagergren P (2017) Oesophageal cancer. Lancet 390(10110):2383–2396. https://doi.org/10.1016/S0140-6736(17)31462-9
3. Smyth EC, Lagergren J, Fitzgerald RC, Lordick F, Shah MA, Lagergren P, Cunningham D (2017) Oesophageal cancer. Nat Rev Dis Primers 3:17048. https://doi.org/10.1038/nrdp.2017.48
4. Prabhu A, Obi KO, Rubenstein JH (2014) The synergistic effects of alcohol and tobacco

consumption on the risk of esophageal squamous cell carcinoma: a meta-analysis. Am J Gastroenterol 109(6):822–827. https://doi.org/10.1038/ajg.2014.71

5. Chiu PWY, Uedo N, Singh R, Gotoda T, Ng EKW, Yao K, Ang TL, Ho SH, Kikuchi D, Yao F, Pittayanon R, Goda K, Lau JYW, Tajiri H, Inoue H (2019) An Asian consensus on standards of diagnostic upper endoscopy for neoplasia. Gut 68(2):186–197. https://doi.org/10.1136/gutjnl-2018-317111
6. Kaltenbach T, Sano Y, Friedland S, Soetikno R, American Gastroenterological A (2008) American Gastroenterological Association (AGA) Institute technology assessment on image-enhanced endoscopy. Gastroenterology 134 (1):327–340. https://doi.org/10.1053/j.gastro.2007.10.062
7. Lal N, Bhasin DK, Malik AK, Gupta NM, Singh K, Mehta SK (1992) Optimal number of biopsy specimens in the diagnosis of carcinoma of the oesophagus. Gut 33(6):724–726. https://doi.org/10.1136/gut.33.6.724
8. Pech O, Gunter E, Dusemund F, Origer J, Lorenz D, Ell C (2010) Accuracy of endoscopic ultrasound in preoperative staging of esophageal cancer: results from a referral center for early esophageal cancer. Endoscopy 42 (6):456–461. https://doi.org/10.1055/s-0029-1244022
9. Rampado S, Bocus P, Battaglia G, Ruol A, Portale G, Ancona E (2008) Endoscopic ultrasound: accuracy in staging superficial carcinomas of the esophagus. Ann Thorac Surg 85 (1):251–256. https://doi.org/10.1016/j.athoracsur.2007.08.021
10. Yip HC, Chiu PW (2017) Endoscopic diagnosis and management of early squamous cell carcinoma of esophagus. J Thorac Dis 9(Suppl 8):S689–S696. https://doi.org/10.21037/jtd.2017.06.57
11. Draganov PV, Wang AY, Othman MO, Fukami N (2019) AGA institute clinical practice update: endoscopic submucosal dissection in the United States. Clin Gastroenterol Hepatol 17(1):16–25 e11. https://doi.org/10.1016/j.cgh.2018.07.041
12. Barret M, Prat F (2018) Diagnosis and treatment of superficial esophageal cancer. Ann Gastroenterol 31(3):256–265. https://doi.org/10.20524/aog.2018.0252
13. Muto M, Minashi K, Yano T, Saito Y, Oda I, Nonaka S, Omori T, Sugiura H, Goda K, Kaise M, Inoue H, Ishikawa H, Ochiai A, Shimoda T, Watanabe H, Tajiri H, Saito D (2010) Early detection of superficial squamous cell carcinoma in the head and neck region and esophagus by narrow band imaging: a multicenter randomized controlled trial. J Clin Oncol 28(9):1566–1572. https://doi.org/10.1200/JCO.2009.25.4680
14. Shiozaki H, Tahara H, Kobayashi K, Yano H, Tamura S, Imamoto H, Yano T, Oku K, Miyata M, Nishiyama K et al (1990) Endoscopic screening of early esophageal cancer with the Lugol dye method in patients with head and neck cancers. Cancer 66 (10):2068–2071. https://doi.org/10.1002/1097-0142(19901115)66:10<2068::aid-cncr2820661005>3.0.co;2-w
15. Dubuc J, Legoux J, Winnock M, Seyrig J, Barbier J, Barrioz T, Laugier R, Boulay G, Grasset D, Sautereau D, Grigoresco D, Butel J, Scoazec J, Ponchon T, Societe Francaise d'Endoscopie D (2006) Endoscopic screening for esophageal squamous-cell carcinoma in high-risk patients: a prospective study conducted in 62 French endoscopy centers. Endoscopy 38(7):690–695
16. McQuaid KR, Laine L (2008) A systematic review and meta-analysis of randomized, controlled trials of moderate sedation for routine endoscopic procedures. Gastrointest Endosc 67(6):910–923. https://doi.org/10.1016/j.gie.2007.12.046
17. Hiki N, Kaminishi M, Yasuda K, Uedo N, Honjo H, Matsuhashi N, Hiratsuka T, Sekine C, Nomura S, Yahagi N, Tajiri H, Suzuki H (2011) Antiperistaltic effect and safety of L-menthol sprayed on the gastric mucosa for upper GI endoscopy: a phase III, multicenter, randomized, double-blind, placebo-controlled study. Gastrointest Endosc 73(5):932–941. https://doi.org/10.1016/j.gie.2010.12.013
18. Fujishiro M, Kaminishi M, Hiki N, Oda I, Fujisaki J, Uedo N, Kaise M, Tanabe S, Iguchi M, Matsuhashi N, Nomura S, Tajiri H, Yahagi N, Suzuki H (2014) Efficacy of spraying l-menthol solution during endoscopic treatment of early gastric cancer: a phase III, multicenter, randomized, double-blind, placebo-controlled study. J Gastroenterol 49 (3):446–454. https://doi.org/10.1007/s00535-013-0856-4
19. Chen HW, Hsu HC, Hsieh TY, Yeh MK, Chang WK (2014) Pre-medication to improve esophagogastroduodenoscopic visibility: a meta-analysis and systemic review. Hepato-Gastroenterology 61(134):1642–1648
20. Araki K, Ohno S, Egashira A, Saeki H, Kawaguchi H, Sugimachi K (2002) Pathologic features of superficial esophageal squamous cell carcinoma with lymph node and distal metastasis. Cancer 94(2):570–575. https://doi.org/10.1002/cncr.10190

21. Yamashina T, Ishihara R, Nagai K, Matsuura N, Matsui F, Ito T, Fujii M, Yamamoto S, Hanaoka N, Takeuchi Y, Higashino K, Uedo N, Iishi H (2013) Long-term outcome and metastatic risk after endoscopic resection of superficial esophageal squamous cell carcinoma. Am J Gastroenterol 108(4):544–551. https://doi.org/10.1038/ajg.2013.8
22. Nakagawa K, Koike T, Iijima K, Shinkai H, Hatta W, Endo H, Ara N, Uno K, Asano N, Imatani A, Shimosegawa T (2014) Comparison of the long-term outcomes of endoscopic resection for superficial squamous cell carcinoma and adenocarcinoma of the esophagus in Japan. Am J Gastroenterol 109(3):348–356. https://doi.org/10.1038/ajg.2013.450
23. Merkow RP, Bilimoria KY, Keswani RN, Chung J, Sherman KL, Knab LM, Posner MC, Bentrem DJ (2014) Treatment trends, risk of lymph node metastasis, and outcomes for localized esophageal cancer. J Natl Cancer Inst 106(7):dju133. https://doi.org/10.1093/jnci/dju133
24. Hulscher JB, van Sandick JW, de Boer AG, Wijnhoven BP, Tijssen JG, Fockens P, Stalmeier PF, ten Kate FJ, van Dekken H, Obertop H, Tilanus HW, van Lanschot JJ (2002) Extended transthoracic resection compared with limited transhiatal resection for adenocarcinoma of the esophagus. N Engl J Med 347(21):1662–1669. https://doi.org/10.1056/NEJMoa022343
25. Yoshida T, Inoue H, Usui S, Satodate H, Fukami N, Kudo SE (2004) Narrow-band imaging system with magnifying endoscopy for superficial esophageal lesions. Gastrointest Endosc 59(2):288–295. https://doi.org/10.1016/s0016-5107(03)02532-x
26. Kumagai Y, Toi M, Inoue H (2002) Dynamism of tumour vasculature in the early phase of cancer progression: outcomes from oesophageal cancer research. Lancet Oncol 3(10):604–610
27. Inoue H, Honda T, Nagai K, Kawano T, Yoshino K, Takeshita K, Endo M (1997) Ultra-high magnification endoscopic observation of carcinoma in situ of the esophagus. Dig Endosc 9(1):16–18. https://doi.org/10.1111/j.1443-1661.1997.tb00453.x
28. Inoue H, Kaga M, Ikeda H, Sato C, Sato H, Minami H, Santi EG, Hayee B, Eleftheriadis N (2015) Magnification endoscopy in esophageal squamous cell carcinoma: a review of the intrapapillary capillary loop classification. Ann Gastroenterol 28(1):41–48
29. Oyama T, Inoue H, Arima M, Momma K, Omori T, Ishihara R, Hirasawa D, Takeuchi M, Tomori A, Goda K (2017) Prediction of the invasion depth of superficial squamous cell carcinoma based on microvessel morphology: magnifying endoscopic classification of the Japan Esophageal Society. Esophagus 14(2):105–112. https://doi.org/10.1007/s10388-016-0527-7
30. Morita FH, Bernardo WM, Ide E, Rocha RS, Aquino JC, Minata MK, Yamazaki K, Marques SB, Sakai P, de Moura EG (2017) Narrow band imaging versus lugol chromoendoscopy to diagnose squamous cell carcinoma of the esophagus: a systematic review and meta-analysis. BMC Cancer 17(1):54. https://doi.org/10.1186/s12885-016-3011-9
31. Nagami Y, Tominaga K, Machida H, Nakatani M, Kameda N, Sugimori S, Okazaki H, Tanigawa T, Yamagami H, Kubo N, Shiba M, Watanabe K, Watanabe T, Iguchi H, Fujiwara Y, Ohira M, Hirakawa K, Arakawa T (2014) Usefulness of non-magnifying narrow-band imaging in screening of early esophageal squamous cell carcinoma: a prospective comparative study using propensity score matching. Am J Gastroenterol 109(6):845–854. https://doi.org/10.1038/ajg.2014.94
32. Sharma P, Wani S, Bansal A, Hall S, Puli S, Mathur S, Rastogi A (2007) A feasibility trial of narrow band imaging endoscopy in patients with gastroesophageal reflux disease. Gastroenterology 133(2):454–464; quiz 674. https://doi.org/10.1053/j.gastro.2007.06.006
33. Mori M, Adachi Y, Matsushima T, Matsuda H, Kuwano H, Sugimachi K (1993) Lugol staining pattern and histology of esophageal lesions. Am J Gastroenterol 88(5):701–705
34. Dawsey SM, Fleischer DE, Wang GQ, Zhou B, Kidwell JA, Lu N, Lewin KJ, Roth MJ, Tio TL, Taylor PR (1998) Mucosal iodine staining improves endoscopic visualization of squamous dysplasia and squamous cell carcinoma of the esophagus in Linxian, China. Cancer 83(2):220–231
35. Lee YC, Wang CP, Chen CC, Chiu HM, Ko JY, Lou PJ, Yang TL, Huang HY, Wu MS, Lin JT, Hsiu-Hsi Chen T, Wang HP (2009) Transnasal endoscopy with narrow-band imaging and Lugol staining to screen patients with head and neck cancer whose condition limits oral intubation with standard endoscope (with video). Gastrointest Endosc 69(3 Pt 1):408–417. https://doi.org/10.1016/j.gie.2008.05.033
36. Takenaka R, Kawahara Y, Okada H, Hori K, Inoue M, Kawano S, Tanioka D, Tsuzuki T, Uemura M, Ohara N, Tominaga S, Onoda T, Yamamoto K (2009) Narrow-band imaging

provides reliable screening for esophageal malignancy in patients with head and neck cancers. Am J Gastroenterol 104(12):2942–2948. https://doi.org/10.1038/ajg.2009.426

37. Kondo H, Fukuda H, Ono H, Gotoda T, Saito D, Takahiro K, Shirao K, Yamaguchi H, Yoshida S (2001) Sodium thiosulfate solution spray for relief of irritation caused by Lugol's stain in chromoendoscopy. Gastrointest Endosc 53(2):199–202. https://doi.org/10.1067/mge.2001.110730
38. Stevens PD, Lightdale CJ, Green PH, Siegel LM, Garcia-Carrasquillo RJ, Rotterdam H (1994) Combined magnification endoscopy with chromoendoscopy for the evaluation of Barrett's esophagus. Gastrointest Endosc 40(6):747–749
39. Thuler FP, de Paulo GA, Ferrari AP (2004) Chemical esophagitis after chromoendoscopy with Lugol's solution for esophageal cancer: case report. Gastrointest Endosc 59(7):925–926. https://doi.org/10.1016/s0016-5107(04)00173-7
40. Sreedharan A, Rembacken BJ, Rotimi O (2005) Acute toxic gastric mucosal damage induced by Lugol's iodine spray during chromoendoscopy. Gut 54(6):886–887. https://doi.org/10.1136/gut.2004.061739
41. Sgourakis G, Gockel I, Lyros O, Hansen T, Mildenberger P, Lang H (2011) Detection of lymph node metastases in esophageal cancer. Expert Rev Anticancer Ther 11(4):601–612. https://doi.org/10.1586/era.10.150
42. Pech O, May A, Gunter E, Gossner L, Ell C (2006) The impact of endoscopic ultrasound and computed tomography on the TNM staging of early cancer in Barrett's esophagus. Am J Gastroenterol 101(10):2223–2229. https://doi.org/10.1111/j.1572-0241.2006.00718.x
43. Thosani N, Singh H, Kapadia A, Ochi N, Lee JH, Ajani J, Swisher SG, Hofstetter WL, Guha S, Bhutani MS (2012) Diagnostic accuracy of EUS in differentiating mucosal versus submucosal invasion of superficial esophageal cancers: a systematic review and meta-analysis. Gastrointest Endosc 75(2):242–253. https://doi.org/10.1016/j.gie.2011.09.016
44. Findlay JM, Bradley KM, Maile EJ, Braden B, Maw J, Phillips-Hughes J, Gillies RS, Maynard ND, Middleton MR (2015) Pragmatic staging of oesophageal cancer using decision theory involving selective endoscopic ultrasonography, PET and laparoscopy. Br J Surg 102(12):1488–1499. https://doi.org/10.1002/bjs.9905
45. Vazquez-Sequeiros E, Norton ID, Clain JE, Wang KK, Affi A, Allen M, Deschamps C, Miller D, Salomao D, Wiersema MJ (2001) Impact of EUS-guided fine-needle aspiration on lymph node staging in patients with esophageal carcinoma. Gastrointest Endosc 53(7):751–757. https://doi.org/10.1067/mge.2001.112741
46. Yoshii T, Ohkawa S, Tamai S, Kameda Y (2013) Clinical outcome of endoscopic mucosal resection for esophageal squamous cell cancer invading muscularis mucosa and submucosal layer. Dis Esophagus 26(5):496–502. https://doi.org/10.1111/j.1442-2050.2012.01370.x
47. Katada C, Muto M, Momma K, Arima M, Tajiri H, Kanamaru C, Ooyanagi H, Endo H, Michida T, Hasuike N, Oda I, Fujii T, Saito D (2007) Clinical outcome after endoscopic mucosal resection for esophageal squamous cell carcinoma invading the muscularis mucosae—a multicenter retrospective cohort study. Endoscopy 39(9):779–783. https://doi.org/10.1055/s-2007-966761
48. Teoh AY, Chiu PW, Yu Ngo DK, Wong SK, Lau JY, Ng EK (2010) Outcomes of endoscopic submucosal dissection versus endoscopic mucosal resection in management of superficial squamous esophageal neoplasms outside Japan. J Clin Gastroenterol 44(9):e190–e194. https://doi.org/10.1097/MCG.0b013e3181ce52fb
49. Chiu PW (2006) Endoscopic submucosal dissection-bigger piece, better outcome! Gastrointest Endosc 64(6):884–885. https://doi.org/10.1016/j.gie.2006.06.012
50. Guo HM, Zhang XQ, Chen M, Huang SL, Zou XP (2014) Endoscopic submucosal dissection vs endoscopic mucosal resection for superficial esophageal cancer. World J Gastroenterol 20(18):5540–5547. https://doi.org/10.3748/wjg.v20.i18.5540
51. Ishihara R, Iishi H, Uedo N, Takeuchi Y, Yamamoto S, Yamada T, Masuda E, Higashino K, Kato M, Narahara H, Tatsuta M (2008) Comparison of EMR and endoscopic submucosal dissection for en bloc resection of early esophageal cancers in Japan. Gastrointest Endosc 68(6):1066–1072. https://doi.org/10.1016/j.gie.2008.03.1114
52. Takahashi H, Arimura Y, Masao H, Okahara S, Tanuma T, Kodaira J, Kagaya H, Shimizu Y, Hokari K, Tsukagoshi H, Shinomura Y, Fujita M (2010) Endoscopic submucosal dissection is superior to conventional endoscopic resection as a curative treatment for early squamous cell carcinoma of the esophagus (with video). Gastrointest Endosc 72(2):255–264, 264 e251–252. https://doi.org/10.1016/j.gie.2010.02.040

53. Pimentel-Nunes P, Dinis-Ribeiro M, Ponchon T, Repici A, Vieth M, De Ceglie A, Amato A, Berr F, Bhandari P, Bialek A, Conio M, Haringsma J, Langner C, Meisner S, Messmann H, Morino M, Neuhaus H, Piessevaux H, Rugge M, Saunders BP, Robaszkiewicz M, Seewald S, Kashin S, Dumonceau JM, Hassan C, Deprez PH (2015) Endoscopic submucosal dissection: European Society of Gastrointestinal Endoscopy (ESGE) Guideline. Endoscopy 47 (9):829–854. https://doi.org/10.1055/s-0034-1392882
54. Muguruma N, Okamoto K, Kimura T, Kishi K, Okahisa T, Okamura S, Takayama T (2012) Endoscopic ablation therapy for gastrointestinal superficial neoplasia. Dig Endosc 24 (3):139–149. https://doi.org/10.1111/j.1443-1661.2011.01227.x
55. Lal P, Thota PN (2018) Cryotherapy in the management of premalignant and malignant conditions of the esophagus. World J Gastroenterol 24(43):4862–4869. https://doi.org/10.3748/wjg.v24.i43.4862
56. Min BH, Kim ER, Lee JH, Kang KJ, Rhee PL, Kim JJ, Rhee JC (2013) Feasibility and efficacy of argon plasma coagulation for early esophageal squamous cell neoplasia. Endoscopy 45 (7):575–578. https://doi.org/10.1055/s-0033-1344025
57. Tanaka T, Matono S, Nagano T, Murata K, Sueyoshi S, Yamana H, Shirouzu K, Fujita H (2011) Photodynamic therapy for large superficial squamous cell carcinoma of the esophagus. Gastrointest Endosc 73(1):1–6. https://doi.org/10.1016/j.gie.2010.08.049
58. He S, Bergman J, Zhang Y, Weusten B, Xue L, Qin X, Dou L, Liu Y, Fleischer D, Lu N, Dawsey SM, Wang GQ (2015) Endoscopic radiofrequency ablation for early esophageal squamous cell neoplasia: report of safety and effectiveness from a large prospective trial. Endoscopy 47(5):398–408. https://doi.org/10.1055/s-0034-1391285
59. Bergman JJ, Zhang YM, He S, Weusten B, Xue L, Fleischer DE, Lu N, Dawsey SM, Wang GQ (2011) Outcomes from a prospective trial of endoscopic radiofrequency ablation of early squamous cell neoplasia of the esophagus. Gastrointest Endosc 74(6):1181–1190. https://doi.org/10.1016/j.gie.2011.05.024
60. Haidry RJ, Butt MA, Dunn J, Banks M, Gupta A, Smart H, Bhandari P, Smith LA, Willert R, Fullarton G, John M, Di Pietro M, Penman I, Novelli M, Lovat LB (2013) Radiofrequency ablation for early oesophageal squamous neoplasia: outcomes form United Kingdom registry. World J Gastroenterol 19 (36):6011–6019. https://doi.org/10.3748/wjg.v19.i36.6011
61. Jansen M, Scholvinck DW, Kushima R, Sekine S, Weusten BL, Wang GQ, Fleischer DE, Yoshinaga S, Dawsey SM, Meijer SL, Bergman JJ, Oda I (2014) Is it justified to ablate flat-type esophageal squamous cancer? An analysis of endoscopic submucosal dissection specimens of lesions meeting the selection criteria of radiofrequency studies. Gastrointest Endosc 80(6):995–1002. https://doi.org/10.1016/j.gie.2014.09.004
62. Zhang YM, Boerwinkel DF, Qin X, He S, Xue L, Weusten BL, Dawsey SM, Fleischer DE, Dou LZ, Liu Y, Lu N, Bergman JJ, Wang GQ (2016) A randomized trial comparing multiband mucosectomy and cap-assisted endoscopic resection for endoscopic piecemeal resection of early squamous neoplasia of the esophagus. Endoscopy 48(4):330–338. https://doi.org/10.1055/s-0034-1393358
63. Katada C, Muto M, Manabe T, Boku N, Ohtsu A, Yoshida S (2003) Esophageal stenosis after endoscopic mucosal resection of superficial esophageal lesions. Gastrointest Endosc 57 (2):165–169. https://doi.org/10.1067/mge.2003.73
64. Yamamoto H, Kawata H, Sunada K, Sasaki A, Nakazawa K, Miyata T, Sekine Y, Yano T, Satoh K, Ido K, Sugano K (2003) Successful en-bloc resection of large superficial tumors in the stomach and colon using sodium hyaluronate and small-caliber-tip transparent hood. Endoscopy 35(8):690–694. https://doi.org/10.1055/s-2003-41516
65. Repici A, Hassan C, Carlino A, Pagano N, Zullo A, Rando G, Strangio G, Romeo F, Nicita R, Rosati R, Malesci A (2010) Endoscopic submucosal dissection in patients with early esophageal squamous cell carcinoma: results from a prospective Western series. Gastrointest Endosc 71(4):715–721. https://doi.org/10.1016/j.gie.2009.11.020
66. Kim JS, Kim BW, Shin IS (2014) Efficacy and safety of endoscopic submucosal dissection for superficial squamous esophageal neoplasia: a meta-analysis. Dig Dis Sci 59(8):1862–1869. https://doi.org/10.1007/s10620-014-3098-2
67. Oyama T, Tomori A, Hotta K, Morita S, Kominato K, Tanaka M, Miyata Y (2005) Endoscopic submucosal dissection of early esophageal cancer. Clin Gastroenterol Hepatol 3(7 Suppl 1):S67–S70
68. Fujishiro M, Yahagi N, Kakushima N, Kodashima S, Muraki Y, Ono S, Yamamichi N, Tateishi A, Shimizu Y, Oka M, Ogura K, Kawabe T, Ichinose M, Omata M

(2006) Endoscopic submucosal dissection of esophageal squamous cell neoplasms. Clin Gastroenterol Hepatol 4(6):688–694. https://doi.org/10.1016/j.cgh.2006.03.024

69. Committee AT, Maple JT, Abu Dayyeh BK, Chauhan SS, Hwang JH, Komanduri S, Manfredi M, Konda V, Murad FM, Siddiqui UD, Banerjee S (2015) Endoscopic submucosal dissection. Gastrointest Endosc 81 (6):1311–1325. https://doi.org/10.1016/j.gie.2014.12.010
70. Suzuki S, Gotoda T, Kobayashi Y, Kono S, Iwatsuka K, Yagi-Kuwata N, Kusano C, Fukuzawa M, Moriyasu F (2016) Usefulness of a traction method using dental floss and a hemoclip for gastric endoscopic submucosal dissection: a propensity score matching analysis (with videos). Gastrointest Endosc 83 (2):337–346. https://doi.org/10.1016/j.gie.2015.07.014
71. Takezawa T, Hayashi Y, Shinozaki S, Sagara Y, Okada M, Kobayashi Y, Sakamoto H, Miura Y, Sunada K, Lefor AK, Yamamoto H (2019) The pocket-creation method facilitates colonic endoscopic submucosal dissection (with video). Gastrointest Endosc 89 (5):1045–1053. https://doi.org/10.1016/j.gie.2019.01.022

Chapter 6

Macroscopic Assessment and Sampling of Endoscopic Resection Specimens for Squamous Epithelial Malignancies with Superficial Involvement of Esophagus

Satoshi Fujii and Alfred K. Lam

Abstract

Endoscopic resection is commonly used for superficial squamous cell carcinoma or high-grade dysplasia of esophageal squamous cell carcinoma. The depth of invasion, clearance from resection margins, and other pathological parameters are important parameters to be examined. The depth of invasion by carcinoma is associated with the risk of lymph node metastases. In endoscopic resection of superficial squamous malignancies of the esophagus, proper pathological examination of the resected specimen could guide the management of the patients in terms of the need for additional treatment, including lymph node dissection, chemotherapy, and radiation therapies.

Key words Endoscopic resection, Pathology, Dysplasia, Esophageal, Early squamous carcinoma

1 Introduction

In the recent years, there are improvements in endoscopic diagnostic technology that combines narrowband imaging (NBI) and magnifying endoscope as well as awareness of need of screening for patients with high risk of having esophageal squamous cell carcinoma such as those with high alcohol consumption and smoking [1, 2]. These resulted in detection of some superficial esophageal epithelial malignancies including high-grade squamous dysplasia and squamous cell carcinoma of early stages [3].

Early-stage squamous cell carcinoma and high-grade squamous dysplasia could be treated by endoscopic resection (*see* Chapter 5). After endoscopic resection of the early esophageal squamous malignancy, additional treatment, including esophagectomy accompanied with lymph node dissection, chemotherapy, or radiotherapy, is necessary to properly examine specimens of endoscopically resected superficial esophageal squamous malignancy to access the possibility of advanced disease status.

Alfred K. Lam (ed.), *Esophageal Squamous Cell Carcinoma: Methods and Protocols*, Methods in Molecular Biology, vol. 2129, https://doi.org/10.1007/978-1-0716-0377-2_6,

Superficial esophageal squamous carcinoma, though indolent in clinical behavior, has risk of spread to lymph node depending on the depth of involvement of the malignancy [4–11]. In pathological T1b stage esophageal squamous carcinoma (involvement of the submucosa), the Japanese Society for Esophageal Diseases divided the stage into the upper one third of the submucosa (sm1), middle one third (sm2), or lower one third (sm3). The prevalence of lymph node metastases is 0% if the squamous malignancy is confined to the mucosa, 5.3% in the lamina propria, 17.7% in the muscularis mucosae, and 26.3% in sm1. In carcinoma located in sm2/3, the frequency of lymph node infiltration increases to 45.3%. The depth of invasion to submucosa could also be measured by SID (submucosal invasive depth) [9]. Multivariate analysis showed that SID of 2000 μm found by drawing ROC (receiver operating characteristic) curve, tumor diameter of 35 mm, and lymphatic infiltration were independent risk factors for lymph node metastasis in superficial esophageal squamous carcinoma. In addition, SID of 2000 μm is reported to be a reduction factor for recurrence-free survival.

Tumor size larger than 20 mm [6] and lymphatic and venous infiltration [8, 12] have been reported as risk factors for lymph node metastasis. In addition, large tumor size [13, 14], larger circumferential spread [13], and deeper invasive depth [13, 14] are associated with increased local recurrence after endoscopic resection.

Since patients with superficial squamous cell carcinoma treated with endoscopic resection had not received lymph node dissection at the same time, it is difficult to evaluate risk factors for lymph node metastasis according to the invasive depth as in patients who underwent esophagectomy. Like the trend in patients who underwent esophagectomy, the frequency of clinical detection of lymph node metastasis increases with the depth of invasion. Nevertheless, the frequency of lymph node metastasis associated with depth on invasion in each layer of endoscopic resection cases is lower than that reported from esophagectomy cases.

For instances, lymphatic infiltration is positive in 12.5% (9 of 72) of surgically treated patients with stage T1a who have cancer cells infiltrated into muscularis propria [4, 5], whereas it is 8.1% (9 of 111) in patients of identical pathological stage who underwent endoscopic resection [9]. There could be more histopathological factors attributed to lymph node metastasis observed in surgical cases than in endoscopic resection cases.

Salvage endoscopic resection could be conducted as a curative treatment for superficial carcinoma after failure of treatment with chemoradiotherapy for esophageal squamous cell carcinoma. Patients with residual lesions after chemoradiotherapy and lesions with a submucosal tumor-like appearance before salvage endoscopic resection were significantly associated with post-salvage endoscopic resection recurrence [15].

The tissue obtained after endoscopic resected specimen could be fixed in formalin and examined as other biopsy specimen. On the other hand, attention to details in pathological examination and correlation with endoscopic imaging will provide more useful information. In this chapter, we would detail the methodology for pathological examination of endoscopic resected early squamous cell carcinoma to allow proper information to be obtained for management and future research on this group of patients.

2 Materials

1. Endoscopic resection specimen.
2. Sponge.
3. Forceps.
4. Pins.
5. Gauze.
6. Saline.
7. Black rubber board.
8. Large plastic container with saline.
9. Stereoscopic (dissecting) microscope.
10. 5 ml plastic syringe.
11. Lugol's iodine (3%).
12. Digital camera.
13. Endoscopic images of the lesion for comparison.
14. 10% buffered formaldehyde.
15. Dissection tools (forceps, scalpel).
16. Ruler.
17. Tissue cassettes.
18. Sponge for wrapping of specimen in tissue cassette.
19. Histology equipment (embedding machine, microtome, slides, hematoxylin and eosin staining platform).

3 Methods

The specimen is best to send fresh as soon as possible to pathology laboratory.

1. Endoscopically resected specimens separated from the patient should be wrapped in gauze moistened with saline to prevent the specimen from drying out, even for a little while stopping to move to the next procedures (Fig. 1).

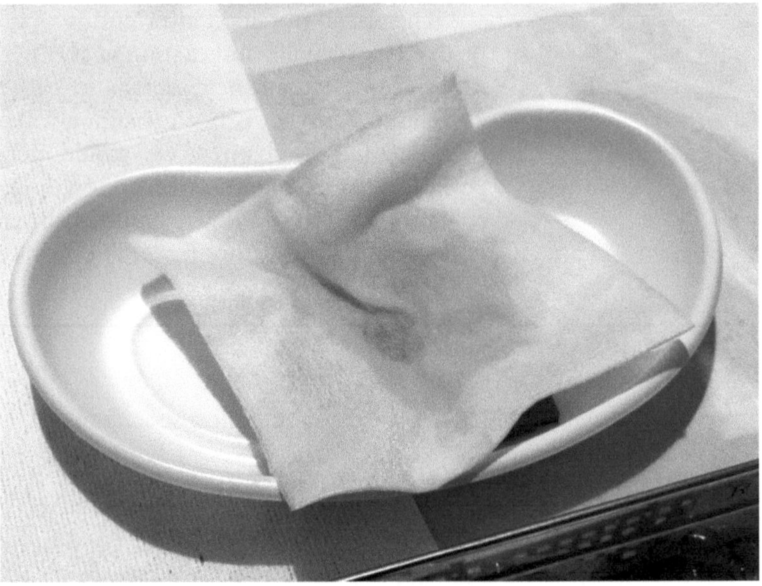

Fig. 1 Endoscopically resected specimen received wrapped in gauze moistened with saline

2. Lay out the specimen flat on a sponge (Fig. 2) (*see* **Note 1**).
3. Pin the specimen on a thin sponge (Fig. 3).
4. Remove clips and deposits (blood, fibrin, etc.) adhering to the surface of specimen gently by applying forceps, filter paper, or gauze. Be gentle as removal is likely to damage the tissue (Fig. 4).
5. Inspect the specimen with an endoscope, and compare with endoscopic images (optional) (Fig. 5).
6. Support the specimen and sponge on a black rubber plate (Fig. 6) (*see* **Note 2**).
7. Immerse the specimen in saline (Fig. 7).
8. Take macroscopic photographs while checking the images taken on the monitor connected to a stereoscopic microscope (Fig. 8).
9. Apply Lugol's iodine staining on the specimen (optional) (Fig. 9).
10. Immerse the specimen in saline, and take macroscopic photographs (*see* **Note 3**) while checking the images taken on the monitor (Fig. 10).
11. Compare the macroscopic photographs and the magnified ones (Fig. 11).

    In the magnified image by the stereoscopic microscope, it is possible to observe the change of the intra-papillary capillary loops (IPCLs) and contrast with the endoscopic image. Iodine

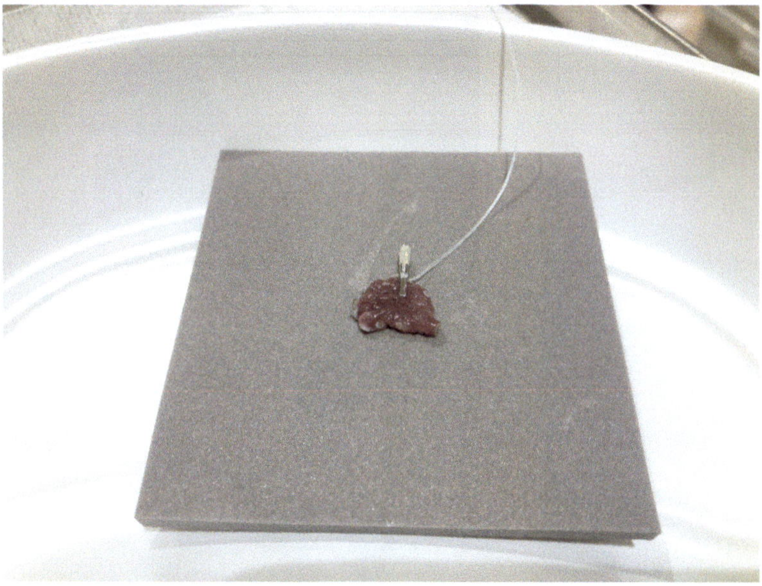

Fig. 2 Layout of endoscopic resection specimen of esophageal squamous cell carcinoma received in fresh

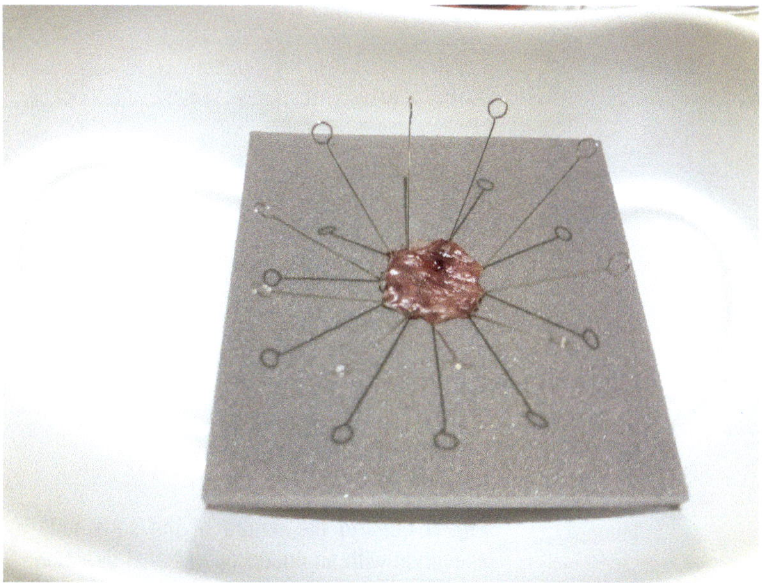

Fig. 3 Pin the specimen to the plastic board with pins on the peripheral of the specimen

stains the non-neoplastic region brown. It is important to thoroughly drop iodine, so false negative of iodine staining does not occur. Good staining is often obtained when slowly spending time using an iodine solution of low concentration (3%). In addition, it could show the distance of the neoplastic

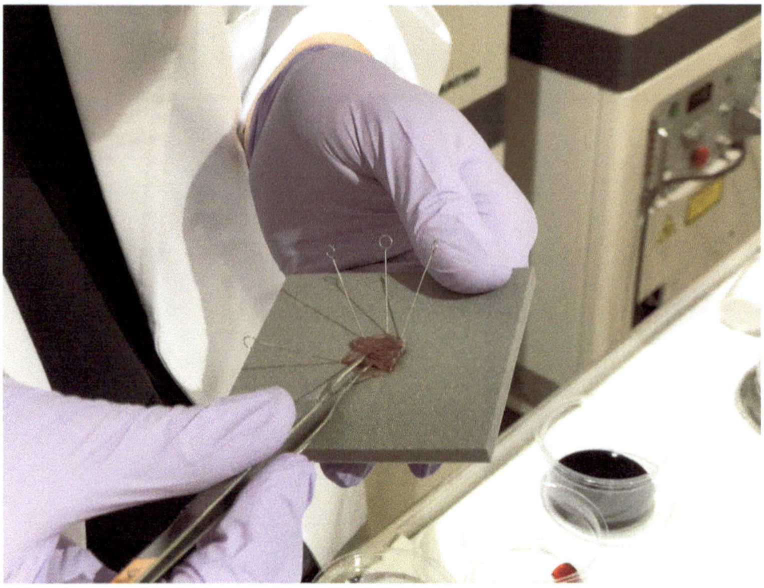

Fig. 4 Removal of blood or debris by forceps

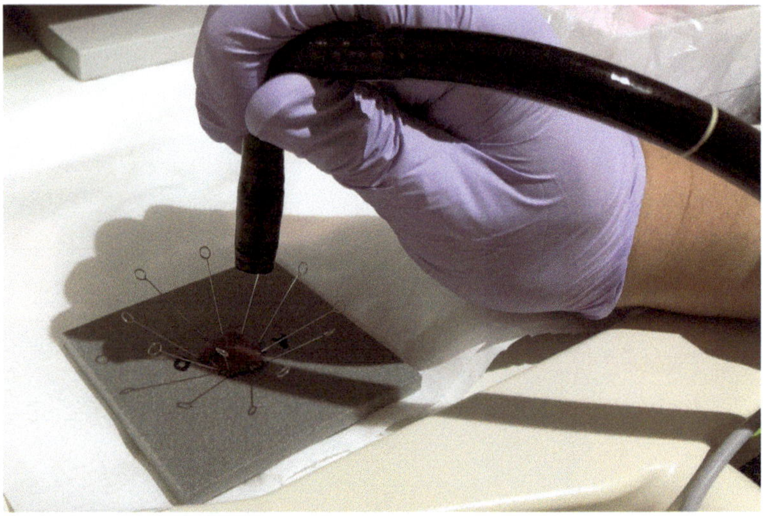

Fig. 5 Confirm the nature of the squamous mucosal lesion in the resected specimen with an endoscope (*A* anal direction, *O* oral direction)

area to the resection margin which is important in histological sampling.

12. Check the endoscopic images and clinical request (Fig. 12).

    Read the clinical request form and understand the characteristics of the lesion. Make sure there are no inconsistencies and deviations between the information on the request document submitted to the pathologist and the clinical and macroscopic findings of the specimen before cutting out a specimen.

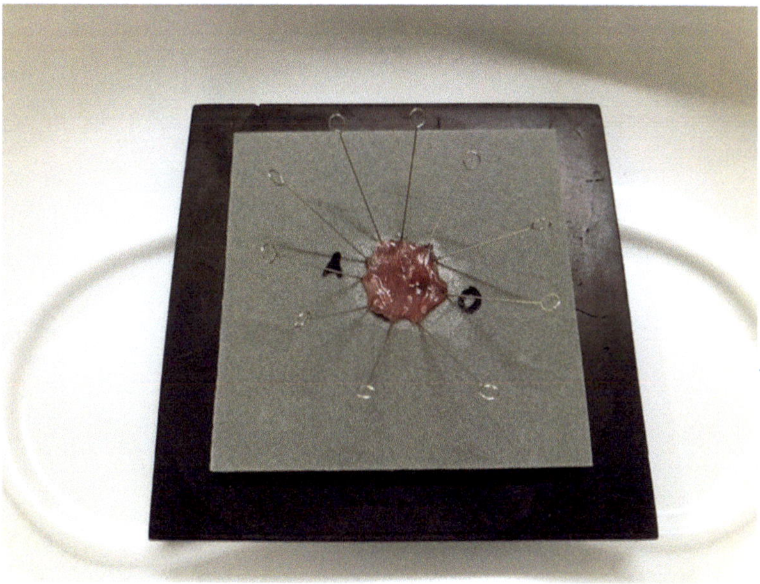

Fig. 6 Place the plastic board on top of the black rubber plate for taking macroscopic photographs of the specimen (*A* anal direction, *O* oral direction)

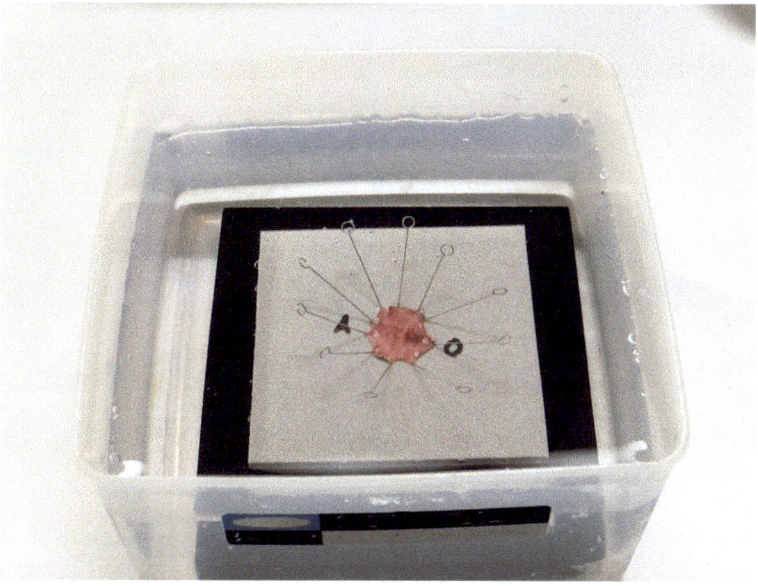

Fig. 7 Immerse the specimen with the boards in container with saline (*A* anal direction, *O* oral direction)

In verifying with the endoscopic findings, it is useful to take a photograph to confirm the orientation of the specimen (*see* **Note 4**).

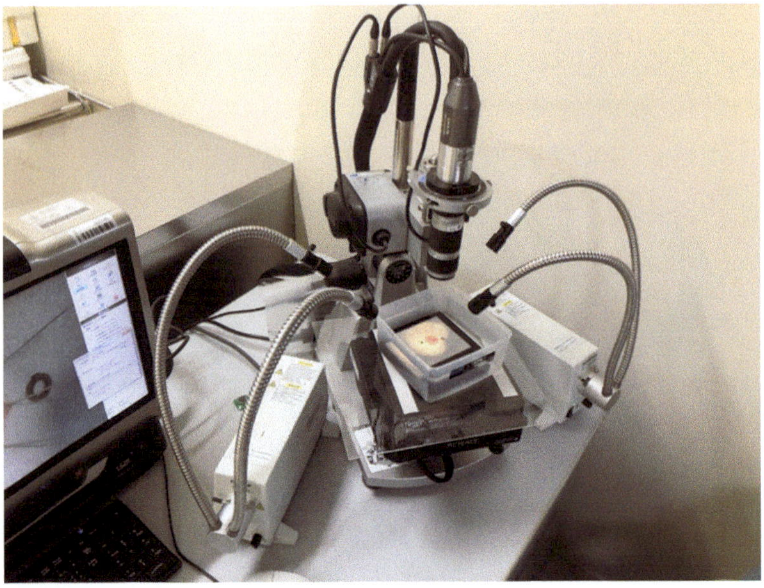

Fig. 8 Place the container on a stereoscopic microscope with connection to computer. Take macroscopic photographs while checking the images taken on the monitor (*A* anal direction, *O* oral direction)

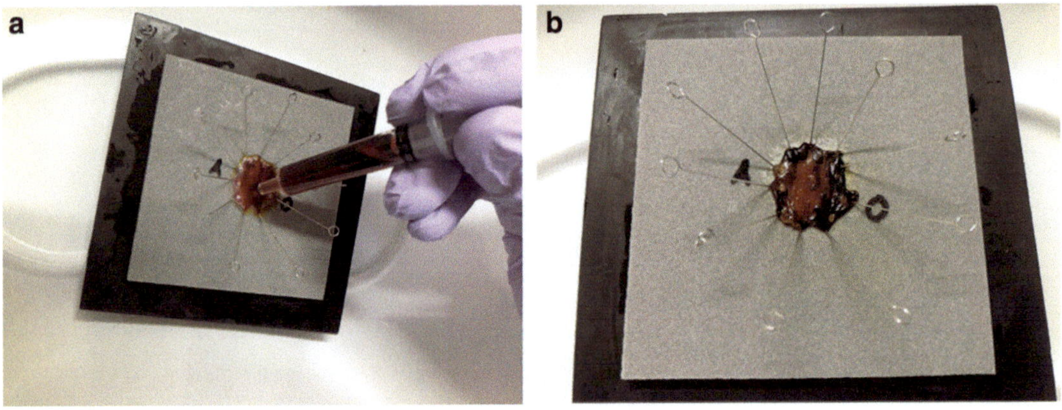

Fig. 9 (**a**) Stain the specimen by pouring approximately 5 ml of iodine using syringe. (**b**) The specimen after stained by iodine

13. Immerse the resected specimen in enough 10% neutral buffered formaldehyde, and fix it for 24–48 h (Fig. 13) (*see* **Note 5**).
14. Carefully remove the needles stuck in the specimen with forceps. Be careful not to damage the specimen by forcibly removing the needles (Fig. 14).
15. Take a macroscopic picture (Fig. 15).
16. Iodine staining of the specimen (Fig. 16) (optional).

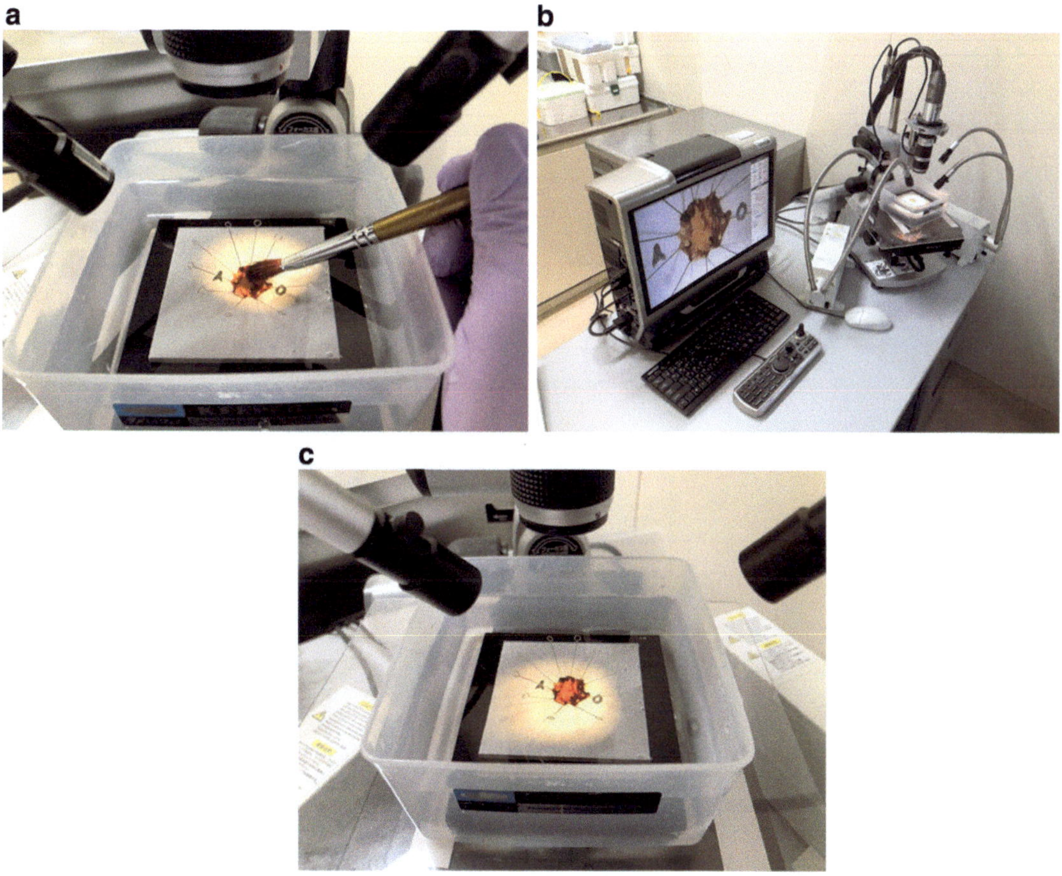

Fig. 10 Immerse the specimen stained with iodine in saline, and take macroscopic photographs (**a–c**)

Iodine staining enhances the recognition of the boundary between the non-tumor area and the tumor area. In the specimen fixed, it may be difficult to recognize the boundary. It is advisable to take another macroscopic photograph as record.

17. Orientate the specimen for dissection (Fig. 17) (*see* **Note 6**).
18. Dissect the specimen (Fig. 18).

    Dissect the whole specimen with cut interval of 2–3 mm.
19. Record on the macroscopic photograph the labelling on the blocks taken (Fig. 19).
20. Lay the serial cut sections in tissue cassette (Fig. 20).

    Wrap the tissue specimen in a sponge, and place in a cassette so that the tissue does not fold up.
21. Histopathological examination of squamous cell carcinoma or squamous dysplasia (*see* Chapter 2) [16, 17] (Fig. 21).

    The parameters should include:

    (a) The largest dimension of the squamous malignancy.

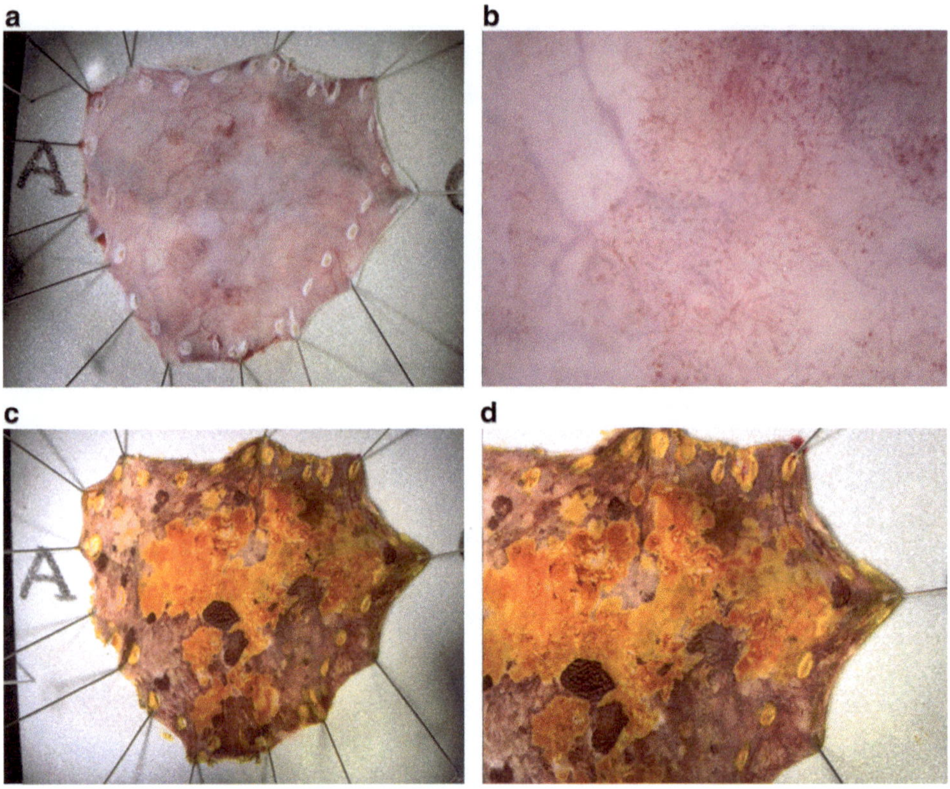

Fig. 11 Macroscopic photos before formalin fixation. (**a**) The macroscopic photograph by stereoscopic microscope of the specimen before formalin fixation (low-power view). (**b**) The macroscopic photograph by stereoscopic microscope of the specimen before formalin fixation (high-power view). Note the proliferation of intra-papillary capillary loops. (**c**) The macroscopic photograph by stereoscopic microscope of the specimen stained with Lugol's iodine (low-power view). (**d**) The macroscopic photograph by stereoscopic microscope of the specimen stained with Lugol's iodine (high-power view). The lesion and resection margins are sufficiently separated, so the way to cut out resected specimens shown in Fig. 3a is chosen for making paraffin-embedded specimens

(b) The depth of esophageal squamous cell carcinoma in the specimen.

(c) Tumor cell infiltration into submucosal layer.

(d) Lymphovascular infiltration by carcinoma.

(e) Perineural infiltration by carcinoma.

(f) Distance of carcinoma as well as squamous dysplasia from horizontal (mucosal) and vertical (deep) resection margins of the specimen.

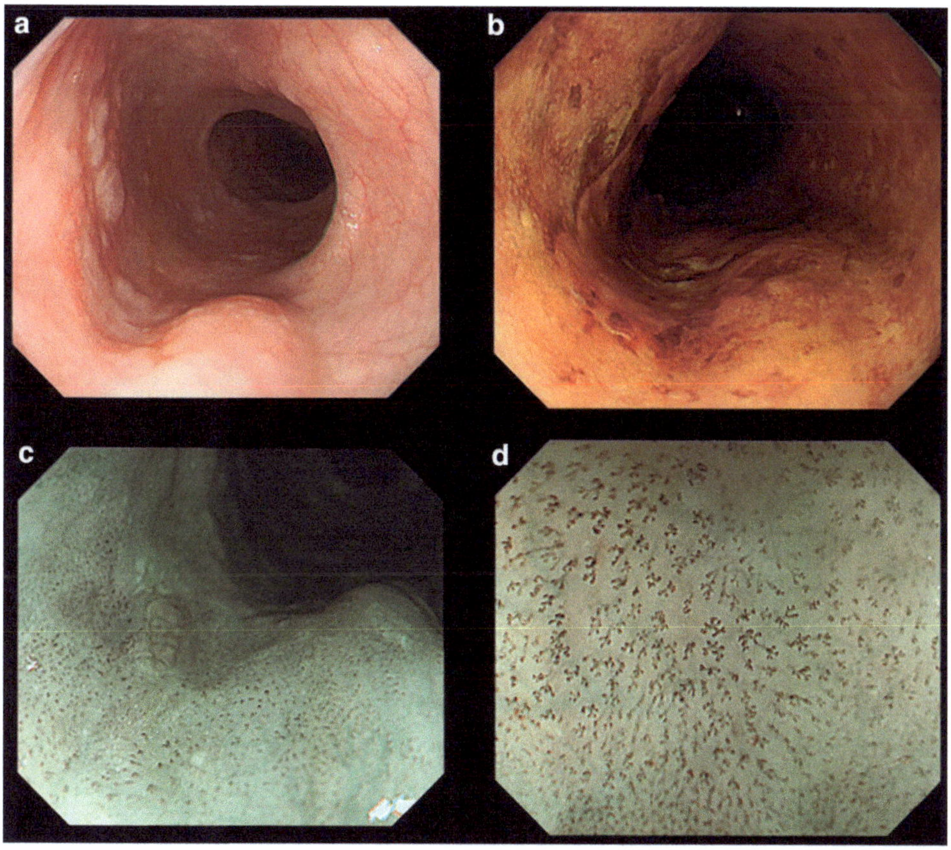

Fig. 12 Endoscopic images. Squamous neoplastic lesions could be identified by combining magnified endoscope with narrowband imaging (NBI) and staining by Lugol's iodine. (**a**) Ordinary endoscope. The lesion is recognized as a flat and slightly depressed lesion with mild redness. (**b**) Iodine-stained image. The lesion is observed as a Lugol's iodine-unstaining area. (**c**) Non-magnifying NBI (narrowband imaging). Non-magnifying NBI detects the vascular pattern of the lesion. (**d**) Magnifying NBI. In the high-power view of NBI, the mucosa between intra-papillary capillary loops is brightly colored and accompanied by proliferation of mildly irregular intra-papillary capillary loops

4 Notes

1. If the specimen is fixed with formalin solution without stretching, the macroscopic shape of the endoscopic resection specimen will be distorted. As a result, the orientation and measurements would be inaccurate. It is best to adhere the specimen to a flat surface carefully so that the muscularis mucosae and the plastic board are parallel. As the esophageal wall is delicate and has small extensibility, it is advisable to take care not to accidentally damage the esophageal wall in this extension process. The pins are stuck on the plastic board at almost equal intervals at the margins of the specimen to avoid damaging the lesion. Take care not to pierce the needle into the

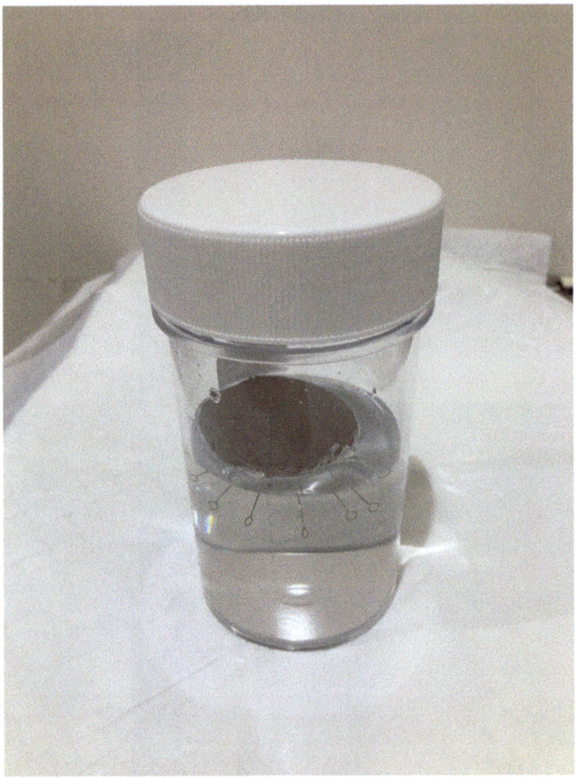

Fig. 13 Immerse the resected specimen in 10% neutral buffered formaldehyde for fixation

lesion which could disturb observation under microscope by artificial formation of pin hole in the lesion. Do not apply excessive load, and pay attention not to stretch the specimen more than necessary.

2. A black or dark-blue background plate is suitable for taking macroscopic photographs. These color backgrounds are low in lightness and reflectance, so color reflection is less likely to occur.
3. There are conditions for good-quality macroscopic photos:
   (a) Can identify the lesion easily in the macroscopic photograph.
   (b) High resolution and focus on the lesion.
   (c) The tone contrast of the lesion and the background is clear.
   (d) Absence of artifact.
   (e) The texture of the lesion is reproduced.

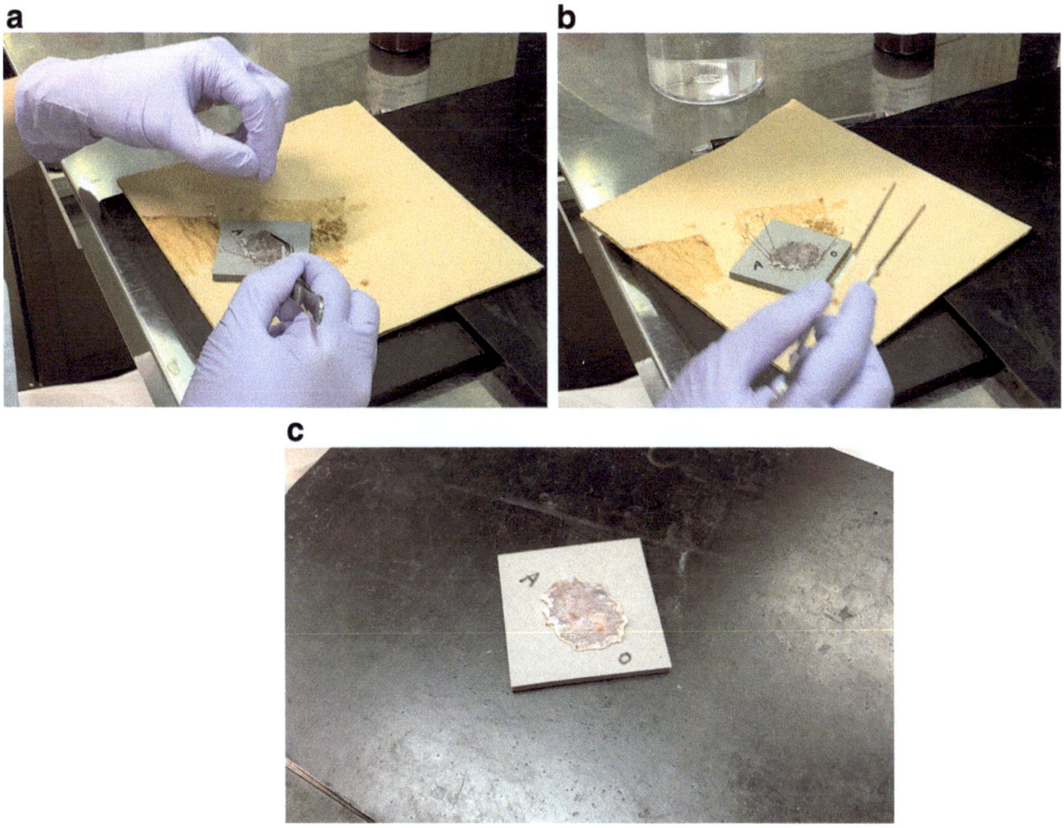

Fig. 14 Carefully remove the needles stuck in the specimen with forceps (*A* anal direction, *O* oral direction). (**a**) Remove the needles stuck in the specimen one by one with forceps carefully. (**b**) Be careful not to damage the specimen in removing the needles. (**c**) Look at the entire specimen to avoid damage or deformation

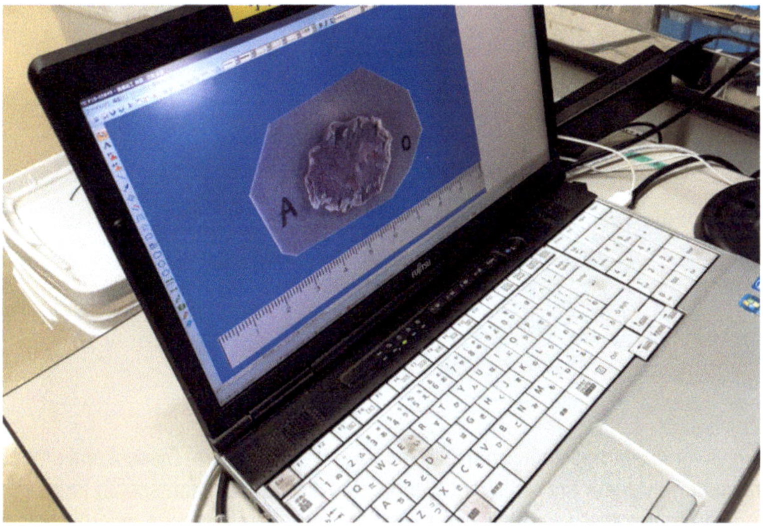

Fig. 15 Take a macroscopic photograph before cutting out the specimen (*A* anal direction, *O* oral direction)

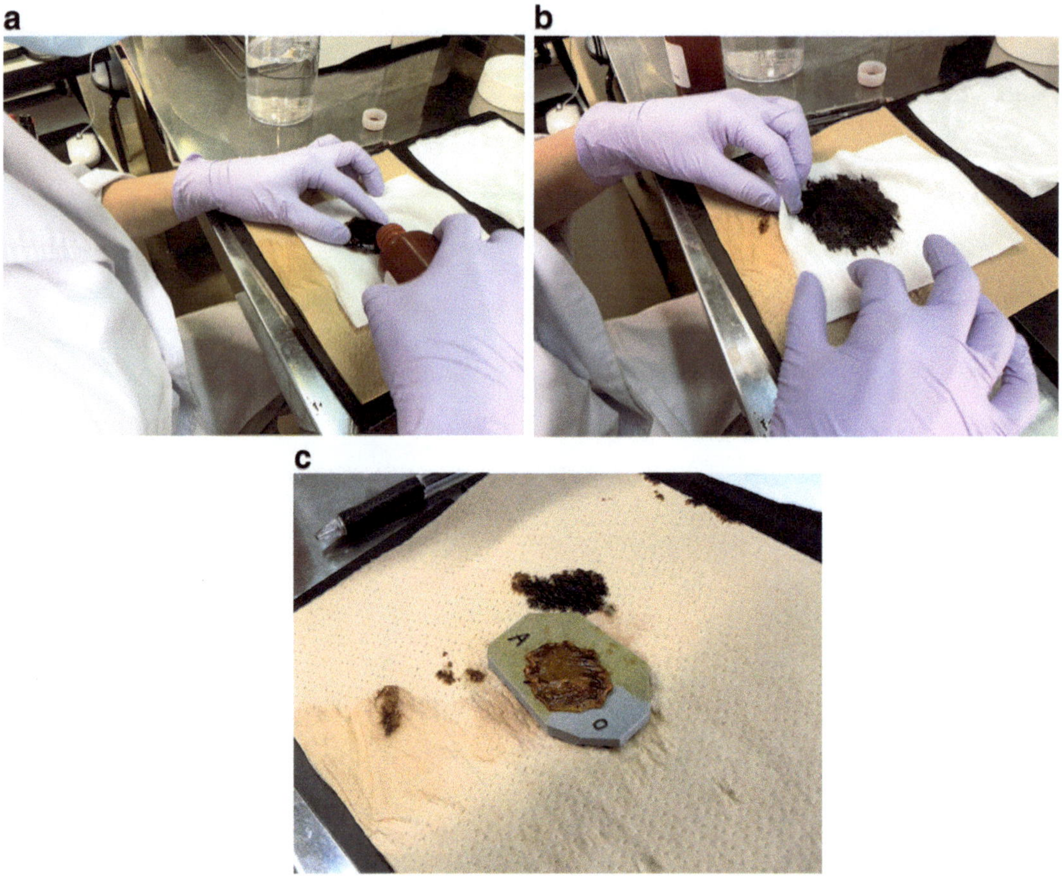

Fig. 16 (*A* anal direction, *O* oral direction). (**a**) Apply 3% iodine solution uniformly to the specimen. (**b**) Wipe off excess dye by wrapping the specimen in gauze. (**c**) Check for uneven iodine staining. Then take a macroscopic photograph as a record

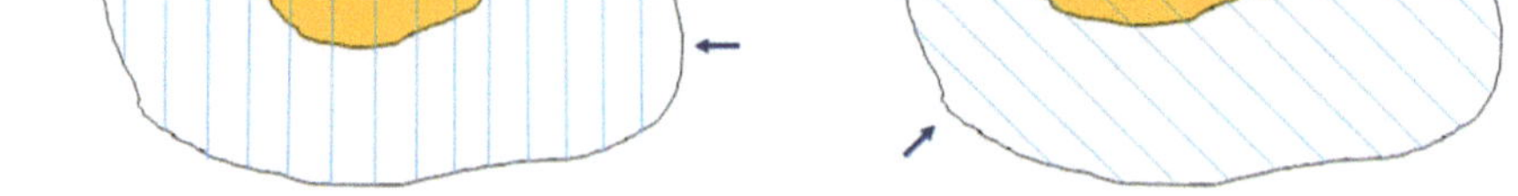

Fig. 17 The two ways for dissecting endoscopically resected specimens. (**a**) Dissect and embed in a way when the lesion and resection margins are sufficiently separated based on macroscopic judging. (**b**) Dissect and embed along a tangent when the lesion is close to resection margin based on macroscopic judging

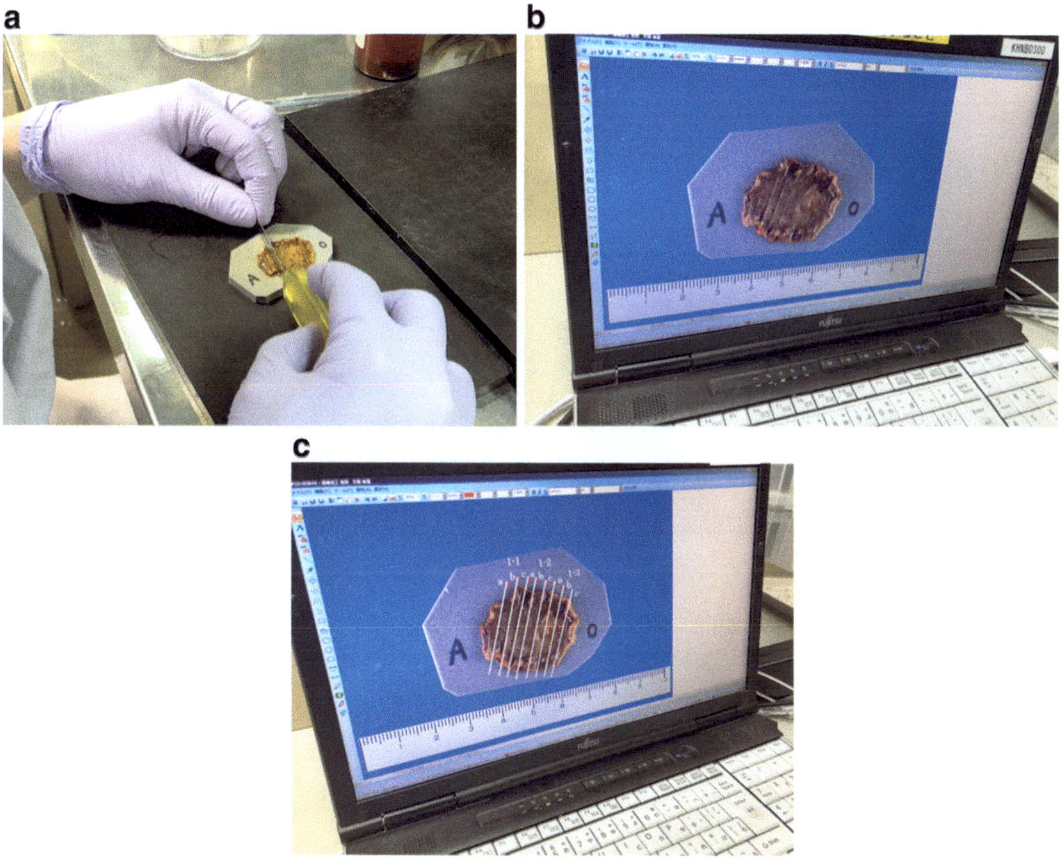

Fig. 18 Cutting out the specimen (*A* anal direction, *O* oral direction). (**a**) Cut the specimen along the long axis of the lesion with an interval of 2–3 mm. (**b**) Take a macroscopic photograph. (**c**) Document information including cassette numbers and cut lines on digital images

(f) The three-dimensional architecture of the lesion is reproduced (e.g., with or without bumps, depressions, or stalks). Take a slide view of the lesion as needed.

(g) The degree of lesion volume is reproduced (e.g., the amount of submucosal component).

(h) Identify the number, location, and distribution of lesions.

(i) Identify the size of the lesion (scale is properly placed).

Overall, a good macroscopic photograph for pathological examination of a specimen could be summarized as a clear picture with a clear message, with the focus properly captured and taken at the best angle. Unlike microscopic photographs, macrophotographs cannot be retaken many times as the specimen has to be further dissected. It is important to choose a camera with high resolution as well as user-friendly. If possible, avoid

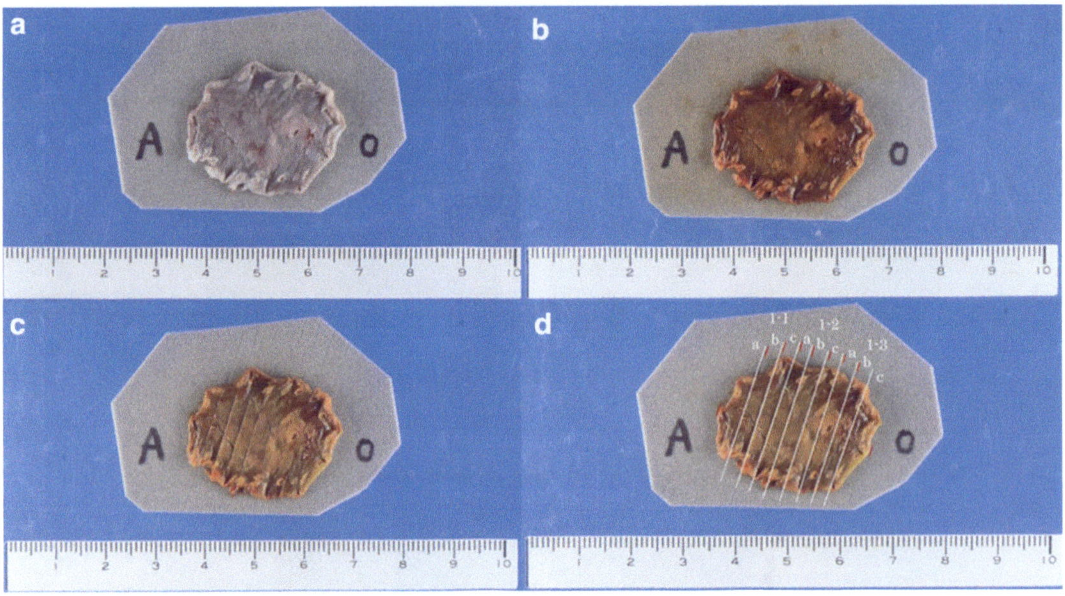

Fig. 19 Preparation of digital images for mapping of tumor cells under microscopic observation (*A* anal direction, *O* oral direction). (**a**) Macroscopic photo of formalin-fixed specimen. (**b**) Macroscopic photo of iodine-stained specimen. (**c**) Macroscopic photo of iodine-stained specimen after cutting. (**d**) Macroscopic photo of iodine-stained specimen after numbering the blocks in the cut specimens

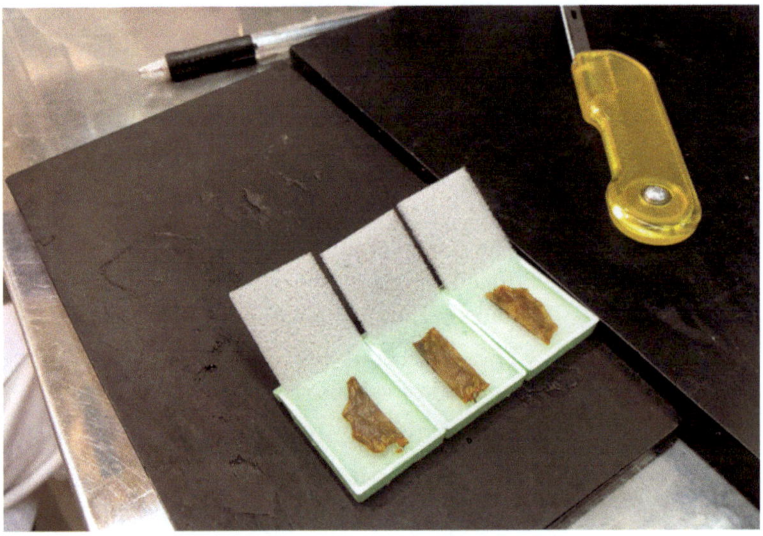

Fig. 20 Put the specimens cut out in tissue cassettes for paraffin embedding

unnecessary vibrations and shadows if the remote release button can be used to release the shutter. It is also useful to have a horizontal platform for taking a picture.

4. It is desirable that extending and fixing the specimen is performed by a doctor who performed or assisted the resection. It

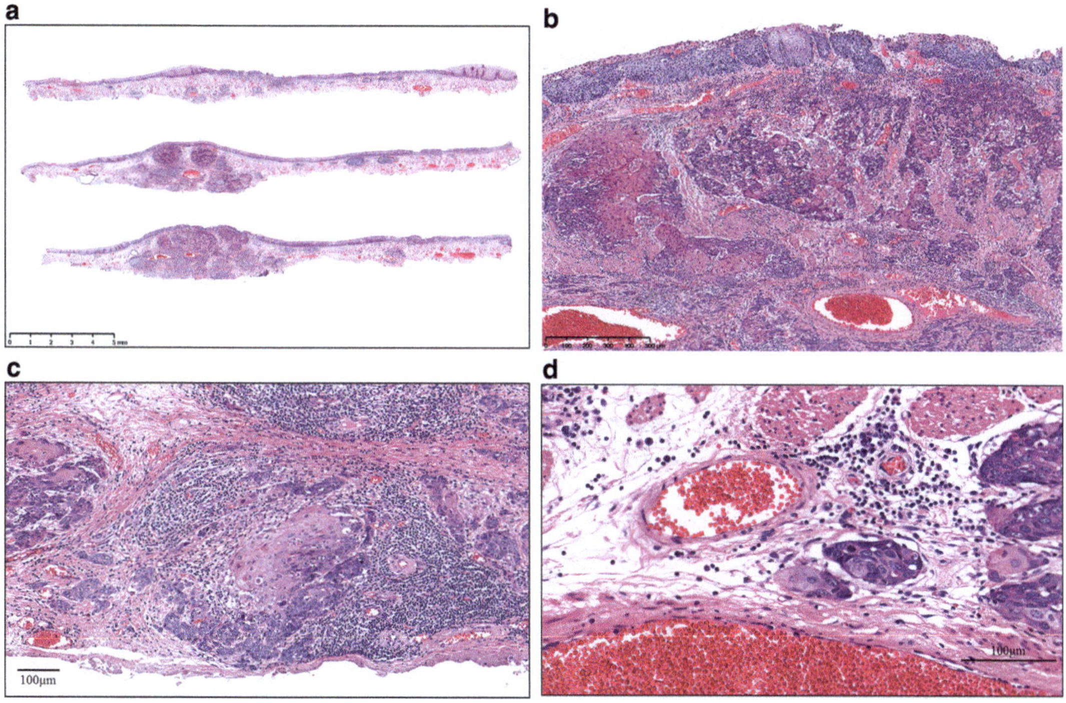

Fig. 21 Micrographs of hematoxylin and eosin-stained sections of endoscopically resected specimens (hematoxylin and eosin stained). (**a**) Low-magnification image of the three serial sections of endoscopic resection of superficial esophageal squamous cell carcinoma. (**b**) Microscopic appearance of squamous cell carcinoma with invasion to submucosa of the esophagus in the endoscopic resection specimen. (**c**) Microscopic appearance showing squamous cell carcinoma close to the deep resection margin. (**d**) Microscopic appearance showing lymphatic infiltration by squamous cell carcinoma cells

is important to specify the orientation of the specimen, the proximal side and the distal side, and the anatomical sub-site as well as stretch and fix the specimen so that the in vivo positional relationship can be reproduced in the resected specimen.

5. 10% neutral buffered formalin is better at fixing the cytoplasm than 15–20% formalin. The specimen retains its antigenicity in immunohistochemical staining, and in the next-generation sequencing era, good results are obtained when performing DNA extracted from the paraffin blocks fixed in this way. Excessive or insufficient fixation of the specimen will also disturb the subsequent histopathological examination and investigations.

6. As a basic principle of composition, the resected specimen is placed to identify the oral side (O, proximal side) and the anal side (A, distal side).

   There are two ways to dissect the resected specimens. Method A is used when the lesion is far away from the resection margin. Insert a cut line perpendicular to the long axis of the lesion with a width of 2–3 mm. Method B is preferred when the lesion is close to the resection margins. In the lesion, first, a tangent line is set to the portion closest to the lesion. And a cut line perpendicular to the tangent line is inserted with a width of 2–3 mm. To accurately reconstruct the lesion, macroscopic photographs must be taken again for the specimens with multiple cut lines so that the lesion mapping showing the areas with cancer cells can be shown accurately. For the outermost side of the specimen, embed the reverse face far from the lesion as a surface of microscopic observation so that the true resection margin can be evaluated.

In case that the lesion is small, set the cut line with enough care so that the lesion is not divided by the cut line and the line does not cause a situation that the lesion is not found on the surface of microscopic observation. In addition, it is important to take note that there may be situations when small lesions discontinuously co-exist with the main lesion.

References

1. Muto M, Minashi K, Yano T, Saito Y, Oda I, Nonaka S, Omori T, Sugiura H, Goda K, Kaise M, Inoue H, Ishikawa H, Ochiai A, Shimoda T, Watanabe H, Tajiri H, Saito D (2010) Early detection of superficial squamous cell carcinoma in the head and neck region and esophagus by narrow band imaging: a multicenter randomized controlled trial. J Clin Oncol 28:1566–1572
2. Katada C, Yokoyama T, Yano T, Kaneko K, Oda I, Shimizu Y, Doyama H, Koike T, Takizawa K, Hirao M, Okada H, Yoshii T, Konishi K, Yamanouchi T, Tsuda T, Omori T, Kobayashi N, Shimoda T, Ochiai A, Amanuma Y, Ohashi S, Matsuda T, Ishikawa H, Yokoyama A, Muto M (2016) Alcohol consumption and multiple dysplastic lesions increase risk of squamous cell carcinoma in the esophagus, Head, and Neck. Gastroenterology 151:860–869
3. Dobashi A, Goda K, Furuhashi H, Matsui H, Hara Y, Kamba S, Kobayashi M, Sumiyama K, Hirooka S, Hamatani S, Rajan E, Ikegami M, Tajiri H (2019) Diagnostic efficacy of dual-focus endoscopy with narrow-band imaging using simplified dyad criteria for superficial esophageal squamous cell carcinoma. J Gastroenterol 154:501–510
4. Araki K, Ohno S, Egashira A, Saeki H, Kawaguchi H, Sugimachi K (2002) Pathological feature of superficial esophageal squamous cell carcinoma with lymph node and distal metastasis. Cancer 94:570–575
5. Eguchi T, Nakanishi Y, Shimoda T, Iwasaki M, Igaki H, Tachimori Y, Kato H, Yamaguchi H, Saito D, Umemura S (2006) Histological criteria for additional treatment after endoscopic mucosal resection for esophageal cancer: analysis of 464 surgically resected cases. Mod Pathol 19:475–480
6. Kim DU, Lee JH, Min BH, Shim SG, Chang DK, Kim YH, Rhee PL, Kim JJ, Rhee JC, Kim KM, Shim YM (2008) Risk factors of lymph node metastasis in T1 esophageal squamous cell carcinoma. J Gastroenterol Hepatol 23:619–625
7. Choi JY, Park YS, Jung HY, Ahn JY, Kim MY, Lee JH, Choi KS, Kim DH, Choi KD, Song HJ, Lee GH, Cho KJ, Kim JH (2011) Feasibility of endoscopic resection in superficial esophageal squamous carcinoma. Gastrointest Endosc 73:881–889
8. Akutsu Y, Uesato M, Shuto K, Kono T, Hoshino I, Horibe D, Sazuka T, Takeshita N, Maruyama T, Isozaki Y, Akanuma N, Matsubara H (2013) The overall prevalence of metastasis in T1 esophageal squamous cell carcinoma: a retrospective analysis of 295 patients. Ann Surg 257:1032–1038
9. Kadota T, Yano T, Fujita T, Daiko H, Fujii S (2017) Submucosal invasive depth predicts lymph node metastasis and poor prognosis in

submucosal invasive esophageal squamous cell carcinoma. Am J Clin Pathol 148:416–426

10. Katada C, Muto M, Momma K, Arima M, Tajiri H, Kanamaru C, Ooyanagi H, Endo H, Michida T, Hasuike N, Oda I, Fujii T, Saito D (2007) Clinical outcome after endoscopic mucosal resection for esophageal squamous cell carcinoma invading the muscularis mucosae—a multicenter retrospective cohort study. Endoscopy 39:779–783
11. Yamashina T, Ishihara R, Nagai K, Matsuura N, Matsui F, Ito T, Fujii M, Yamamoto S, Hanaoka N, Takeuchi Y, Higashino K, Uedo N, Iishi H (2013) Long-term outcome and metastatic risk after endoscopic resection of superficial esophageal squamous cell carcinoma. Am J Gastroenterol 108:544–551
12. Li B, Chen H, Xiang J, Zhang Y, Kong Y, Garfield DH, Li H (2013) Prevalence of lymph node metastases in superficial esophageal squamous cell carcinoma. J Thorac Cardiovasc Surg 146:1198–1203
13. Esaki M, Matsumoto T, Hirakawa K, Nakamura S, Umeno J, Koga H, Yao T, Iida M (2007) Risk factors for local recurrence of superficial esophageal cancer after treatment by endoscopic mucosal resection. Endoscopy 39:41–45
14. Wen J, Linghu E, Yang Y, Liu Q, Wang X, Du H, Wang H, Meng J, Lu Z (2014) Relevant risk factors and prognostic impact of positive resection margins after endoscopic submucosal dissection of superficial esophageal squamous cell neoplasia. Surg Endosc 28:1653–1659
15. Hombu T, Yano T, Hatogai K, Kojima T, Kadota T, Onozawa M, Yoda Y, Hori K, Oono Y, Ikematsu H, Fujii S (2018) Salvage endoscopic resection (ER) after chemoradiotherapy for esophageal squamous cell carcinoma: what are the risk factors for recurrence after salvage ER? Dig Endosc 30:338–346
16. Lam AK, Ochiai A, Odze RD (2019) Tumours of the oesophagus: introduction. In: Odze RD, Lam AK, Ochiai A, Washington MK (eds) Chapter 2: WHO classification of tumours, 5th edn, pp 28–29
17. Brown IS, Fujii S, Kawachi H, Lam AK, Saito T (2019) Oesophageal squamous cell carcinoma NOS. In: Odze RD, Lam AK, Ochiai A, Washington MK (eds) Chapter 2: WHO classification of tumours, 5th edn, pp 48–53

Chapter 7

Roles of Pathological Assessments of Frozen Sections in Esophageal Squamous Cell Carcinoma

Alfred K. Lam

Abstract

Pathological assessment of frozen sections of tissues is important in the clinical management (intraoperative consultation) and research in patients with esophageal squamous cell carcinoma. Frozen sections may be used in the assessment of status of resection margins, extent of cancer metastasis (pathological staging), confirmation of the pathology, and increased volume of cancer cells for tissue banking. However, the applications of frozen sections have many technical limitations. Thus, interpretation of frozen sections needs expertise, collaborations, and attention to proper technical skills in the sectioning.

Key words Esophagus, Frozen section, Squamous carcinoma, Pathology

1 Introduction

Fresh human tissue turns hard after frozen, which favors for cutting of sections for pathological assessment. Pathological interpretation of sections from frozen tissue of esophageal squamous cell carcinoma (ESCC) serves many clinical as well as research purposes. To preserve tissues from ESCC for research purposes, it is important to have the tissues stored in cold (frozen) to prevent degradation (*see* Chapter 8). In studies on the genomic of ESCC, it is best to use fresh frozen cancer tissue [1, 2].

In research, morphological assessments allow confirmation of the presence of cancer taken for tissue biobanking, cell culture, or implantation in mice. In some instances, macroscopic presence of a tumor may not be equivalent to a carcinoma. The tumor could be necrotic tissues or fibrotic stromal tissue without viable cancer cells. This often occurs in tissues sampled from patients who have received adjuvant chemoradiation. On the other hand, macroscopic non-cancer tissue may have squamous dysplasia (pre-invasive) or early invasive squamous cell carcinoma on microscopic examination (Fig. 1). In addition, it is worth to sample the lymph node with cancer metastases in patients with ESCC to study specific genomic

Alfred K. Lam (ed.), *Esophageal Squamous Cell Carcinoma: Methods and Protocols*, Methods in Molecular Biology, vol. 2129, https://doi.org/10.1007/978-1-0716-0377-2_7,

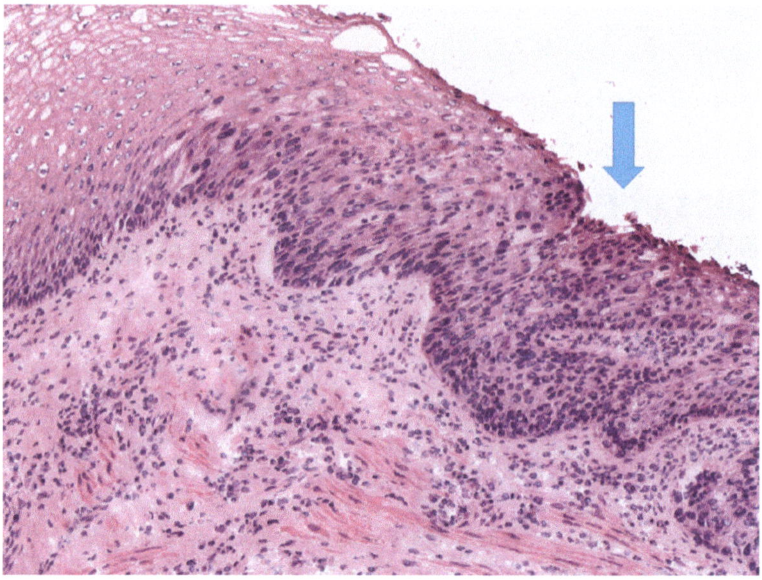

Fig. 1 Frozen section from tissue taken from macroscopic tumor-free esophageal mucosa showing high-grade squamous dysplasia (arrow) (hematoxylin and eosin × 8)

changes in cancer metastases [3]. Sometimes, it is impossible to differentiate lymph node with reactive change from lymph node with metastatic carcinoma on macroscopic sampling of enlarged lymph node. Effects of adjuvant chemoradiation add further difficulty to identify a lymph node with viable metastatic carcinoma. In genomic works, pathological assessment of the sections is essential to estimate the proportion of cancer cells in the tissue before research works such as sequencing [1]. In some instances, with the help of morphological assessment, the portion of the tissues with the cancer could be micro-dissected out from the necrotic/ fibrotic tissues in order to increase the yield of the viable cancer cells (*see* Chapter 8).

Intraoperative pathological consultation by frozen sectioning of fresh tissue is an important means to get a rapid diagnosis for surgeon in making decision for the management in patients with esophageal squamous cell carcinoma at the time of surgery. It is a procedure of high specificity and sensitivity in clinical practice [4]. Making pathological diagnosis using frozen section (s) normally needs a short period (approximately 15–20 min depending on the expertise of the surgeon, scientists, and pathologist, the type of tissue, and the nature of the consultation question). In standard pathological assessment of esophagectomy specimen, the time-determining factors are time for fixation in formalin, sampling for appropriate tissue blocks, paraffin block making, cutting of sections, and pathological interpretation (*see* Chapter 4). Usually, for a standard pathology laboratory, it needs more than

2 days (from the time of receiving the specimen) for making a pathological reporting of an esophagectomy for ESCC.

Frozen section diagnosis is important when there are unexpected findings during operation for ESCC. It is central for pathological staging of ESCC (*see* Chapter 3). The findings may represent examples of metastases in the liver, pleural or peritoneal surfaces, lungs, and non-regional lymph nodes. In some instances, ESCC metastasizes to the heart, spleen, and adrenal gland [5–7]. Findings of cancer in these organs will upstage the cancer. If surgeon found distant metastases at esophagectomy at frozen section, the scope of the operation may change. On the other hand, benign lesions in the liver could mimic liver metastases [8]. Thus, frozen section examination is essential to confirm the nature of unexpected macroscopic abnormal lesions noted at surgery for ESCC.

Sometimes, it is important to decide whether the macroscopic tumor-free margin of resection is free from dysplasia or invasive squamous cell carcinoma. This is for the proximal resection margin, which has a high chance of recurrence of cancer at anastomosis [9]. An extensive macroscopic-free margin is difficult to achieve in patients having ESCC in upper third of the esophagus because of the technical limitations for extensive surgery in the region. Chiu and colleagues demonstrated that in patients having ESCC treated with chemoradiotherapy, positive proximal resection margin occurred in 4.8% [9]. In addition, a macroscopic-free margin of less than 35 mm was a significant predictor of microscopic presence of proximal resection margin (4.473 higher in risk). Intraoperative frozen section analysis could help to assess the patients having ESCC with high risk of residual microscopic disease at surgery.

Lymph node metastasis is a common event in ESCC. In autopsy study, positive lymph node occurred in more than 40% of patients with ESCC [10]. The multidirectional and rich lymphatic also made lymphatic spread and multiple tumors common [11]. Nevertheless, the minimization of lymph node dissection is under consideration for patients with early-stage ESCC. Sentinel node is the draining lymph node associated with primary cancer and should be the first lymph node that cancer metastasizes. If a sentinel lymph node is negative for malignancy (e.g., in patients with melanoma and breast carcinoma) as examined on frozen sections at the time of surgery, the surgeons may not do the lymph node dissection [12]. Sentinel lymph node biopsy for frozen section at the time of operation may be useful in the management of early-stage ESCC. However, the concept of sentinel lymph node biopsy remains controversial in ESCC [13]. One of the reasons for lack of prediction power of lymph node metastases by sentinel lymph node biopsy is the complex anatomy of drainage of lymphatic vessels in the esophagus [14].

There are many limitations on using frozen section to interpret morphology of ESCC in both clinical and research settings. The

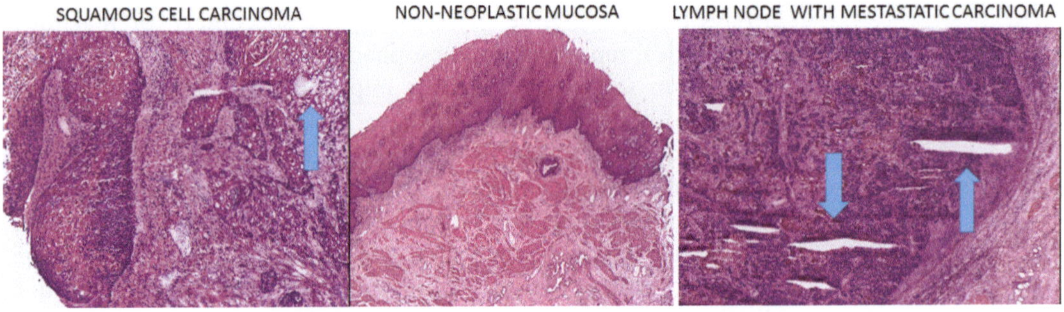

Fig. 2 Frozen sections of a set of sections taken from a patient with esophageal squamous cell carcinoma. These include the carcinoma, the non-neoplastic mucosa, and the lymph node with metastatic carcinoma. Note that the morphology is inferior to formalin-fixed paraffin-embedded sections. There are many artifacts noted (arrows) (hematoxylin and eosin × 4)

quality of frozen section is inferior to formalin-fixed paraffin-embedded sections with reference to pathological assessment (Fig. 2). There could be folding up/wrinkling of sections and various freezing artifacts in cryostat sections. Freezing artifacts are due to chemical property of water in the tissue. The water in the tissue turns into ice when frozen and the ice expanses the tissue resulting in artifacts. The artifacts could cause bubbles in stroma, cells, and nuclei. Artifactual "ballooning" of squamous carcinoma cells may make them appear benign [15]. Clinical history of chemoradiation is important as this makes interpretation of morphology more difficult and prone to give rise to errors in the diagnosis in frozen section interpretation (*see* Chapter 2). Accurate assessments of morphology in frozen sections require knowledge, training, and experience of surgeons, scientists, and pathologists to make diagnosis at frozen section. In addition, all pathology laboratories performing intra-operative frozen section analysis should have quality assurance programs in place. Furthermore, there should be guidelines of workflow to perform intraoperative frozen section analysis at work and taking research material for biobanking at the same time.

2 Materials

1. Biosafety cabinet.
2. Gloves for protection in handling tissue.
3. Dissecting kits for cutting of tissue (includes disposable scalpel blades and blade holders, forceps, sharp scissors, and tissue papers for drying).
4. Measurement and labelling kits (metal rulers, pencil, and camera).
5. Holding units for freezing:

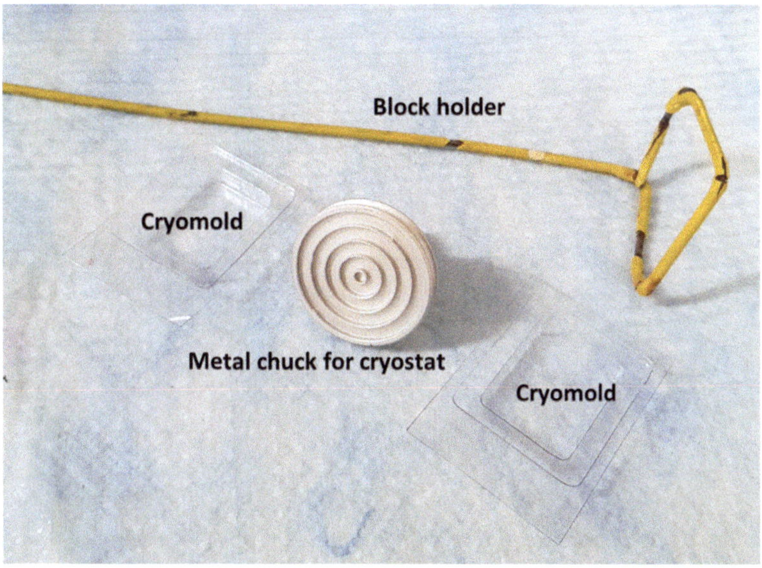

Fig. 3 The tools which include (1) cryomolds (transparent) to hold the tissue, (2) metal chuck to hold the frozen tissue to be cut in the cryostat, and (3) metal block holder to hold the cryomolds and metal chuck in liquid nitrogen

(a) Disposable plastic cryomolds for holding the tissue—can have different sizes; usually the largest one is preferred.

(b) Cryostat chuck (to fit in the hole in the cryostat for orientating the frozen block for cutting by the blade of cryostat).

(c) Holder for tissue in liquid nitrogen (Fig. 3).

6. OCT (optimal cutting temperature) compound—gel-like compound composing of polyvinyl alcohol, polyethylene glycol, and non-reactive ingredients, which is of similar density to human tissue.
7. Liquid nitrogen and metal container for holding liquid nitrogen (for rapid cooling).
8. Cryostat (equipment for cutting frozen sections).
9. Cryogen spray coolant.
10. Positive-charge glass slides.
11. FAA (formalin-acetic acid-alcohol) fixature (from mixing of ethanol [810 ml], water [40 ml], formaldehyde [100 ml], and glacial acetic acid [50 ml]).
12. Hematoxylin and eosin staining workstation (*see* **Note 1**).
13. Tap water (should be near the hematoxylin and eosin staining station).
14. Coverslips and mounting medium.
15. Light microscope.

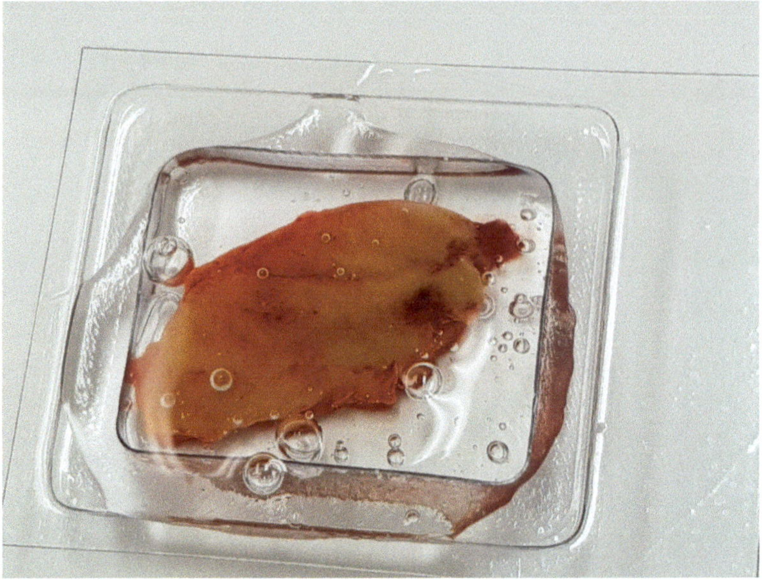

Fig. 4 Cryomold filled with tissue and covered with OCT medium

3 Methods

3.1 Preparation of Frozen Blocks

1. Orient the specimen, and make necessary measurements, recordings, and pictures (*see* Chapters 4 and 8 on macroscopic dissection and biobanking) in the biosafety cabinet.
2. Dissect the fresh tissue obtained at surgery.
3. Fit the tissue in the cryomold(s) (*see* **Note 2**).
4. Blot the surface of the specimen and dry with towel paper to prevent ice crystal artifacts.
5. Put OCT medium to fill up the plastic cryomolds (Fig. 4).
6. Invert the metal cryostat chuck on the plastic cryomolds (Fig. 5a).
7. Using a metal holder, insert the chuck and cryomolds into liquid nitrogen for approximately 15–30 s until the block is frozen (Fig. 5b) (*see* **Note 3**).

3.2 Cutting of Frozen Blocks

1. Label glass slides with pencil with identifications (code number, patient's family name, etc.).
2. Slide open the glass window of the cryostat (*see* **Note 4**).
3. Mount and fix the chuck in the fitting area of the cryostat (Fig. 6).
4. Set the thickness of the cut sections to be 4 μm each (*see* **Note 5**).

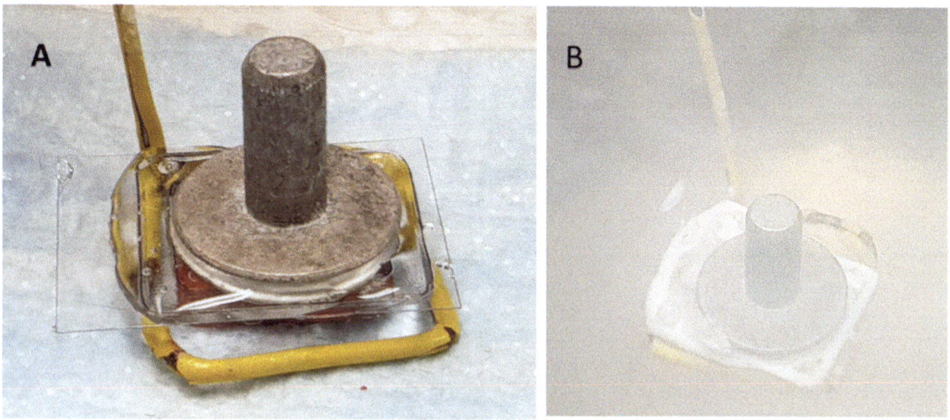

Fig. 5 (**a**) Assemble the cryomold with the surface of the tissue and metal chuck touching each other (so that they will fix together after frozen), and place in the holder to be frozen in liquid nitrogen (**b**)

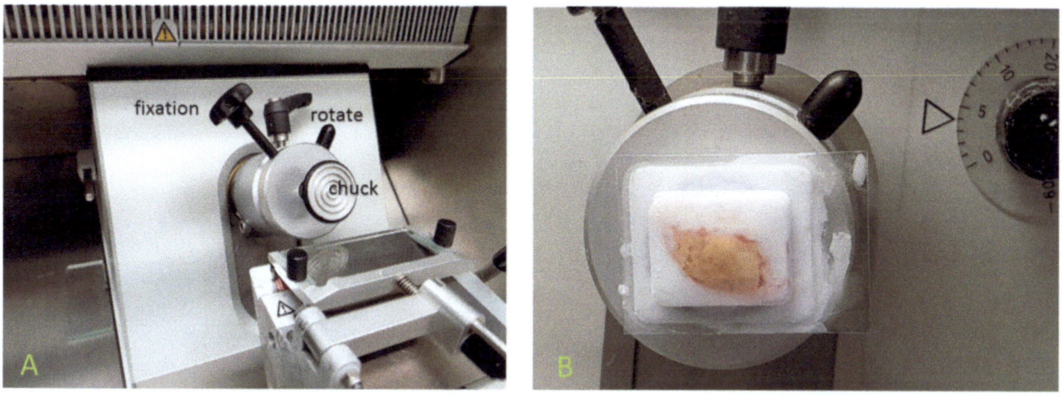

Fig. 6 (**a**) Cryostat showing the area where operator can attach the chuck. The right handle allows rotation of the chuck to different angles, whereas the right handle is to fix the angle and position of the chuck for cutting. (**b**) The tissue with the metal chuck fit to a hole in cryostat. The frozen block is covered by the cryomold on top on the chuck, which will be removed before the start of cutting. Note the knob with arrowhead on the right side in which the operator can choose the thickness of each of the cut sections. The thickness was set at 4 μm

5. Remove the cryomold which cover the frozen tissue block and expose the surface of the frozen block for cutting.
6. Trim the surface of the block, covered with frozen mounting medium (OCT), by advancing the block toward the blade of the cryostat until reaching the tissue surface (*see* **Note 6**) (Fig. 7).
7. Cut whole section from the block when possible (Fig. 8).
8. In some instances, gently hold down the best cut tissue section with a fine brush or forceps to flatten the tissue cut on the blade.
9. Lay the labelled glass slide at room temperature upon the tissue section. The tissue section should stick ("melt") into the slide.

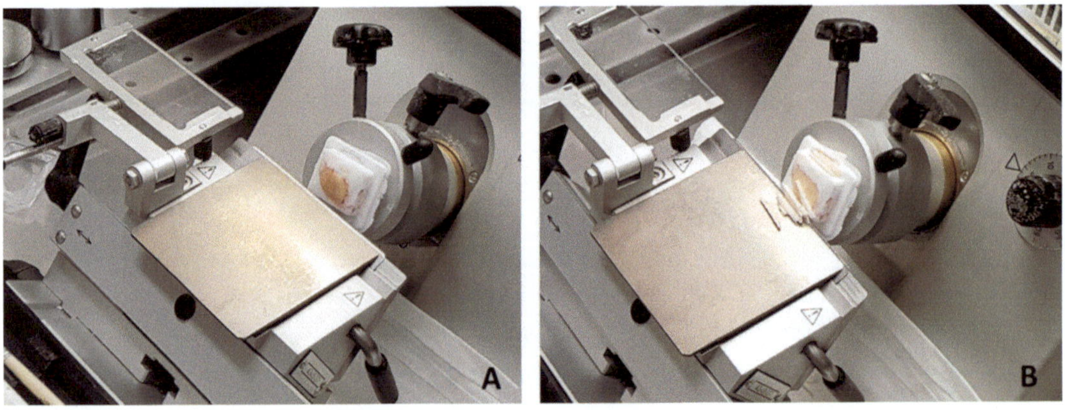

Fig. 7 (**a**) A frozen block advances toward the blade of the cryostat. (**b**) Rolls of attempted sections cut

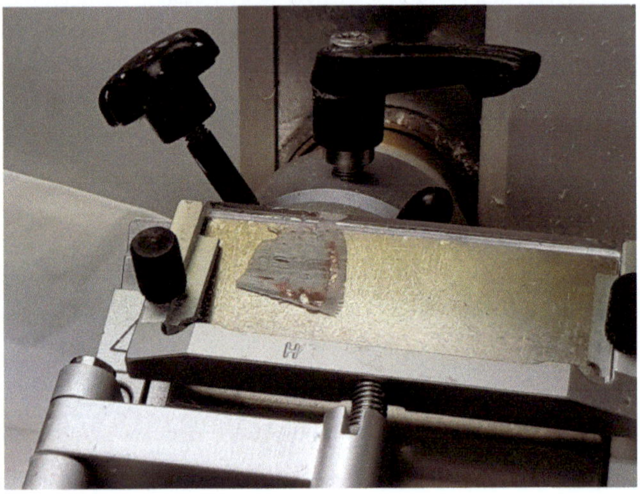

Fig. 8 A full phrase cut section ready to be picked up

3.3 Staining of Frozen Sections

The section(s) then proceed to the hematoxylin and eosin staining station. Different stains (toluidine blue, Giemsa, Oil Red O, etc.) have been used to stain, but the best and most common for interpretation is by hematoxylin and eosin. In addition, pathologists are more familiar with the hematoxylin and eosin stain and could compare the results from frozen sections easily with those from the sections obtained after formalin fixation.

1. Fix the section(s) immediately in acid fixatures (formalin-acetic acid-alcohol (FAA)) for 10–30 s (to prevent drying artifact—air-drying will result in poor stain uptake and "blow-up" of cells).
2. Rinse in tap water.
3. Filter on hematoxylin for 10–15 s.
4. Rinse in tap water.

5. Blue with Scott solution for a few seconds.
6. Rinse in tap water.
7. Rinse in absolute alcohol for a few dips.
8. Put in eosin for 15 s.
9. Wash off excess stain with few dips in absolute alcohol.
10. Pass the slides through three changes of absolute alcohol (few dips each).
11. Clear in two changes of xylene (few dips).
12. Coverslip the slides with mounting medium to allow even thickness for viewing under microscope.

3.4 Interpret the Sections with Microscope by Pathologist (See Note 7)

Section (s) need to be examined under light microscope to detect the presence of tumour. Communications of the reults of interpretation (preliminary diagnosis) with clinician(s) are important. The clinicians may send more tissue to be examined if the diagnosis is in doubt.

3.5 Tissues for Clinical Diagnosis Should Transfer Back to formlin fixation and then embedded in paraffin After Frozen Sectioning to Confirm the Diagnosis (See Note 8)

Definite diagnosis needs to be make on proper hematoxylin and esoin stained section(s) from paraffin embeded tissue after frozen section anlaysis. If the diagnosis of cancer is confirmed, may get some tissue for biobanking at thi stage.

4 Notes

1. The working station for staining should be a series of plastic/glass containers containing FAA, hematoxylin stain, Scott solution (*see* below), eosin stain, alcohols, and xylene (Fig. 9). Hematoxylin dyes nuclei and binds to the histones. It makes the nuclei of cells having blue color. Scott solution could be made by mixing 2000 ml distilled water, 40 g magnesium sulfate, and 7 g sodium bicarbonates. It converts the initial soluble red color of the hematoxylin within the nucleus to an insoluble blue color. The alkaline pH of the bluing solution causes the staining more permanent. Eosin is an acidic dye that is negatively charged. It stains basic (or acidophilic) structures, such as cytoplasm of many tumor cells, pink.
2. Try to remove unnecessary fatty tissue as they can affect rapid freezing. Cryomold standardizes the size of the tissue for cutting in the cryostat. The fresh tissue or frozen tissue from the

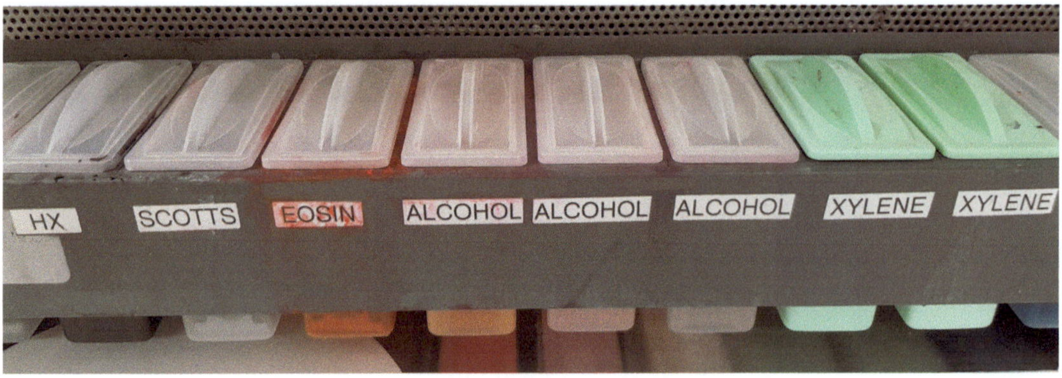

Fig. 9 Containers contain the reagents required for staining the sections. They are lined up in sequential manner so that a section could transfer through them rapidly for staining

biobank should fit in disposable plastic cryomolds. The tissue should not be more than 15 mm × 10 mm in area. In addition, trim the block to a thickness of no more than 3 mm. Orientate the surface of the tissue for cutting.

3. Ice crystals will form when the tissue is frozen. They form more slowly at lower temperatue. Rapid cooling of the tissue is to prevent massive formation of ice crystals. A lower temperature of freezing is required for fat or lipid-rich tissue. Do not put the specimen in liquid nitrogen for too long as the temperature will drop too low and cutting will be impossible.

4. Cryostat comprises of a chamber with freezing temperature at around −20 °C, a microtome with blade for cutting, and a control panel. The control panel allows for advancing and retracting mechanism for cutting the block with cutting blade of the microtome. Cryostat must be defrosted and decontaminated regularly to maintain the optimal function.

5. Thicker sections may be required in some tissues to decrease the artifacts. For instance, for fat or difficult-to-cut tissue, thicker sections are preferred. However, thick sections may be difficult to interpret on microscopic examination. It is better to limit the sections to no more than 8 μm.

6. The temperature of the cryostat is set at −20 °C. The optimal temperature of cutting depends on the tissue and should not be too warm and not too cold. Cryogen spray coolant could cool the tissue block. The block should be orientated so that the cryostat blade could hit perpendicular to it. The handle (wheel) at the side of the cryostat is used to advance the tissue to the blade of the cryotome.

7. If there are a lot of folding and artifacts, repeat the steps to obtain better section(s). In interpretation of the pathology from lymph node, make sure that the lymph node pathology

does not contain infective organisms—e.g., tuberculosis. If mycobacterial infection is found, inform the relative staff to decontaminate the equipment and areas for safety measures.

8. To recover the frozen tissue for formal histopathological examination, leave the frozen tissue in room temperature. This allows the frozen tissue to melt and becomes soft before putting into fixation in formalin. However, many artifacts occur in the FFPE sections when the tissues have been frozen.

References

1. Dai W, Ko JMY, Choi SSA, Yu Z, Ning L, Zheng H, Gopalan V, Chan KT, Lee NP, Chan KW, Law SY, Lam AK, Lung ML (2017) Whole-exome sequencing reveals critical gene underlying metastasis in oesophageal squamous cell carcinoma. J Pathol 242:500–510
2. Kwong D, Lam A, Guan X, Law S, Tai A, Wong J, Sham J (2004) Chromosomal aberrations in esophageal squamous cell carcinoma among Chinese: gain of 12p predicts poor prognosis after surgery. Hum Pathol 35:309–316
3. Haque MH, Gopalan V, Chan KW, Shiddiky MJ, Smith RA, Lam AK (2016) Identification of novel FAM134B (JK1) mutations in oesophageal squamous cell carcinoma. Sci Rep 6:29173
4. Nayanar SK, M AK IMK, Thavarool PSB, Thiagarajan S (2019) Frozen section evaluation in head and neck oncosurgery: an initial experience in a tertiary cancer center. Turk Patoloji Derg 35:46–51
5. Lam KY, Lo CY (2002) Metastatic tumours of the adrenal glands: a 30-year experience in a teaching hospital. Clin Endocrinol 56:95–101
6. Lam KY, Tang V (2000) Metastatic tumors to the spleen: a 25-year clinicopathologic study. Arch Pathol Lab Med 124:526–530
7. Lam KY, Dickens P, Chan AC (1993) Tumors of the heart: a 20-year experience with a review of 12,485 consecutive autopsies. Arch Pathol Lab Med 117:1027–1031
8. Fritz S, Hackert T, Blaker H, Hartwig W, Schneider L, Buchler MW, Werner J (2006) Multiple von Meyenburg complexes mimicking diffuse liver metastases from esophageal squamous cell carcinoma. World J Gastroenterol 12:4250–4252
9. Chiu CH, Chao YK, Wen YW, Chang HK, Tseng CK, Liu YH (2017) Unexpected microscopically positive proximal resection margins in esophageal squamous cell carcinoma after chemoradiotherapy: predictors and prognostic significance. World J Surg 41:191–199
10. Lam KY, Law S, Wong J (2003) Low prevalence of incidentally discovered and early-stage esophageal cancers in a 30-year autopsy study. Dis Esophagus 16:1–3
11. Lam KY, Ma LT, Wong J (1996) Measurement of extent of spread of oesophageal squamous carcinoma by serial sectioning. J Clin Pathol 49:124–129
12. Hagihara T, Uenosono Y, Arigami T, Kozono T, Arima H, Yanagita S, Hirata M, Ehi K, Okumura H, Matsumoto M, Uchikado Y, Ishigami S, Natsugoe S (2013) Assessment of sentinel node concept in esophageal cancer based on lymph node micrometastasis. Ann Surg Oncol 20:3031–3037
13. Akutsu Y, Kato K, Igaki H, Ito Y, Nozaki I, Daiko H, Yano M, Udagawa H, Nakagawa S, Takagi M, Mizusawa J, Kitagawa Y (2016) The prevalence of overall and initial lymph node metastases in clinical t1n0 thoracic esophageal cancer: from the results of jcog0502, a prospective multicenter study. Ann Surg 264:1009–1015
14. Kumakura Y, Yokobori T, Yoshida T, Hara K, Sakai M, Sohda M, Miyazaki T, Yokoo H, Handa T, Oyama T, Yorifuji H, Kuwano H (2018) Elucidation of the anatomical mechanism of nodal skip metastasis in superficial thoracic esophageal squamous cell carcinoma. Ann Surg Oncol 25:1221–1228
15. Thomson AM, Wallace WA (2007) Fixation artefact in an intra-operative frozen section: a potential cause of misinterpretation. J Cardiothorac Surg 2:45

Chapter 8

Biobanking for Esophageal Squamous Cell Carcinoma

Alfred K. Lam

Abstract

Biobanking is important and fundamental for research and personalized medicine in patients with esophageal squamous cell carcinoma. The process often involves prospective collection of surgically obtained tissues (tissue banking) as well as serial blood samples (liquid biopsies) from the patients with esophageal squamous cell carcinoma. Apart from frozen tissues, formalin-fixed paraffin-embedded tissues are important sources of translational research. Careful planning and selection of the region of the paraffin-embedded tissues will maximize the use of tissue for molecular studies. Both cancer and non-cancer samples (controls) could be collected. The success and sustainability of the process needs proper infrastructure, advanced planning, funding, and multidisciplinary collaborations. The understanding of the principles and issues are detrimental for the success of biobanking. The technical procedures involved are standardized, complex, and time-consuming and needs coordinated taskforce.

Key words Esophagus, Tissue banking, Squamous carcinoma, Biobank, Blood

1 Introduction

Biobanking is a storage of biological samples (often from human) for use in research in diverse range of diseases. It normally includes standardized collection of a category of samples with harmonized collection protocols. With the advance of science and technology, scientists started large-scale collections of biological specimens from human in the 1990s. Nowadays, small tissue banks in individuals' laboratories as well as large-scale national or global biobanks are widely available in every continent for researchers (https://specimencentral.com/biobank-directory/) [1].

In the context of cancer research, the most common types of sample that researchers would like to collect are cancer tissues (tissue biopsy) as well as blood samples (liquid biopsy) from the patients. In esophageal cancers, there are tissue banks that contribute to the integrated genomic characterization of the cancer [2, 3]. Healthy people are often asked to donate samples to act as controls. Control samples could be blood samples from healthy person or non-neoplastic tissues from the matched organ removed

Alfred K. Lam (ed.), *Esophageal Squamous Cell Carcinoma: Methods and Protocols*, Methods in Molecular Biology, vol. 2129, https://doi.org/10.1007/978-1-0716-0377-2_8, © Springer Science+Business Media, LLC, part of Springer Nature 2020

for other non-neoplastic diseases. In tissue banking for cancer, control tissue is matched non-neoplastic tissue sampled some distance away from the resected cancer specimen from the same patient.

The purposes of the biobank in cancer research are diverse and well known in scientific research such as drug discovery, development, and validation [4]. In the era of personalized medicine, tracking the changes in the characteristics of biological samples from individual patient is important in prevention, diagnosis, treatment, and monitoring of the cancer. Nevertheless, there are many issues encountered in starting and maintenance of biobanks such as ethical, legal, and social issues related to the biobanks [4]. More importantly, biobanking needs sustainability in terms of infrastructure, funding, labor, collaborations, education, and managements.

Although there are many cancer biobanks globally available to researchers, there is always a need for researchers to collect their own biobanks to target for their special research needs. In some instances, researchers need to collect samples of rare cancers or unique sets of clinical data linked to samples not available in other collections. It is of importance to collect biobank in the personalized medicine where the need is on a unique group of patients with cancer under the care of local multidisciplinary health team.

Biological samples will undergo degeneration after leaving the human body. The cells, DNA, RNA, and proteins will suffer different degree of loss. It is essential to process the collected samples immediately to prevent degeneration or keep to minimum as possible. RNA is one of the most vulnerable components suggestive to decay.

In clinical settings, cancer tissues obtained after surgical biopsy are formalin fixed and embedded in paraffin blocks. Hematoxylin and eosin-stained sections cut from these blocks are for the pathologists to make diagnosis and formulate management advices. This method provides tissue sections best for morphological assessment and immunohistochemical detection of proteins in cancer. Many of the pathology laboratories would store the paraffin blocks for extended period but unlikely to be indefinitely because of limitation of space of storage. Nevertheless, scientists need time and resource to retrieve the blocks for research purposes. It is best to make some paraffin blocks for research purpose at the time of operation.

Formalin-fixed paraffin-embedded blocks are important resources for cancer research. However, the tissues obtained from endoscopic biopsy (*see* Chapter 5) or biopsy at the time of recurrence is usually small in size. Tissues must be preserved for clinical diagnosis and may not have enough remain for research purposes. Thus, biobanking at the time of surgical resection will get tissues big enough to serve many purposes. However, the use of preoperative adjuvant therapy may affect the nature of the cancer as well as decrease the size of the cancer. Overall, it is essential to preserve the

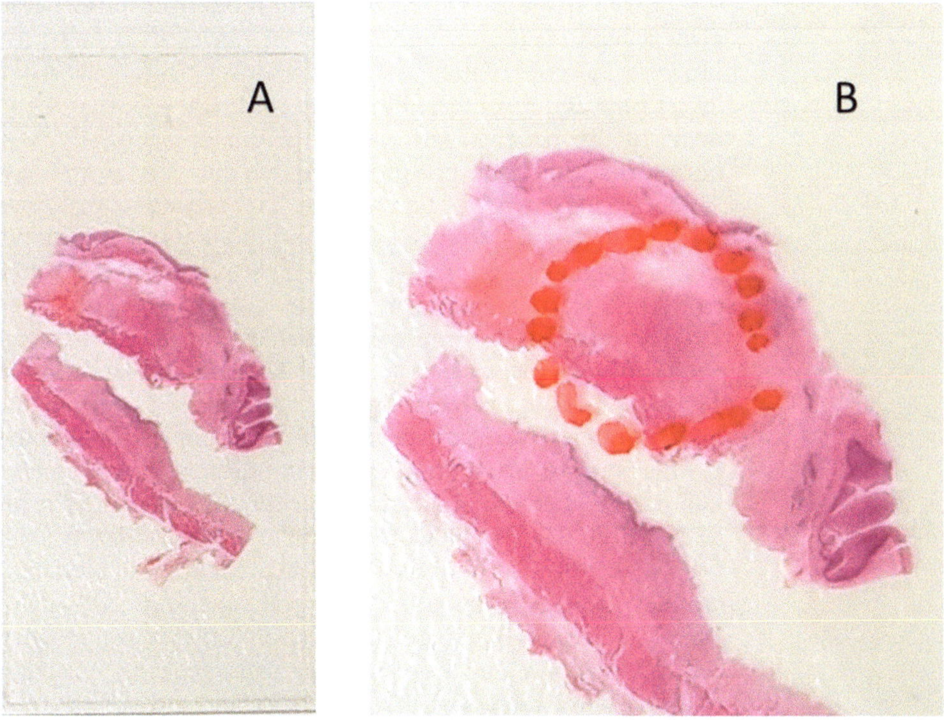

Fig. 1 Selection of area for genomic studies in hematoxylin and eosin section with esophageal squamous cell carcinoma. (**a**) Two sections noted on the blocks from the esophagus with squamous cell carcinoma; (**b**) Circulates the area with esophageal squamous cell carcinoma to be micro-dissected for genomic studies

cancer tissue as much as possible as new tests or useful research for investigation of biomarkers useful for management of esophageal squamous cell carcinoma in the future. One way of preservation of cancer tissue in small biopsy specimen is to plan the number of tests (number of sections cut) required to minimize re-cutting of the block leading to loss of tissues in each cutting of the block.

Microdissection of formalin-fixed paraffin-embedded tissues to select the area with high concentration of tumor cells is often employed to enrich the yield of DNA for genomic tests (Fig. 1). It is better to be done by a pathologist who could select the areas with high proportion of tumor cells with less contamination by necrotic cells and stromal cells. The pathologist could estimate the percentage of tumor cells. The information could feed back to the molecular biologists. Low percentage of tumor cells will give rise to false negative in detection mutation in genomic studies.

It is worth noting that cancer cells, though of small amount, obtained by fine needle aspiration biopsy may also be a source for immunohistochemical and genomic tests. The supernatant from cell block in fine needle aspiration may contain cell-free DNA for genomic tests.

Frozen tissue is favored for many modern testings because it gives a high yield and high quality of nuclei acids and proteins. However, to collect and bank frozen cancer tissue, scientists must invest time and resources. Blood are routinely collected for assessment of the patients with cancer before operation. It is worth noting that they were not processed, adequate, or stored in a way for the requirements of biobanking. The recommended temperature for long-term storage of the components of the blood and frozen samples is −80 °C [4]. Nevertheless, reduced RNA integrity could still occur in long-term storage.

The technical procedure of biobanking is time-consuming and needs advance planning in terms of funding and labor resources. The samples could come at unexpected time (e.g., surgery may be more complicated than expected and the samples could come late in afternoon or in evening). More importantly, the samples need immediate or urgent processing after they are out from the human body before they can be stored under optimal conditions.

This chapter outlines the technical procedures of biobanking of samples from patients with esophageal squamous cell carcinoma. There are decades of research publications on esophageal squamous cell carcinoma arising from samples from biobank reflecting the usefulness and success of the process in the study of DNA, RNA, and proteins in tissue and blood of patients with esophageal squamous cell carcinoma [5–10] as well as raising esophageal squamous carcinoma cell lines and mouse models [11–14].

2 Materials

2.1 Raw Materials

1. Signed consent forms from the patients with tissue and blood collection.
2. Tissues and blood samples of patients.

2.2 Reagents and Consumables

1. Plastic tissue embedding cassette.
2. Ethylenediaminetetraacetic acid (EDTA)/heparin-containing blood collection tubes.
3. RNAlater stabilization solution (to stabilize and protect cellular RNA by inactivation of RNase).
4. Dissecting tools for pathologist (scalpel blades and handles, rulers, digital camera).
5. Gloves (for protection).
6. Freeze spray or liquid nitrogen (for rapid cooling).
7. 10% formaldehyde solution/formalin (for fixing the tissues).
8. Phosphate-buffered saline (PBS) solution.
9. Histopaque solution (isolation of blood components).

10. 15 ml Falcon tubes.
11. 2 ml Eppendorf tubes.
12. Stocking solution (comprises 60% Roswell Park Memorial Institute [RPMI] medium, 30% fetal bovine serum [FBS] for growth of human lymphocytes and cells, and 10% dimethyl sulfoxide [DMSO] for freezing of cells to prevent formation of ice crystals during freezing process).

2.3 Equipment

1. Biosafety cabinet (for processing blood and tissue samples).
2. −80 freezer (for storage).
3. Centrifuge.

3 Method

Handing of the samples is with gloves and in biosafety cabinet.

3.1 Collection Procedures

1. Prepare and obtain written consents from patients (*see* **Note 1**).
2. Collect the blood samples in tubes (coated with chemical for anticoagulation) before or at the time of operation as well as planned periods after (*see* **Note 2**).

3.2 Tissue Handing Protocol

1. Collect the tissue samples at the time of operation in fresh (*see* **Note 3**).
2. Snap freeze the tissue samples, put in container, label properly, and store them in freezer of −80 °C (*see* **Note 4**).
3. Dissect the tissues with scalpels (taken adjacent to each of the frozen tissue blocks), put in plastic tissue embedding cassette, close the cassette, label the cassette, and put in container containing 10% formaldehyde for fixation (*see* **Note 5**).

3.3 Blood Handling Protocol

1. For the collected blood samples, prepare 7 ml of Histopaque solution, and then gently add 7 ml of collected blood on top of the Histopaque solution in a 15 ml Falcon tube so that they do not mix (*see* **Note 6**).
2. Centrifuge at 400 × *g* at room temperature for 30 min (*see* **Note** 7).
3. Pipette up the thin portion (buffy coat) into a new 15 ml tube.
4. Collect the plasma and store at −80 °C.
5. Add 10 ml PBS to the buffy coat to wash. Shake it vigorously.
6. Centrifuge at 250 × *g*, 10 min at room temperature.
7. Collect the pellet and discard supernatant.
8. Repeat **steps 5–17**, but this time with 5 ml PBS instead.

9. Resuspend pellet in 500 μl stocking solution.
10. Transfer to 2 ml Eppendorf tube and store in −80 °C.

3.4 Data Management Protocol

1. Proper record of the patient details and labelling of the samples collected.
2. Collect the demographical, clinical, and pathological information of the patient with the sample taken (*see* **Note 8**).
3. Review the information and link together in a database (*see* **Note 9**).

4 Notes

1. It is essential to prepare the time required for the process of research ethical approval, build up the multidisciplinary team, as well as obtain consents from patients. In addition, the research team should file the consent forms obtained from the patients properly. Furthermore, we need a code to label each of the tubes containing the patient's sample. One of the purposes of coding is to de-identify the patients involved in the research according to the human ethics requirements.
2. The tubes used are either heparin or ethylenediaminetetraacetic acid (EDTA)-coated tubes to prevent clotting of the blood. The blood could be collected at any time before the operation of the cancer. In addition, blood samples are to be obtained before and after adjuvant therapy if the researchers would like to see the changes in biomarkers before surgery. In addition, blood samples should be collected at a scheduled time from the patients after operations depending on the purpose of the project. For example, researchers could obtain blood samples after postoperative chemotherapy, routine clinical follow-up, or detection of cancer recurrence. It is best to obtain and process the tissues as soon as possible after removal of blood supply. Tissue ischemia could occur soon leading to degradation of tissue. There is significant reduction in immunohistochemistry staining of protein in cancer tissue in ischemia. In breast cancer, cold ischemia time (tissue kept at 4 °C) should be of less than 1 h [15].
3. There are different ways to collect the samples. One common way is to transfer the whole specimen to a pathologist as soon as possible. It is better to transport the specimen in low temperature (on wet ice) during the short transit time to the laboratory to decrease the chance of degradation. The pathologist should open the esophagectomy specimen and dissect macroscopically as described in Chapter 4. The advantages of collection of the samples by pathologist are (1) to better orientate and dissect

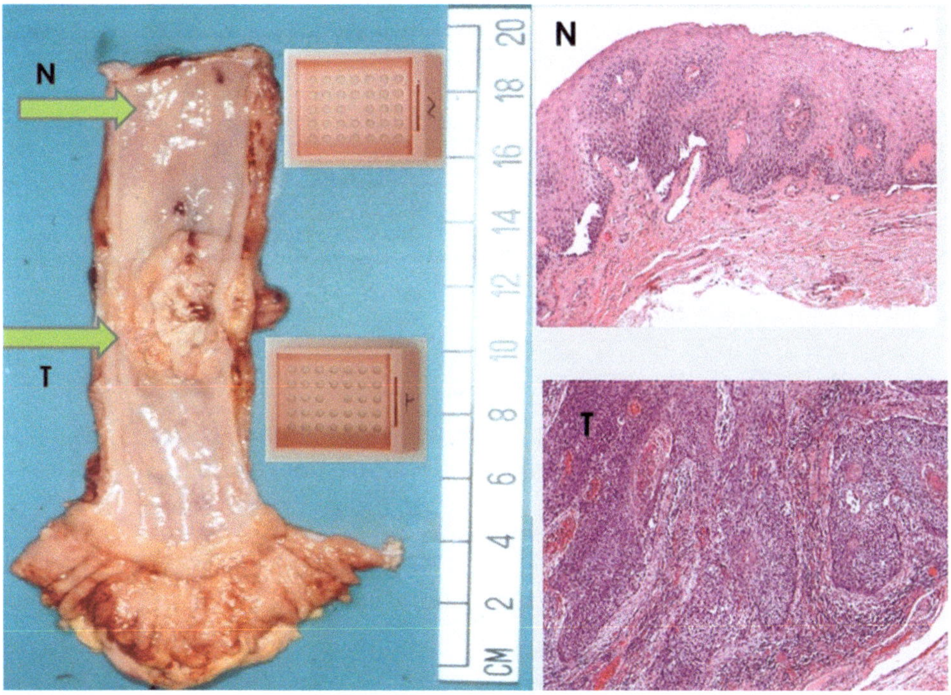

Fig. 2 The esophagogastrectomy specimen showing the sites for taking the blocks for biobanks. T stands for the tumor and N stands for non-neoplastic mucosa. Note that the site of taking of N block should be as far away from T as possible

the specimen for histological examination and biobanking and (2) to be able to perform additional complex laboratory procedures in the laboratory setting. The second way is the sampling of research tissues by a surgeon. The tissue samples are in tubes with RNAlater stabilization solution to prevent degeneration during transport to laboratory. The advantage of this step is the better-preserved tissues obtained as the tissues are in RNAlater before transporting to laboratory for further processing. Tissue blocks taken are from (1) the carcinoma, (2) the non-neoplastic mucosa, and (3) any detected lymph node positive for carcinoma (Fig. 2). For specimen (2), the best area for sample should be esophageal mucosa close to the proximal resection margin. For specimen (3), look for enlarged lymph node that may be found in the peri-esophageal fatty tissue. This procedure needs the expertise of a pathologist. Tissues can be triage in this stage for making esophageal squamous cell carcinoma cell lines and patient-derived xenograft (PDX) in mice (*see* Chapter 11).

4. Spray the tissues with Lab freeze, or put the tissues in liquid nitrogen for approximately 15–30 s. The tissues should turn hard (Fig. 3). Frozen tissues could be in Eppendorf tubes with RNAlater stabilization solution. Alternatively, wrap larger

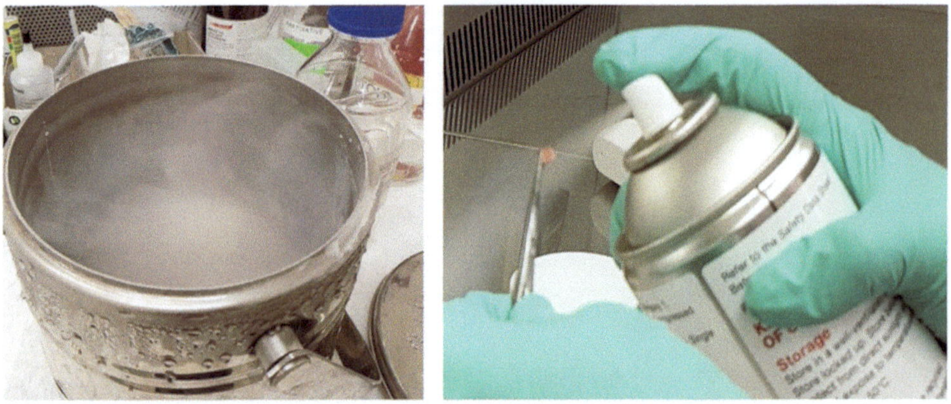

Fig. 3 Two ways to snap freeze the tissues. The right side shows container with freshly prepared liquid nitrogen. Insert the tissue with forceps into the container to freeze the tissue. The left side shows the freezing of tissue by freezing spray

tissue blocks in foil so that cryostat sections can be obtained later to check the histology of the collected tissues.

5. The histology of frozen tissue section is inferior to formalin-fixed paraffin-embedded (FFPE) section for microscopic analyses (Fig. 4). The FFPE sections are useful to test the morphology as well as immunohistochemical detection of paraffin. The cross-linking of the protein may be a problem in FFPE sections. However, modern immunohistochemical techniques (e.g., antigen retrieval methods) largely overcome this problem. In addition, storage of paraffin blocks is easy and needs to be at room temperature. Thus, it is important to have both FFPE and frozen blocks. After the initial blocking, the pathologist needs to process the whole esophagectomy (as described in Chapter 4) for providing diagnosis and staging information. The tissues should be placed in formalin as quick as possible, preferably less than 30 min. The formaldehyde-fixed tissue should be processed in paraffin within a day [16]. The pathologist should check the hematoxylin and eosin-stained sections of the research blocks.
6. Histopaque contains polysucrose and sodium diatrizoate adjusted to a density for a density gradient to separate the components of the blood (Fig. 5).
7. After centrifuge, there will be layers of different colors. The top layer is yellow and is the plasma for storage (Fig. 6). There is then a thin layer—buffy coat—which is a concentrated white blood cells and platelets as wells as circulating tumor cells if present. The buffy coat is so called because it is usually buff in hue. It is of golden color and around 3 ml. The next big layer is the Histopaque and the red blood cells in the bottom. These bottom two layers are discarded.

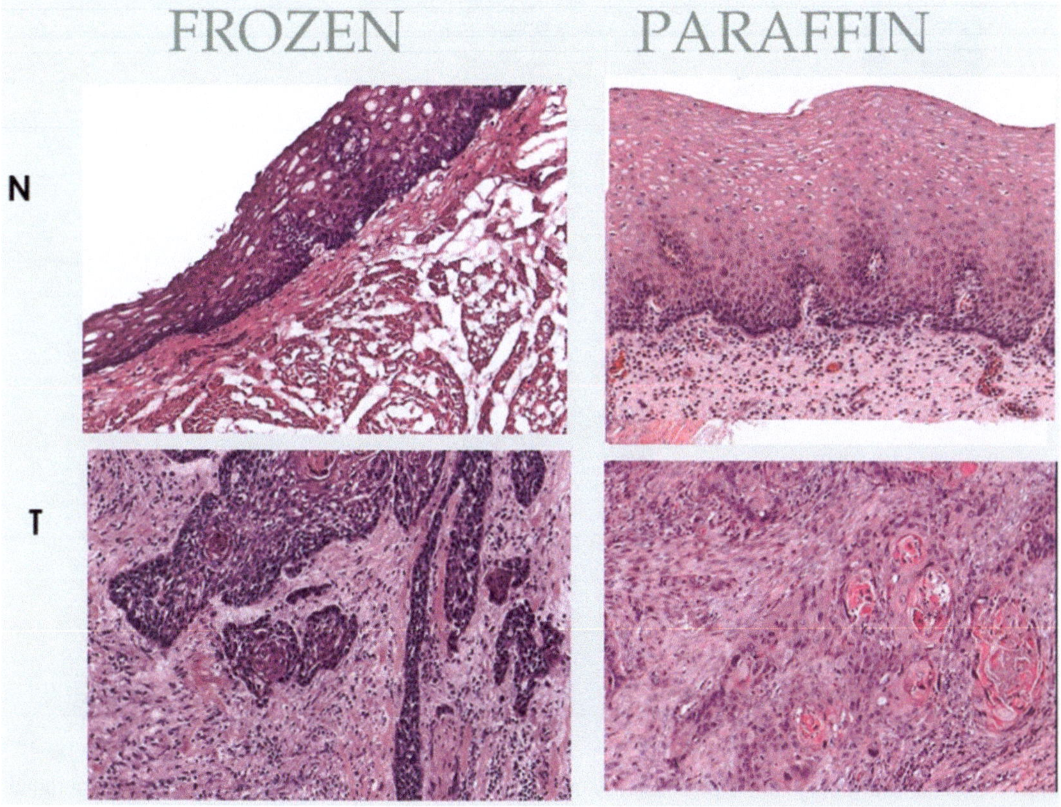

Fig. 4 The comparison of morphology of sections from formalin-fixed paraffin-embedded (FFPE) tissue versus frozen sections. The histological features of tumor block (T) of esophageal squamous cell carcinoma and non-neoplastic esophageal mucosa (N) in the FFPE sections are of better quality to be interpretable. The frozen sections show more artifacts such as artificial gaps in stroma and unclear nuclear features

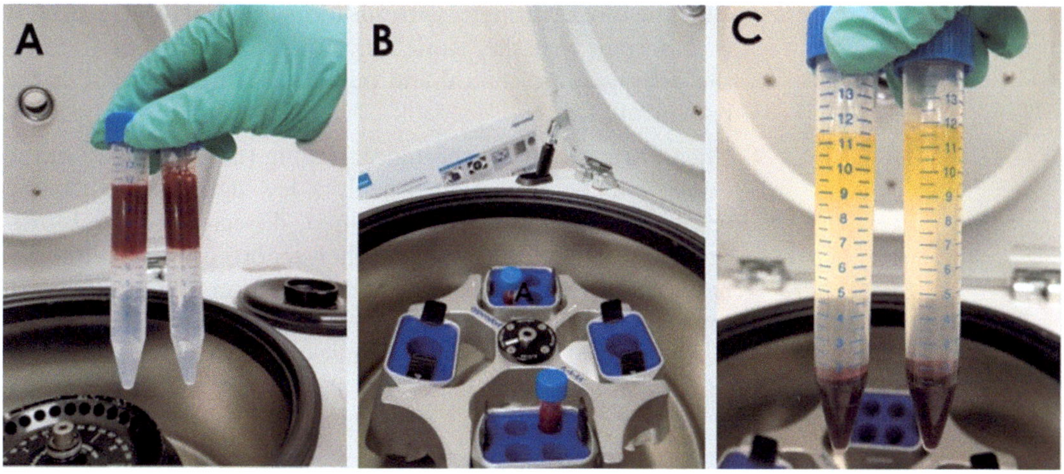

Fig. 5 The procedures of processing the blood samples from patients with cancer. (**a**) Blood samples add on top on Histopaque. (**b**) Centrifuge the samples. (**c**) Different levels noted after centrifugation

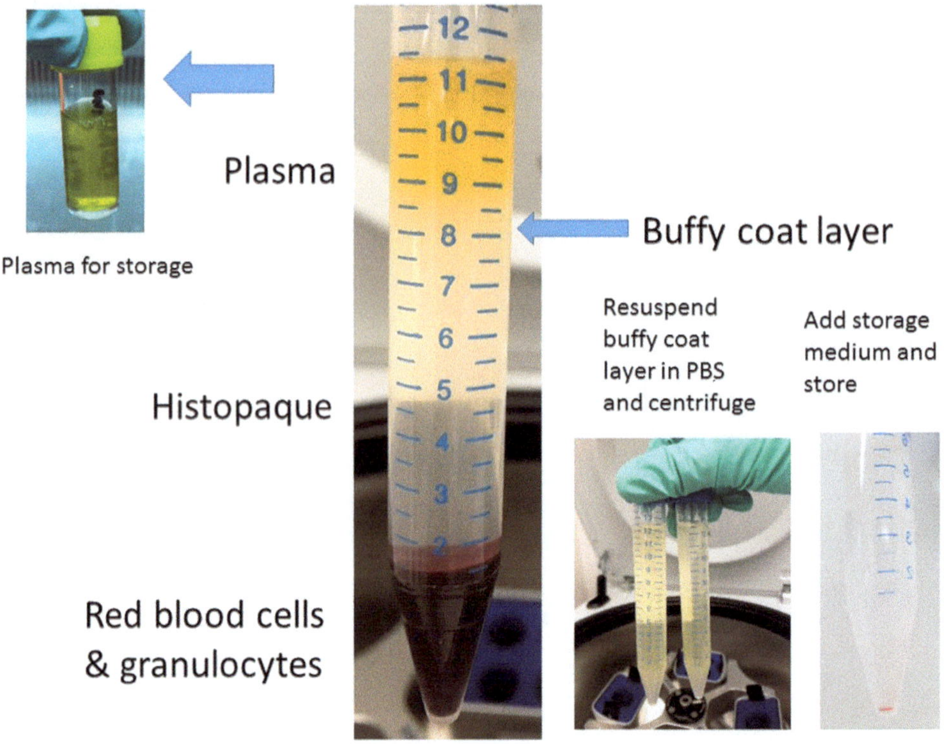

Fig. 6 Collection and storage of the processed blood. The top level is plasma that is collected in the first round. The thin layer of buffy coat needs to be resuspended in phosphate-buffered saline (PBS) and centrifuged for two times. The bottom two layers (red blood cells and Histopaque) are discarded. The resulting pellet contains cells (including white blood cells, circulating cancer cells) that should be collected with storage medium

8. The paraffin-embedded blocks should have hematoxylin and eosin sections checked to confirm the histology. In addition, label the blocks properly with additional clinical information. It is important that the "code" given to the sample can decode the demographic clinical and pathological information of the patient.
9. The information of pathological staging (*see* Chapter 3) of the cancer will be available normally a few days later when the whole specimen has been examined, dissected, blocked, processed, cutting of sections and then reported by a pathologist (*see* Chapter 4) as well as having information in multidisciplinary team meeting for management of the cancer. The database needs to update with the changes of disease status of the patients in follow-up.

References

1. Kinkorová J, Topolčan O (2018) Biobanks in Horizon 2020: sustainability and attractive perspectives. EPMA J 9:345–353
2. Cancer Genome Atlas Research Network; Analysis Working Group: Asan University; BC Cancer Agency; Brigham and Women's Hospital; Broad Institute; Brown University; Case Western Reserve University et al (2017) Integrated genomic characterization of oesophageal carcinoma. Nature 541:169–175
3. Ennis DP, Pidgeon GP, Millar N, Ravi N, Reynolds JV (2010) Building a bioresource for esophageal research: lessons from the early experience of an academic medical center. Dis Esophagus 23:1–7
4. Shabihkhani M, Lucey GM, Wei B, Mareninov S, Lou JJ, Vinters HV, Singer EJ, Cloughesy TF, Yong WH (2014) The procurement, storage, and quality assurance of frozen blood and tissue biospecimens in pathology, biorepository, and biobank settings. Clin Biochem 47:258–266
5. Ng HY, Li J, Tao L, Lam AK, Chan KW, Ko JMY, Yu VZ, Wong M, Li B, Lung ML (2018) Chemotherapeutic treatments increase pd-l1 expression in esophageal squamous cell carcinoma through EGFR/ERK Activation. Transl Oncol 11:1323–1333
6. Dai W, Ko JMY, Choi SSA, Yu Z, Ning L, Zheng H, Gopalan V, Chan KT, Lee NP, Chan KW, Law SY, Lam AK, Lung ML (2017) Whole-exome sequencing reveals critical genes underlying metastasis in oesophageal squamous cell carcinoma. J Pathol 242:500–510
7. Haque MH, Gopalan V, Islam MN, Masud MK, Bhattacharjee R, Hossain MSA, Nguyen NT, Lam AK, Shiddiky MJA (2017) Quantification of gene-specific DNA methylation in oesophageal cancer via electrochemistry. Anal Chim Acta 976:84–93
8. Islam F, Gopalan V, Law S, Tang JC, Chan KW, Lam AK (2017) MiR-498 in esophageal squamous cell carcinoma: clinicopathological impacts and functional interactions. Hum Pathol 62:141–151
9. Gopalan V, Islam F, Pillai S, Tang JC, Tong DK, Law S, Chan KW, Lam AK (2016) Overexpression of microRNA-1288 in oesophageal squamous cell carcinoma. Exp Cell Res 348:146–154
10. Haque MH, Gopalan V, Chan KW, Shiddiky MJ, Smith RA, Lam AK (2016) Identification of novel FAM134B (JK1) mutations in oesophageal squamous cell carcinoma. Sci Rep 6:29173
11. Pun IH, Chan D, Chan SH, Chung PY, Zhou YY, Law S, Lam AK, Chui CH, Chan AS, Lam KH, Tang JC (2017) Anti-cancer effects of a novel quinoline derivative 83b1 on human esophageal squamous cell carcinoma through down-regulation of COX-2 mRNA and PGE (2). Cancer Res Treat 49:219–229
12. Ip JC, Ko JM, Yu VZ, Chan KW, Lam AK, Law S, Tong DK, Lung ML (2015) A versatile orthotopic nude mouse model for study of esophageal squamous cell carcinoma. Biomed Res Int 2015:910715
13. Tang JC, Wan TS, Wong N, Pang E, Lam KY, Law SY, Chow LM, Ma ES, Chan LC, Wong J, Srivastava G (2001) Establishment and characterization of a new xenograft-derived human esophageal squamous cell carcinoma cell line SLMT-1 of Chinese origin. Cancer Genet Cytogenet 124:36–41
14. Hu Y, Lam KY, Wan TS, Fang W, Ma ES, Chan LC, Srivastava G (2000) Establishment and characterization of HKESC-1, a new cancer cell line from human esophageal squamous cell carcinoma. Cancer Genet Cytogenet 118:112–120
15. Yildiz-Aktas IZ, Dabbs DJ, Bhargava R (2012) The effect of cold ischemic time on the immunohistochemical evaluation of estrogen receptor, progesterone receptor, and HER2 expression in invasive breast carcinoma. Mod Pathol 25:1098–1105
16. Thompson SM, Craven RA, Nirmalan NJ, Harnden P, Selby PJ, Banks RE (2013) Impact of pre-analytical factors on the proteomic analysis of formalin-fixed paraffin-embedded tissue. Proteomics Clin Appl 7:241–251

Chapter 9

Whole-Slide Imaging of Esophageal Squamous Cell Carcinoma

Alfred K. Lam and Melissa Leung

Abstract

Whole-slide imaging (WSI) contributes to medical education, collaboration, quality assurance, examination, and consultation in pathology. The images obtained from WSI are of high quality and could be stored indefinitely. In research involving esophageal squamous cell carcinoma, the combination of WSI and image processing program allows effective interpretations of expressions of various immunomarkers related to pathogenesis, prognosis, and response to therapy in tissue microarray sections. The operation and basic principles of whole-slide imaging of esophageal squamous cell carcinoma are also presented. Common use of WSI will occur with modifications of the whole-slide imaging scanners to adapt to the workflows in diagnostic and research laboratories.

Key words Whole-slide imaging, Scanning, Ki-67, Esophageal, Squamous carcinoma, Image analysis, TMA

1 Introduction

Whole-slide imaging is a technique for digitization of the whole glass slide by a scanner. Initially, this revolutionized approach in pathology imaging support resulted in changes in practice in medical education, research, and collaboration [1–3]. In the recent years, applications of whole-slide imaging are adopted in anatomical pathology practices. Images from whole-slide imaging have long been used for quality assurance programs (QAP) which are important to support scientific and medical communities in Australia [4]. In addition, whole-slide imaging scanner has been approved by the Food and Drug Administration in the USA to be use as primary diagnosis in surgical pathology in 2017 [5]. In Australia, whole-slide imaging is used for anatomical pathology specialist examination starting from 2015 (https://www.rcpa.edu.au/Library/Practising-Pathology/DM). Furthermore, validations of pathology consultation and intraoperative consultation of frozen section (*see* Chapter 7) by whole-slide imaging have been studied

Alfred K. Lam (ed.), *Esophageal Squamous Cell Carcinoma: Methods and Protocols*, Methods in Molecular Biology, vol. 2129, https://doi.org/10.1007/978-1-0716-0377-2_9, © Springer Science+Business Media, LLC, part of Springer Nature 2020

[6]. WSI of consultation slides could help to keep documentations before returning original slides to the referring laboratories.

However, there are still some obstacles for replacement of glass slides and light microscopy in diagnostic pathology. One of the major limitations for use is the time required to scan a slide (including the preparation time), which added to the turnaround time in the diagnostic laboratory. The new models of whole-slide imaging scanner have been designed to target to the workflows of the busy anatomical pathology laboratory. In future, WSI is likely to be incorporated into the workflows of the anatomical pathology.

The other barriers to use WSI are the large size and cost of the whole-slide imaging scanner. With the increasing use of the technology, the cost of the equipment will certainly come down. Portable models of whole-slide imaging scanner are also available in the market. A portable whole-slide imaging scanner could be very useful for an individual pathologist or researcher working on limited number of microscopic slides.

Whole-slide scanned images have many advantages over traditional static digitized images. Whole-slide imaging has the advantage of providing higher-quality and better focused images when compared with the static images taken by the standard digital camera. The staining in histological sections often fades after years of storage. Whole-slide imaging of the histological sections allows permanent storage of the invaluable histological information of esophageal squamous cell carcinoma. The digital storages greatly decrease the demand of space required for storing large number of glass slides. In addition, taking whole-slide scanned images (compared to cutting the paraffin block for more sections for education, consultation, quality assurance, and examination purposes) allows the preserving of the precious biopsy tissue for additional tests such as immunohistochemistry and other molecular biology tests (*see* Chapters 17 and 21).

In research and collaborations in esophageal squamous cell carcinoma, digitalizing of the sections by whole-slide imaging from esophageal squamous cell carcinoma allows the capturing of multiple fields of the images for image analysis. Depending on the complexity of the analysis one needs, there are many image analysis programs in the market to suit the need of the researchers. ImageJ, a complementary Java-based image processing program, developed at the National Institutes of Health and the Laboratory for Optical and Computational Instrumentation in the USA is the most frequently employed by researchers.

One of the most common research analyses in esophageal squamous cell carcinoma that requires the image analysis on whole scanned images is the study of proliferative index. Proliferative index, measured by Ki-67 (MIB-1), could be used to assess and predict the biological aggressiveness or the survival of patients with esophageal squamous cell carcinoma [7–9]. The assessment of proliferative index involves counting the portion of Ki-67 positively stained carcinoma nuclei which may involve at least counting over 500 to thousands of cancer cells to get an accurate value. Image analysis system is needed to reduce the subjective, tedious, and inaccurate manual counting of nuclei staining [10]. In addition, using image analysis system, it was shown to involve less time in obtaining the Ki-67 index than manual counting in esophageal squamous cell carcinoma [10]. Whole-slide scanning allows to capture multiple fields of the Ki-67-stained esophageal squamous cell carcinoma to allow for more accurate representation of the sections to be analyzed by image analysis system.

The most important role for whole-slide scanning in research on esophageal squamous cell carcinoma is to help in the assessment of immunostaining of large number of esophageal squamous cell carcinomas on a tissue microarray section (*see* Chapter 10). Immunohistochemical study of esophageal squamous cell carcinoma allows the detection of expression of proteins related to pathogenesis and prognosis [11–16]. Examples include assessments of tumor suppressor gene—FAM134B (family with sequence similarity 134 member B) JK1/reticulophagy regulator 1 (RETREG1); markers of metastases, NID2 (nidogen 2) and p-AKT (protein kinase B); and markers of angiogenesis, VEGFR-1 (vascular endothelial growth factor-1) and VEGFR-2 (vascular endothelial growth factor-2). In addition, nuclear expression of DNAJB6 (DnaJ heat shock protein family (Hsp40) member B6) and cytoplasmic expression of CAPN10 (calpain 10) were shown to be associated with survival of patients with esophageal squamous cell carcinoma. Recently, there was a report of upregulation of PD-L1 (maker for immunotherapy) by chemotherapy in esophageal squamous cell carcinoma [17].

Tissue microarray (TMA) technology allows dozens of tissue samples to be put on a section [18]. This allows evaluation of cancer tissues from large number of ESCCs in a rapid and economical way (*see* Chapter 10). However, with numerous sections under small eye fields of a light microscope, it is stressful, tedious, and almost impossible for a pathologist to navigate to make accurate scoring of the immunostaining. With the help of whole-slide imaging, pathologists could transfer the act of viewing the sections in front of the small microscope eye fields to the computer monitor. In front of the monitor, the small tissue sections in the TMA sections could be zoomed to larger size for assessment (Fig. 1). This allows better assessment and documentation of the scoring of the tiny tissue microarray sections stained by immunohistochemical methods.

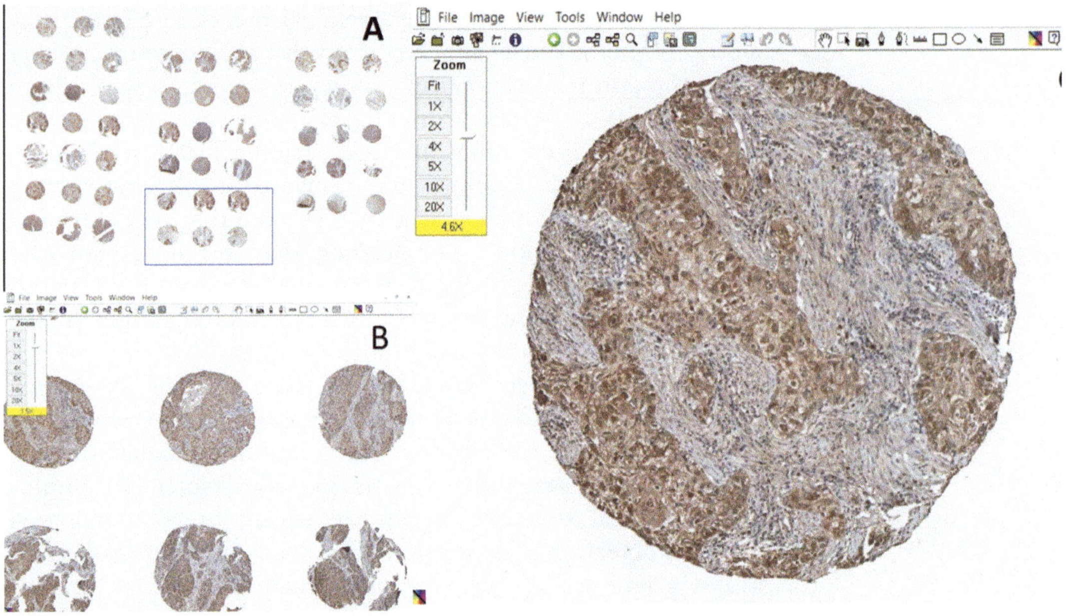

Fig. 1 Assessment of immunostaining in tissue microarray section. (**a**) Whole-scanned image of immunohistochemical staining in a tissue microarray section. (**b**) The selected region in (**a**) are zoomed up. (**c**) One of the tissues is further zoomed to large size so as to be able to score the cellular location and intensity of the immunohistochemical staining

2 Materials

1. A well-prepared glass slide holding histological section of esophageal squamous cell carcinoma with coverslip is important for the success of scanning.
2. Cleaning tools for the slides (ethanol, xylene, hand sanitizer, cotton cloth or tissue towel, razor blade).
3. Whole-slide scanner (*see* **Note 1**).
4. Computer (link with the scanner).
5. Hard disc or other computer storage system (need high storage capacity as the approximate size of one scanned image is 1 GB).
6. Software (to view the scanned image and as well as analyze the images).

3 Methods

3.1 Prepare the Slides Before Scanning

1. Prepare the label of the slides (*see* **Note 2**).
2. Arrange the slides in order, and record the order of the label number (as well as other information, e.g., type of stain) of the slides to be scanned.

3. Make sure all the slides for scanning have coverslips and are dry and not sticky. In addition, the labels are not sticky or overhanging.
4. With excessive glass coverslip on slide, it can be resolved by trimming the slide edge with razor blade.
5. Clean the slides (*see* **Note 3**).

3.2 System Start-Up

1. Turn on the power of scanner.
2. Switch on computer monitor.
3. Log in to the system with password (if there is a pre-set password).

3.3 Loading the Slides for Scanning (Fig. 2)

1. Open the door of the scan.
2. Get the autoloader slide rack.
3. Load the slides to autoloader slide racks. Make sure the slides are in right position (i.e., glass coverslip face up and slide label up to the front) and in good order (*see* **Note 4**).
4. Put back the slide rack in scanner.
5. Close the scanner door.

3.4 Set Up the Scanning Field

1. The program should show up the images of the slide rack.
2. Select the racks with the slides placed for scanning (Fig. 3).
3. Make snapshots for these slides using autofocusing—this will select the areas with the tissue.
4. Review the snapshots captured.
5. Design the setting of the scanning: select the designed scan magnification (5×, 10×, 20×, or 40×). The best is to select 40×.
6. Data entry step (image labelling): label the image according to designed label number of the slide (*see* **Note 5**).
7. Adjust the pre-selected areas in each slide to be scanned (*see* **Note 6**).
8. Make sure the areas to be scanned have the calibration point. The calibration point should be on a clear area.
9. Setting up the focus points – there are some focus points automatically set up by the scanner. The operator needs to add some more focus points to achieve better results in focusing the fine details. If the focus point is not enough, the scanned images could be fainted or dark (*see* **Note 7**).
10. Review the snapshot setting to avoid any missing in settings and enable fine-tuning for successful scan.

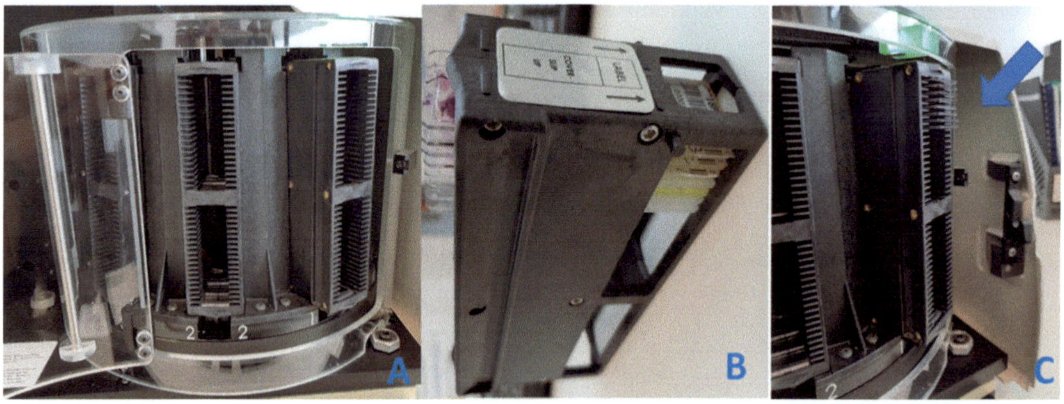

Fig. 2 (**a**) A scanner opened to show the empty slide racks. (**b**) A slide rack was taken out from the scanner in (**a**) and loaded with slides to be scanned. Note that there are arrows to make sure the slides were loaded in correct orientation. (**c**) The slide rack in (**b**) was loaded in the scanner (arrow)

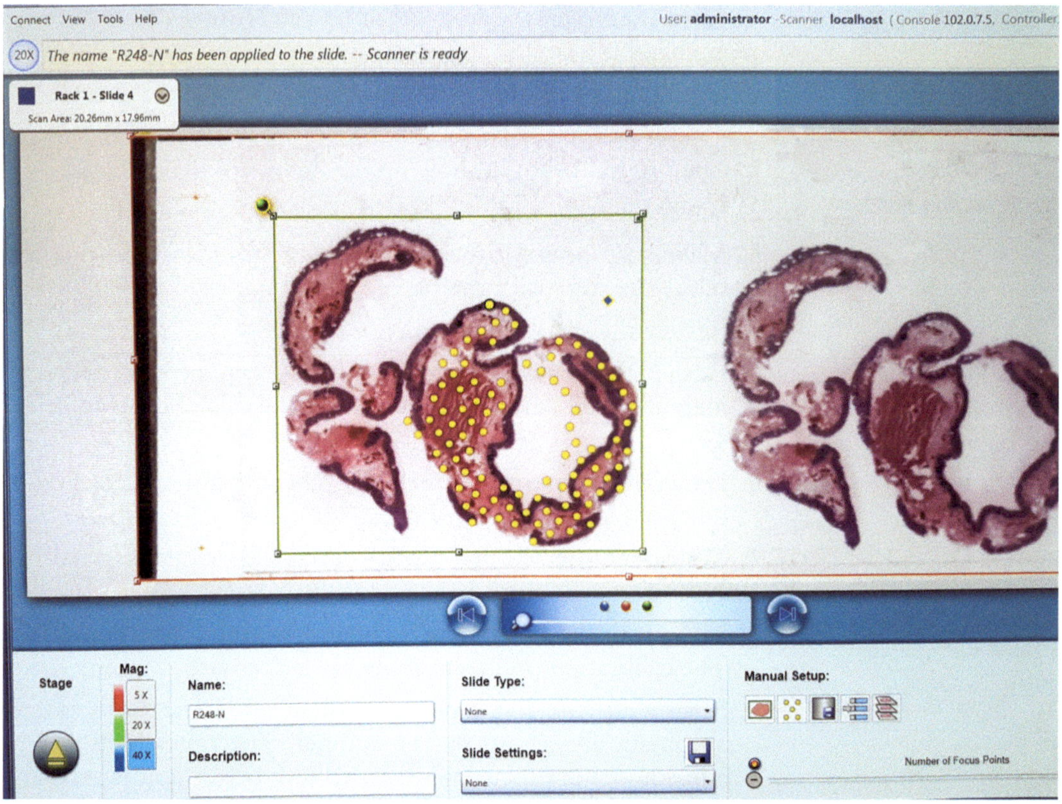

Fig. 3 Operation in the computer screen before the scanning: The green rectangle delineated the selected area of interest for scanning. The yellow spots are the focus points. The more focus points allow precise focusing of the image. If there are only a few yellow spots, more focus points should be added. The toolbar in the lower portion of the screen have the option of choosing magnification of scanning and entering of identities of the slide such as label of the slide (name)

3.5 Scanning

1. Click the Scan button to progress the scanning. The time for scanning depends on the magnification, nature of slide (staining quality and use of tissue microarray sections), and size of the area of interest (*see* **Note 8**).
2. During the process, monitor any error messages that occurred. Occasionally, some of the slides may need to be re-scanned.
3. After the completion of scanning, the slide(s) with error message should be reloaded to the scanner to repeat the procedure.

3.6 Completion

1. Check the scanned images.
2. Copy and save the image files from computer to hard disc or portable devices.
3. Press the Eject button.
4. Open the Scanner door.
5. Collect the slides from the autoloader slide rack.
6. Put back the slide rack into the Scanner.
7. Log off the system, switch off the computer, and turn off the scanner.

3.7 Work with the Images (See Note 9)

Download the softwares for working with the whole-slide scanned image. Saved the image in your decided format.

4 Notes

1. There are many models of whole-slide scanner available in the market. All the scanners could suit the purpose of scanning slides at good resolution. One practical factor for choice of scanner that suits the individual laboratory is the speed of scanning of the scanner. The speed of scanning depends primarily on the resolution of images needed as well as the logistics of the operation. Scanning at lower resolution is faster than scanning at higher solution. The logistics of operation depends largely on the capacity (how many slides the scanner could hold for each run of the scanning) of the scanner. In the past, imaging scanning equipment could scan one or a few slides in a run. The operator has to perform the task of loading and scanning frequently for a few slides. Advanced and more expensive models of whole-slide scanner have the capacity to hold and scan hundreds of slides at one time. This allows smooth running of the workflow for diagnostic and research laboratory. Thus, researcher could choose the capacity of the scanner depending on the budget as well as the required volume of slides to be scanned in the laboratory. In addition, scientific

researchers may need a whole mount section of an organ affected by cancer. The slide could be up to 6″ × 8″ instead of the conventional size of 1″ × 3″. Scanner with slide holders to accommodate different size of glass slides is available in the market.

2. Glass slide may have barcodes with patient information as well as automatic labelling. If the slide label has sensitive information (e.g., patient's identity) not to be shown, make sure that the label was covered before the scanning.
3. The slides should be in clean and good condition. Dirty slide can cause scanning artifacts. Make sure that the slides have no dirt, fingerprints, excessive adhesion, glue, or scratches around. Use solvent lens cleaner to clean coverslip of glass slides. Felt pen or ink marking on the glass slide could be wiped with solvents such as hand sanitizer or 70% ethanol. Xylene could be used to remove glue on the coverslip (caution is needed to prevent coverslip from detachment). Avoid using strong cleansing agent as this may wipe away slide labelling. The slides could be dried by cotton cloth or tissue towel. Allow time for drying of the slides before scanning is started.
4. Avoid broken slides and slides with excessive labelling. These features may cause disruption to the automation during image acquisition. If the slide is sitting on a non-flat position after lodging or rocking while scanning, individual strips of scanned image will be poorly focused. If this happen, the slides should be repositioned in the slide rack and redone the scanning.
5. Different types of sections could need different setup for better scanning. The typical setup is for a standard hematoxylin and eosin-stained section. However, the setting (Slide type) could be different for tissue section such as a tissue microarray (TMA), serial section, cytology, blood smear, very faintly stained section, in situ hybridization, etc. To save time, the operator could pre-set some of the chosen setting (Slide setting) suitable for use in the research group and use the same setting in future.
6. The pre-selected area in the slide for scanning needs to be adjusted manually because there are some portions of the slides that the operator may want to exclude. This will reduce the area needed to scan and hence increase the speed of scanning.
7. If the glass cover is too thick, use manual focusing to select additional focus points in the tissue area. In addition, if there are slides with air pockets (bubbles) under glass coverslip, perform a manual scan, and avoid selecting the area of interest with air pockets. When scanner fails to capture a calibrated image from scanned slides or it fails in capture focus points

from the image, it may need to reset line camera gains. To perform this, place a clean slide (no scratches or markings) on the stage.

8. Although the scanning is automatic, manual work is required for setup (as listed in above sections). The time requirement of scanning depends on the operator's experience, the scanner, the size and type of images, as well as the resolution required. The most common setting for scanning of hematoxylin and eosin-stained (H&E) sections is at 40-× magnification. According to experience, we have calculated that the average time for scanning of H&E slide in this setting was approximately 12 min per slide (including the time in preparation). In future, the use of models of scanners which adapt to the workflows of diagnostic pathology laboratory will certainly decrease the average scanning time.

9. The dynamic images obtained by scanner are in special digital format. Different scanners used different image formats. Each image format could be read by complimentary program provided by the scanner's company. Normally, the various portions of the virtual images can be modified to make smaller virtual slides.

   Labels (such as scale bar, arrows, etc.) could be added to the whole-scanned virtual images of the histological section (Fig. 4). The region(s) of interest could be captured into classical image files (such as .jpg [Joint Photographic Experts

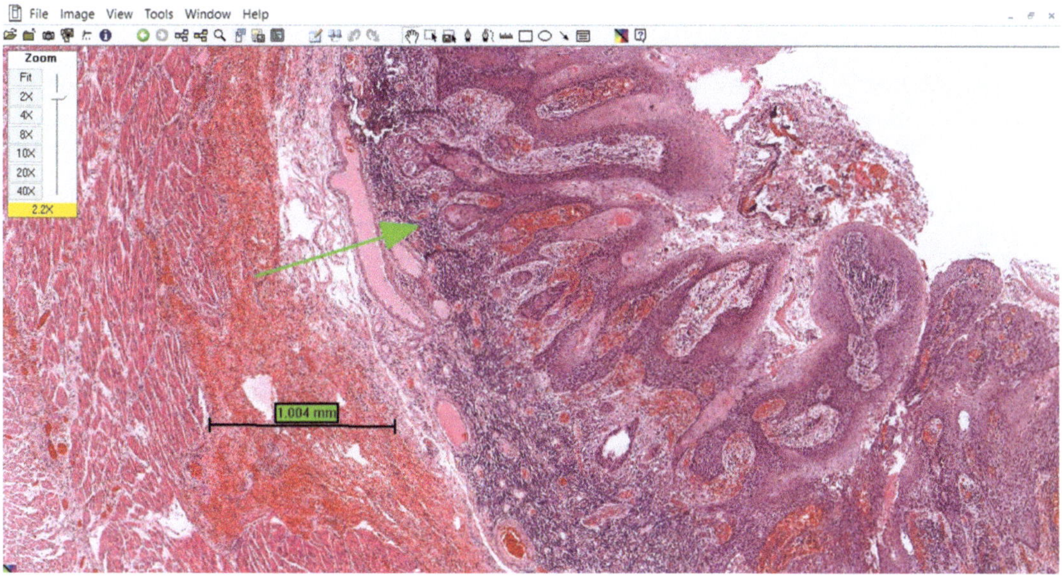

Fig. 4 An example of whole-scanned image of esophageal squamous cell carcinoma. The slide was scanned at 40× magnification and could be zoomed into different magnifications (left upper corner). The scale and arrow could be added to the selected area before downloading the image into format such as .jpg

Group] or .tiff [Tagged Image File Format]). These images could be used for presentation as well as loaded into programs for image analysis.

References

1. Zarella MD, Bowman D, Aeffner F, Farahani N, Xthona A, Absar SF, Parwani A, Bui M, Hartman DJ (2019) A practical guide to whole slide imaging: a white paper from the digital pathology association. Arch Pathol Lab Med 143:222–234. https://doi.org/10.5858/arpa.2018-0343-RA
2. Lam AK, Leung M (2018) Whole-slide imaging for esophageal adenocarcinoma. Methods Mol Biol 1756:135–142. https://doi.org/10.1007/978-1-4939-7734-5_12.
3. Gopalan V, Kasem K, Pillai S, Olveda D, Ariana A, Leung M, Lam AKY (2018) Evaluation of multidisciplinary strategies and traditional approaches in teaching pathology in medical students. Pathol Int 68:459–466. https://doi.org/10.1111/pin.12706
4. Van Es SL (2019) Digital pathology: semper ad meliora. Pathology 51:1–10. https://doi.org/10.1016/j.pathol.2018.10.011
5. Evans AJ, Bauer TW, Bui MM, Cornish TC, Duncan H, Glassy EF, Hipp J, McGee RS, Murphy D, Myers C, O'Neill DG, Parwani AV, Rampy BA, Salama ME, Pantanowitz L (2018) US food and drug administration approval of whole slide imaging for primary diagnosis: a key milestone is reached and new questions are raised. Arch Pathol Lab Med 142:1383–1387. https://doi.org/10.5858/arpa.2017-0496-CP
6. Cima L, Brunelli M, Parwani A, Girolami I, Ciangherotti A, Riva G, Novelli L, Vanzo F, Sorio A, Cirielli V, Barbareschi M, D'Errico A, Scarpa A, Bovo C, Fraggetta F, Pantanowitz L, Eccher A (2018) Validation of remote digital frozen sections for cancer and transplant intraoperative services. J Pathol Inform 9:34. https://doi.org/10.4103/jpi.jpi_52_18
7. Wang H, Zhou Y, Liu Q, Xu J, Ma Y (2018) Prognostic value of SOX2, Cyclin D1, P53, and ki-67 in patients with esophageal squamous cell carcinoma. Onco Targets Ther 11:5171–5181. https://doi.org/10.2147/OTT.S160066.
8. Sunpaweravong S, Puttawibul P, Sunpaweravong P, Nitiruangjaras A, Boonyaphiphat P, Kemapanmanus M (2016) Correlation between serum SCCA and CYFRA 2 1-1, tissue Ki-67, and clinicopathological factors in patients with esophageal squamous cell carcinoma. J Med Assoc Thail 99:331–337
9. Lam KY, Law SY, So MK, Fok M, Ma LT, Wong J (1996) Prognostic implication of proliferative markers MIB-1 and PC10 in esophageal squamous cell carcinoma. Cancer 77:7–13
10. Law AK, Lam KY, Lam FK, Wong TK, Poon JL, Chan FH (2003) Image analysis system for assessment of immunohistochemically stained proliferative marker (MIB-1) in oesophageal squamous cell carcinoma. Comput Methods Prog Biomed 70:37–45
11. Islam F, Gopalan V, Law S, Tang JC, Lam AK (2019) FAM134B promotes esophageal squamous cell carcinoma in vitro and its correlations with clinicopathologic features. Hum Pathol 87:1–10. https://doi.org/10.1016/j.humpath.2018.11.033
12. Yu VZ, Wong VC, Dai W, Ko JM, Lam AK, Chan KW, Samant RS, Lung HL, Shuen WH, Law S, Chan YP, Lee NP, Tong DK, Law TT, Lee VH, Lung ML (2015) Nuclear localization of dnajb6 is associated with survival of patients with esophageal cancer and reduces AKT signaling and proliferation of cancer cells. Gastroenterology 149:1825–1836. https://doi.org/10.1053/j.gastro.2015.08.025
13. Li B, Xu WW, Lam AKY, Wang Y, Hu HF, Guan XY, Qin YR, Saremi N, Tsao SW, He QY, Cheung ALM (2017) Significance of PI3K/AKT signaling pathway in metastasis of esophageal squamous cell carcinoma and its potential as a target for anti-metastasis therapy. Oncotarget 8:38755–38766. https://doi.org/10.18632/oncotarget.16333
14. Chai AW, Cheung AK, Dai W, Ko JM, Ip JC, Chan KW, Kwong DL, Ng WT, Lee AW, Ngan RK, Yau CC, Tung SY, Lee VH, Lam AK, Pillai S, Law S, Lung ML (2016) Metastasis-suppressing NID2, an epigenetically-silenced gene, in the pathogenesis of nasopharyngeal carcinoma and esophageal squamous cell carcinoma. Oncotarget 7:78859–78871. https://doi.org/10.18632/oncotarget.12889
15. Xu WW, Li B, Lam AK, Tsao SW, Law SY, Chan KW, Yuan QJ, Cheung AL (2015) Targeting VEGFR1- and VEGFR2-expressing non-tumor cells is essential for esophageal cancer therapy. Oncotarget 6:1790–1805

16. Chan D, Tsoi MY, Liu CD, Chan SH, Law SY, Chan KW, Chan YP, Gopalan V, Lam AK, Tang JC (2013) Oncogene GAEC1 regulates CAPN10 expression which predicts survival in esophageal squamous cell carcinoma. World J Gastroenterol 19:2772–2780. https://doi.org/10.3748/wjg.v19.i18.2772.
17. Ng HY, Li J, Tao L, Lam AK, Chan KW, Ko JMY, Yu VZ, Wong M, Li B, Lung ML (2018) Chemotherapeutic treatments increase PD-L1 expression in esophageal squamous cell carcinoma through EGFR/ERK activation. Transl Oncol 11:1323–1333. https://doi.org/10.1016/j.tranon.2018.08.005
18. Saremi N, Lam AK (2018) Application of tissue microarray in esophageal adenocarcinoma. Methods Mol Biol 1756:105–118. https://doi.org/10.1007/978-1-4939-7734-5_10

Chapter 10

Use of Tissue Microarray in Esophageal Squamous Cell Carcinoma

Alfred K. Lam and David K. Lor

Abstract

Tissue microarray (TMA) is widely used for identifying the expression of markers in many tissues from patients with esophageal squamous cell carcinoma. The technology is mostly used in immunohistochemical studies to test the expression of markers and oncoproteins in signalling pathway as well as targeting proteins involved in therapies for esophageal squamous cell carcinoma. Appropriate use of TMA sections needs consideration of labor, planning, and expertise involved. For the best performance, it is important to design the layout of the TMA as well as use whole-slide scanning for interpretation of the TMA sections.

Key words Tissue microarray, TMA, Esophageal, Squamous carcinoma

1 Introduction

A tissue microarray (TMA) block contains many small tissue samples on single paraffin block. The tissue samples in the TMA block are normally taken from the standard paraffin-embedded tissues, most often resected cancer tissues [1]. The primary purpose of the technology is to allow tests to be done on a large number of samples with the advantages of saving reagent cost, labor, and time as well as under identical experimental conditions. TMA blocks are very useful in research for validation of markers from cancer tissues in a large number of patients. They can be comprised of tissues of different organs for use as controls in immunohistochemistry. In addition, the blocks could be used by external quality assurance program (QAP) in pathology for assessment of staining techniques [2].

In the research on esophageal squamous cell carcinoma, there are hundreds of studies using tissue microarray sections to test the expression of markers by immunohistochemistry (*see* Chapter 21).

Alfred K. Lam and David K. Lor are contributed equally to this work.

Alfred K. Lam (ed.), *Esophageal Squamous Cell Carcinoma: Methods and Protocols*, Methods in Molecular Biology, vol. 2129,
https://doi.org/10.1007/978-1-0716-0377-2_10,

The TMA sections are most often used to study the expression of markers and oncoproteins in signalling pathway and to correlate with the clinicopathological features as well as prognosis of the patients with esophageal squamous cell carcinoma [3–7]. In addition, they could be used to test the expression of receptors, e.g., VEGFR for therapy of the cancer [8]. Recently, TMA technology is used to study the expression of programmed death-ligand 1 (PD-L1) in large number of esophageal squamous cell carcinoma for assessment of the role of immunotherapy in the cancer [9, 10].

Apart from immunohistochemical studies, in situ hybridization has been applied on TMA sections to study the identification of micro-RNA (miR-1) as a biomarker of patient survival in esophageal squamous cell carcinoma [11]. Also, using fluorescence in situ hybridization (FISH) on TMA sections, *TP53* deletions were shown to be related to advanced cancer stages and presence of lymph node metastasis in esophageal squamous cell carcinoma [12].

Tumor heterogeneity is a challenge for making assessment in testing markers on TMA sections. It is hard to make sure the small tissue samples from a single tumor block (approximately 4 mm^2 in area) represent the whole tumor of esophageal squamous cell carcinoma (often 50 mm in length). A recommendation is to use three tissue cores from each tumor to tackle this problem [1]. In addition, to improve the presentation of the research data, we could add the test(s) of the protein markers in a few whole-slide sections in addition to the TMA sections in the experiments. In good hands, TMA technology could be used effectively in immunohistochemistry with minimal discrepancy in staining between whole-slide sections and TMA sections [2].

Although TMA could save time and money, there are initial costs in term of money and labor. There are different tissue microarrayer machines available commercially capable of constructing the TMA. The machine purchased could be manual or automatic (or semi-automatic) depending on the budget of the researcher (s) and purpose of the project. No matter which method to use, it is essential to devote time for pathologist, scientist, and technicians to design the type and number of tissues in the TMA block, to construct the block, to cut histological sections, and to peform immunohistochemical staining [1]. It is worth noting that cutting of TMA sections requires more technical skills, and time is needed for training of staff to acquire the techniques to obtain the sections.

Unstained TMA sections of esophageal squamous cell carcinoma could be obtained from commercial sources [8]. However, in the era of precision medicine, it is important to research on the tissues obtained from the populations of patients with clinical and pathological characteristics known to the researchers. Thus, many researchers choose to design and construct their own TMA blocks. In this chapter, we present two methods of making TMA blocks for the study of esophageal squamous cell carcinoma.

2 Materials

2.1 "Recipient" Paraffin Block

"Recipient" paraffin block is the block that received multiple tissue cores from "donor" blocks. It is composed of blank paraffin. The quality of blank paraffin block should be examined for air bubbles and cracks. Some companies provide premade "recipient" block with an array of holes ready for insertion of tissues. However, this premade block may not be in line with the design of the individual researcher.

1. The mold for embedding "recipient" block should be at least 1 mm thicker than the "donor" blocks. The mold with a larger surface area is preferable. Large embedding mold can be used to ensure enough thickness of the recipient block (Fig. 1). More space under the tissue column after insertion can avoid delayed popping up because of air compression underneath.
2. The cassettes of the "recipient" block are placed on the heater plate at 60 °C for 5 min before putting it on top of the mold. This can avoid air trapped between mold and cassette while pouring paraffin.
3. Put the mold on the heating plate at 60 °C while pouring liquefied paraffin.
4. To decrease the viscosity of liquefied paraffin, the temperature of the heater is set at 2 °C above the melting point of the paraffin. Some may prefer a mixture of paraffin at a different melting point for better performance of sectioning (*see* **Note 1**).

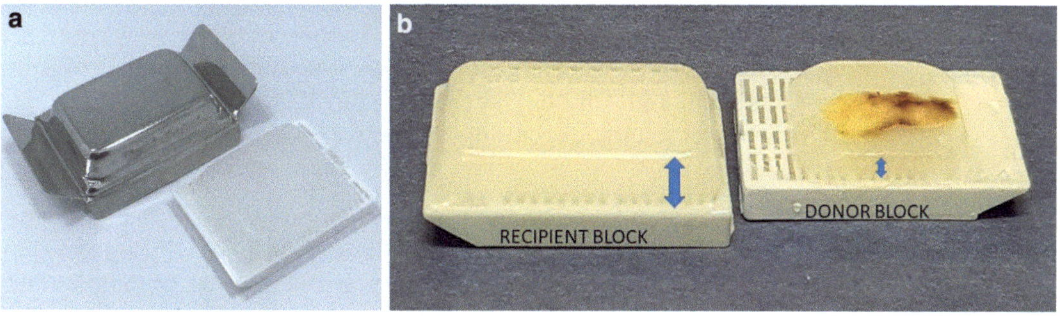

Fig. 1 (**a**) Large metal mold for constructing "recipient" block and the "recipient" block, (**b**) thickness comparison (note the length of the arrows) between "donor" block (left side) and "recipient" block (right side)

5. The procedure for embedding "recipient" block is the same as for the "donor" block without tissue. Place the cassette on top of the mold with the label facing upward.
6. Pour an adequate amount of liquefied paraffin on top of the cassette while heating the mold. The mold should hold the paraffin more than enough to cover the bottom of the cassette. This can avoid detachment of paraffin and cassette after punching large number of cores on the "recipient" block.
7. For achieving better quality, the surface of "recipient" block could be trimmed with microtome before carrying on with the protocol of making TMA block (*see* **Note 2**).

2.2 "Donor" Paraffin Blocks

"Donor" blocks are the source of tissues being transferred to the "recipient" block. In order to include the proper tissue cores in the study of TMA, histopathologists may need to examine the corresponding pathology report as well as hematoxylin and eosin (H&E)-stained sections of the esophageal squamous cell carcinoma. While there is no restriction in including "donor" blocks, some can be more difficult to extract than others due to the nature or preservation of the specimens (*see* **Note 3**).

1. The "donor" blocks usually have their tissue identity handwritten or printed on the cassettes. Many laboratories use barcode scanner to identify and to retrieve the information of the tissue. The technician must pay extra attention not to misplace the tissue samples in the wrong position.
2. Warm up the "donor" blocks to soften the tissue at 37–40 °C. Overnight incubation may solve some difficult cases.
3. Preparing a database of "donor" blocks for the "recipient" block. Database made up of Excel file is preferable for loading up in some systems.
4. Line up the "donor" blocks of esophageal squamous cell carcinoma. Select the areas with cancer to be sampled into the "recipient" block by pathologist (Fig. 2).

2.3 TMA Layout Design

The principal investigator designs the content of the array based on the aims of the study. Although there is no limit in numbers of rows and columns on the "recipient" block, the amount of data is however greatly depending on the following factors of the layout design:

1. The standard diameters of core sizes are 0.6, 1.0, 1.5, 2.0, and 2.5 mm. Core size is perhaps mostly evaluated during the step of planning in terms of balancing the number of samples and coverage of tissue heterogeneity (*see* **Note 4**).

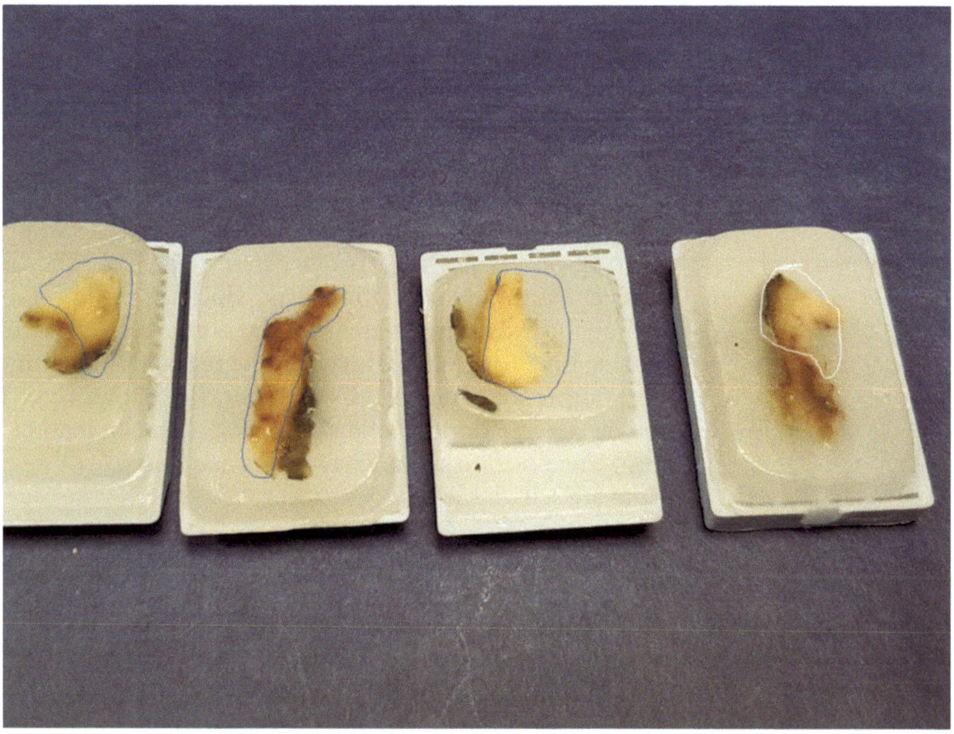

Fig. 2 The "donor" block of esophageal squamous cell carcinoma is lined up in the sequence according to the pattern that would like to be inserted in the "recipient block." In each of the "donor" block, mark the area of the tumor that the puncher could be inserted to obtain a core of tissue from the carcinoma

2. Another factor is the number of "donor" blocks included in the study. Smaller core sizes allow more samples from "donor" blocks. The automatic method may have higher density because of precise alignment and evenly spaced cores. The maximum number of samples with core size of 0.6 mm on 40 × 25 mm area can be up to 550 cores. Precautions should be taken to avoid cracking (*see* **Note 5**).
3. The asymmetrical design of array can preserve the orientation when preparing the slide for the TMA blocks. For example, try to omit the top and/or bottom rows of tissues (*see* Subheading 3.3). Alternatively, non-neoplastic tissues from different organs could be used to create an asymmetrical design. Different non-neoplastic tissues could act as controls when using the TMA block for immunohistochemical studies.

2.4 Tools and Punchers

1. Two punchers for the manual method: manual punchers—for each core size, there are two sets of manual punchers, one for punching holes on the recipient block and another one for extracting tissue from the donor blocks. Each set of punchers is paired with one metallic tube for extraction and one plunger

for repelling the tissue or the blank paraffin inside the tube. The inner diameter of the donor puncher matches the outer diameter of the recipient puncher so that the tissue tube can fit in the recipient hole. There are drawbacks of using two punchers in the automatic method (*see* **Note 6**).

2. Coaxial punchers for the automatic method: Some advanced system uses one coaxial puncher (Fig. 4) instead of two punchers to resolve issues with two separate punchers. The coaxial puncher has three consecutive parts, which are the lower metallic tube for extracting tissue from the donor block, the middle metallic tube for creating holes on the recipient block, and the top plunger for repelling. Coaxial puncher allows tight junction between "donor" and "recipient" for eliminating core drop. The position of punching holes and position of inserting tissue are self-aligned by design.

3 Methods

Tissue microarray can be created by the manual method or automatic method. Each method has many models, and some may prefer one over another. In the following subsections, we will introduce the manual method using alignment mold as well as automatic method using coaxial puncher and computer vision.

3.1 Manual Method by Alignment Mold

The manual system with the use of alignment mold has the advantage of easier transfer of the tissue from the "donor" block compared to premade "recipient" block. For making a tissue microarray block, it is required to follow the following steps:

1. Place the "recipient" block under the alignment mold (Fig. 3a).
2. Place the alignment mold together with the "recipient" block in a heating oven at a temperature of 55–60 °C for 15 min to tightly attach the paraffin to the mold.
3. Use the "recipient" puncher to punch the holes on the "recipient" blocks (Fig. 3b).
4. Repel the paraffin out of the puncher by pushing the plunger (Fig. 3c).
5. Extract tissue from the "donor" block using "donor" puncher (Fig. 3d).
6. Transfer the tissue to the "recipient" block (Fig. 3e).
7. Repeat the steps for every sample.

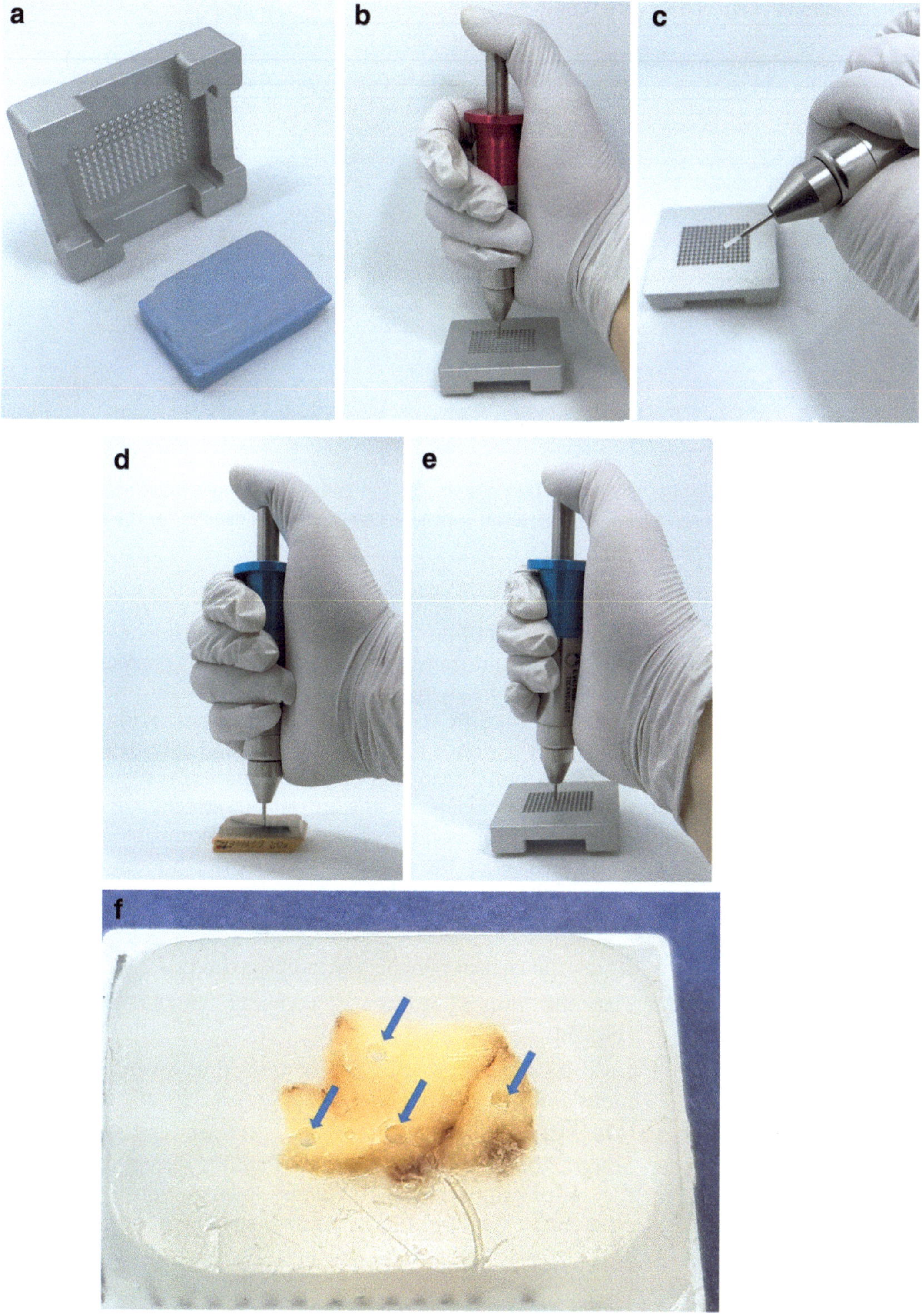

Fig. 3 Manual TMA using alignment mold. (**a**) The alignment mold has holes to guide the process. It should be on top of "recipient" block. (**b**) Use the "recipient" puncher to punch the holes on the "recipient" blocks under the guidance of the alignment mold. (**c**) Repelling the paraffin out of the puncher after each punch. (**d**) "Donor" puncher is used to extract tissue from the "donor" block. (**e**) Transferring the tissue (extracted in the process above) to the "recipient" block. (**f**) One of the "donor" blocks with holes (arrows) showing the tissue samples have been taken

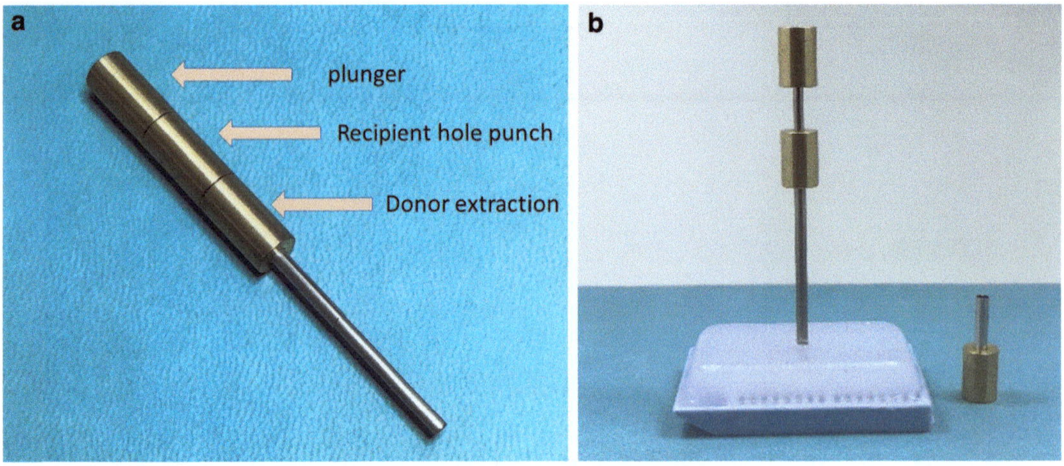

Fig. 4 Coaxial punchers for the automated TMA system. (**a**) Top portion = plunger (solid needle); middle portion = recipient hole punch (hollow needle); lower = donor extraction (hollow needle). (**b**) The action on the puncher shown on a paraffin block

3.2 Automatic Method by Coaxial Puncher

The basic concept of automatic TMA is like the manual method, except the process of punching the holes in "recipient" block and "donor" blocks and transfer of the tissue to the "recipient" blocks are executed by mechanical gadgets. The delicate maneuver of punching holes on the recipient blocks and transferring the tissue samples from the donor blocks to the assigned cores is carried out by moving the puncher up and down automatically. When inserting the tissue into the recipient, the automated system will adjust the inserting depth based on the thickness of the donor blocks, and all tissue should level up the surface discarding the difference in thickness among the donor blocks (*see* **Note 7**). The procedures of the fully automated TMA are as follows:

1. Install the coaxial punchers with designated core size (Fig. 4).
2. Place the "donor" blocks and "recipient" block in their holder (Fig. 5a).
3. Load coding information of the individual esophageal squamous cell carcinoma tissue of the donors from the database (Fig. 5b).
4. Scan the barcode on the cassettes. Barcode system can prevent the misplacement of the "donor" blocks, while technician replaces the "donor" blocks in each batch (Fig. 5b).
5. Measure the "donor" blocks before the process using laser height sensor (Fig. 5b).
6. Capture the macroscopic overview of the "donor" blocks, the "recipient" block, and the slide of the "donor." The automated system is also equipped with the built-in digital camera to guide

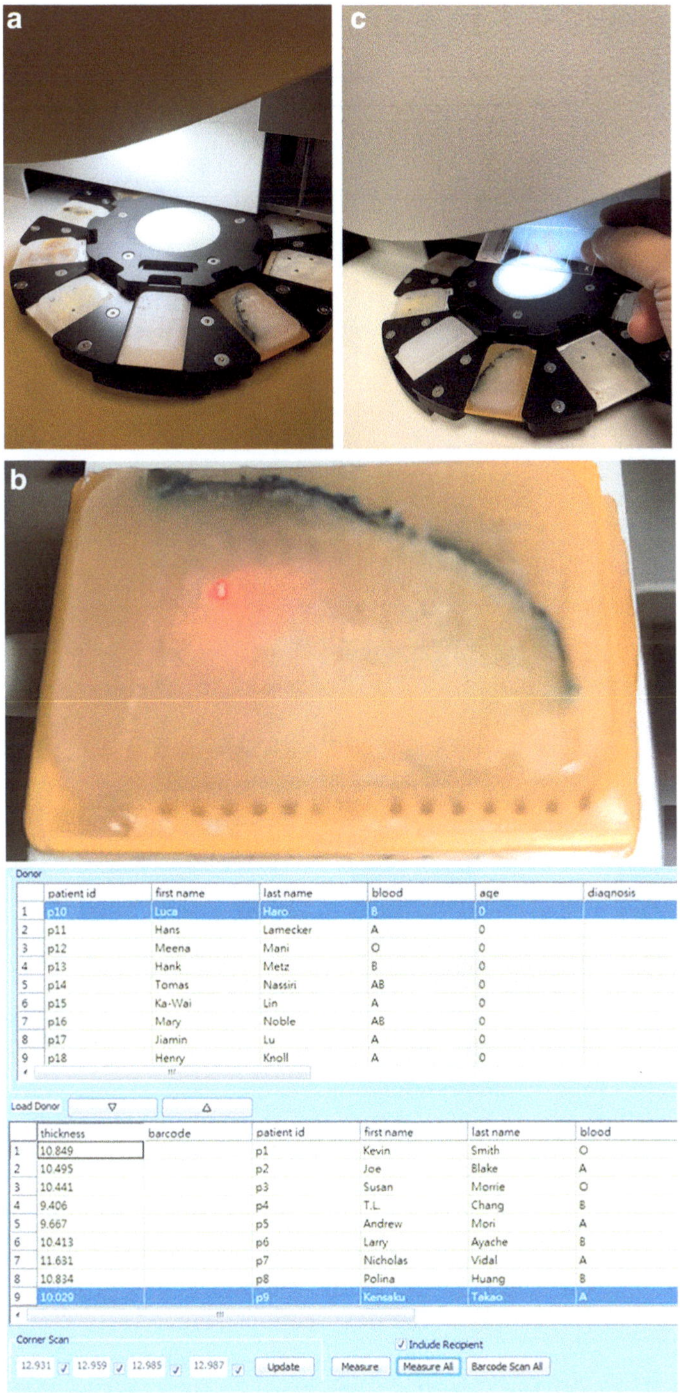

Fig. 5 Automatic TMA using coaxial puncher. (**a**) Insert "recipient" block and "donor" blocks to the holder according to layout design. (**b**) Load donor block identification information from the database, and measure the thickness of each block by the laser (red spot). (**c**) Place the corresponding slide to the stage for taking snapshot. (**d**) The lower image shows the schematic array on the recipient block; the upper right image shows the designated positions in the "donor" tissue assigning to the spots of the array, and the upper left image is the magnified image of the upper right image in real time. (**e**) Punching holes on the "recipient" blocks using the middle metallic tube. (**f**) Repelling the paraffin using the top plunger. (**g**) Extracting tissue from the "donor" block using the lower tube, and (**h**) transferring the tissue to the "recipient" block, and use top two parts of the coaxial needle as the plunger to insert the tissue into the hole

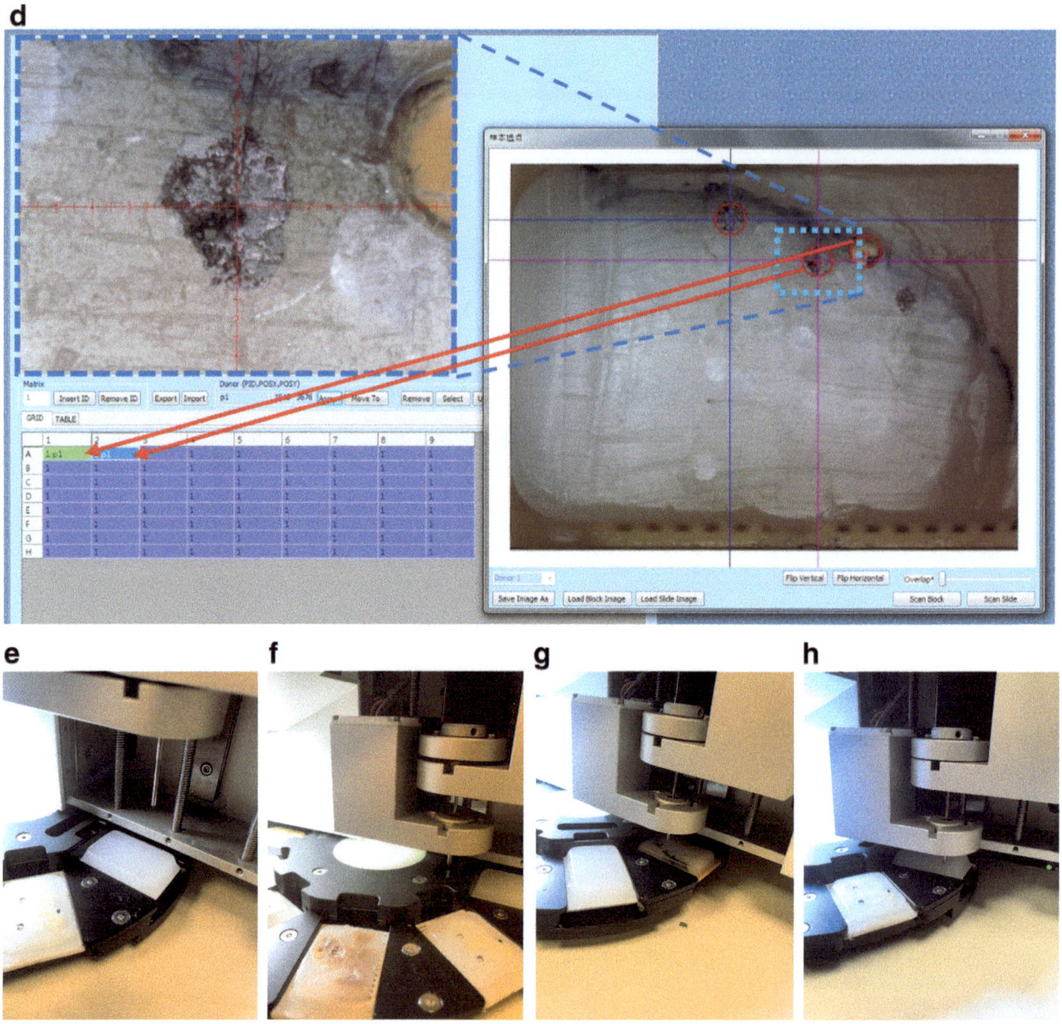

Fig. 5 (continued)

the layout design of the array on the "recipient" block and to assist the selection of the targeting positions on the "donor" blocks in the next sections (Fig. 5c).

7. Users define the number of columns and rows and the pitch between the cores. There is the advantage of viewing on the computer screen in this step (*see* **Note 8**).
8. Remove a core at the corner or add an extra core to the last row. Creating asymmetrical TMA design can preserve the orientation when preparing the slide for the TMA block (Fig. 5d).

9. Overlay the "donor" block image with "donor" slide image to align the region of interest. The automated system can perform shape deformation and transformation to achieve optimal matching (Fig. 5d). The image of the slide can be image captured from the setup or the image file imported from the digital slide scanner (*see* Chapter 9). There is the advantage of using computer screen in this step (*see* **Note 9**).
10. Select targeting positions on "donor" block. Some advanced system also installs the magnifier lens for the digital camera to capture the close-up image of the "donor" blocks. Inspecting the high-resolution image, the technician can observe the tissue and adjust the targeting positions directly from the screen (Fig. 5d).
11. Assign the positions to the designated spot of the array (Fig. 5d).
12. Start the operation.
13. Create holes on the "recipient" block using the middle needle (Fig. 5e).
14. Repel the paraffin extracted from "recipient" block to the collecting bin (Fig. 5f).
15. Pick and place the tissue column from "donor" block to spot on the "recipient" block using the lower needle (Fig. 5g).
16. Adjust the inserting depth of the "donor" tissue automatically. When inserting the tissue into the "recipient" block, the automated system will adjust the inserting depth based on the thickness of the "donor" blocks, and all tissue should level up the surface discarding the difference in thickness among the "donor" blocks (Fig. 5h).
17. Update the status and export the Excel files. This file can be imported to repeat the procedure or to be modified for correction.

3.3 Preparation for Sectioning

1. A TMA block made would best to have (a) control tissues, (b) multiple cores of each patient, and (c) asymmetrical display of the cores (Fig. 6).
2. Place a blank slide on top of the TMA block. Press it down firmly and gently (Fig. 7).
3. Flip the "recipient" block together with the slide upside down, and put it in the oven at 48 °C for 15 min. A longer time of baking may improve adhesion of tissue and paraffin.
4. After baking the "recipient" block, cool it down at room temperature for 15 min before placing it on a cold plate for sectioning by the microtome. Putting it in the freezer after cooling it down at room temperature may also help to avoid

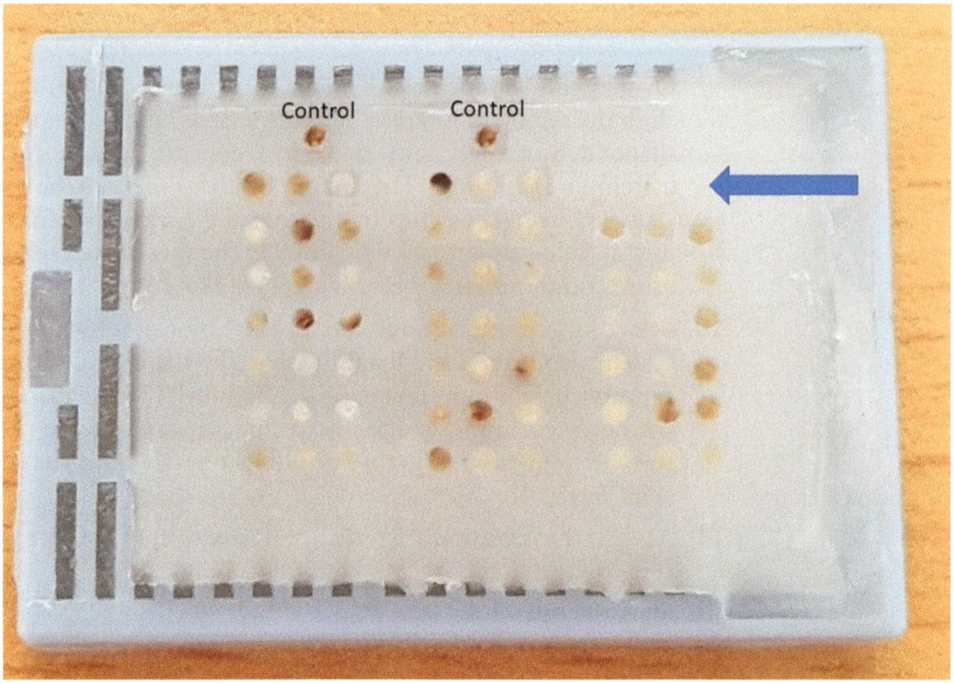

Fig. 6 An example of a TMA block of tissues from many patients with esophageal squamous cell carcinoma. Note that the block contains two cores of control tissue at the top. The control tissues used could be non-neoplastic liver, colon, etc. The other important feature is the absence of tissue in one row (arrow). This help the pathologist to orientate the TMA section for microscopic examination. In addition, 3 cores of tissue from each patient were put in 1 row (tissues from 20 patients were included in the block)

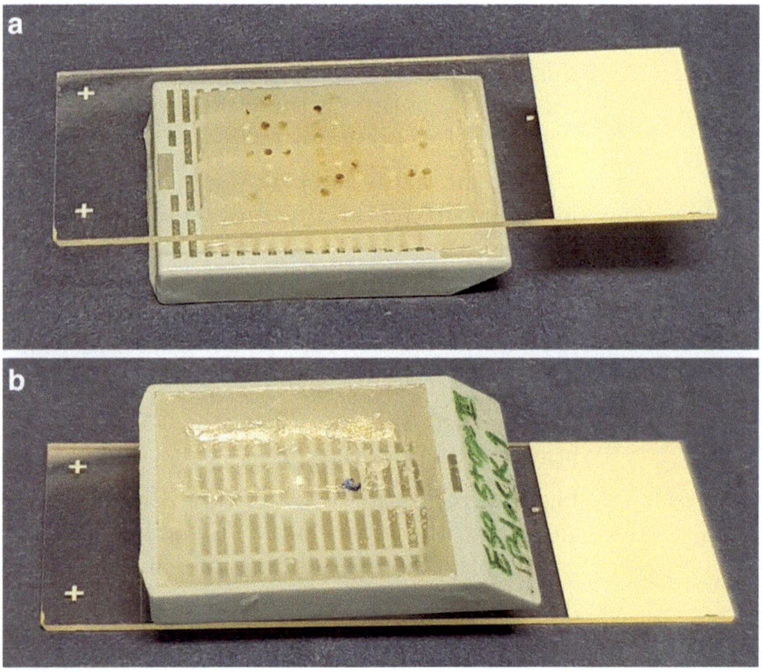

Fig. 7 Preparation of the TMA block: (**a**) Gently pressing slide to the top of the TMA block. (**b**) Flipping the TMA block upside down and leaving it in an incubator for the paraffin tissue fusion for some time

wrinkle sections. One must be aware not to have dramatic temperature change for the "recipient" block. A sudden dramatic temperature change such as moving to freezer after baking will cause cracks and tissues falling off.

5. The thickness of 4 μm is ideal for thin sectioning of esophageal squamous cell carcinoma. The temperature for the water bath is 37–39 °C.

3.4 Image Processing

1. After sectioning by microtome, the TMA sections can be stained with hematoxylin and eosin stain (Fig. 8).
2. Scan the TMA section with the digital slide scanner for further investigation and image analysis (Fig. 9). It is worth noting that in the presence of large number of sections from different cancers, examination by light microscopy would be difficult and increase the chance of error. Scanning of the TMA section to interpret the section in front of the monitor will make the task easier for pathologist.

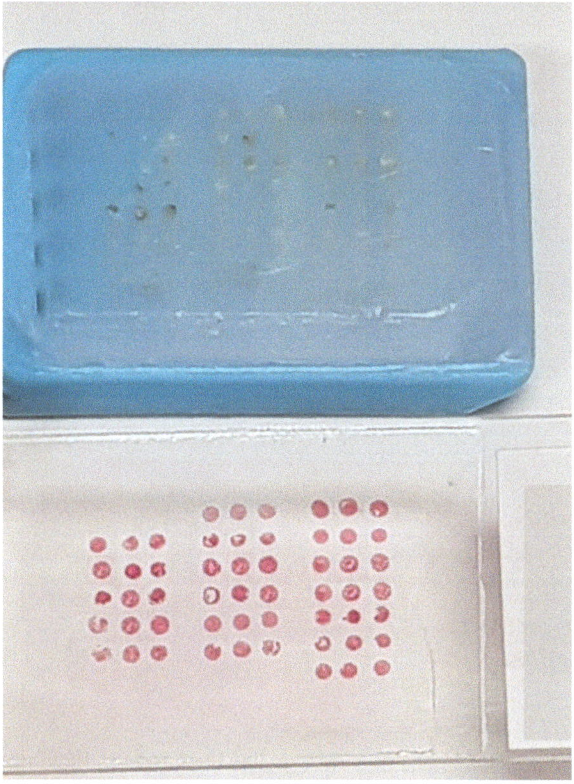

Fig. 8 A hematoxylin and eosin-stained section of a TMA block of 18 cases of esophageal squamous cell carcinoma. Note the asymmetry of the tumor tissues in the section. Each case has three cores of tumor tissues in a row

a

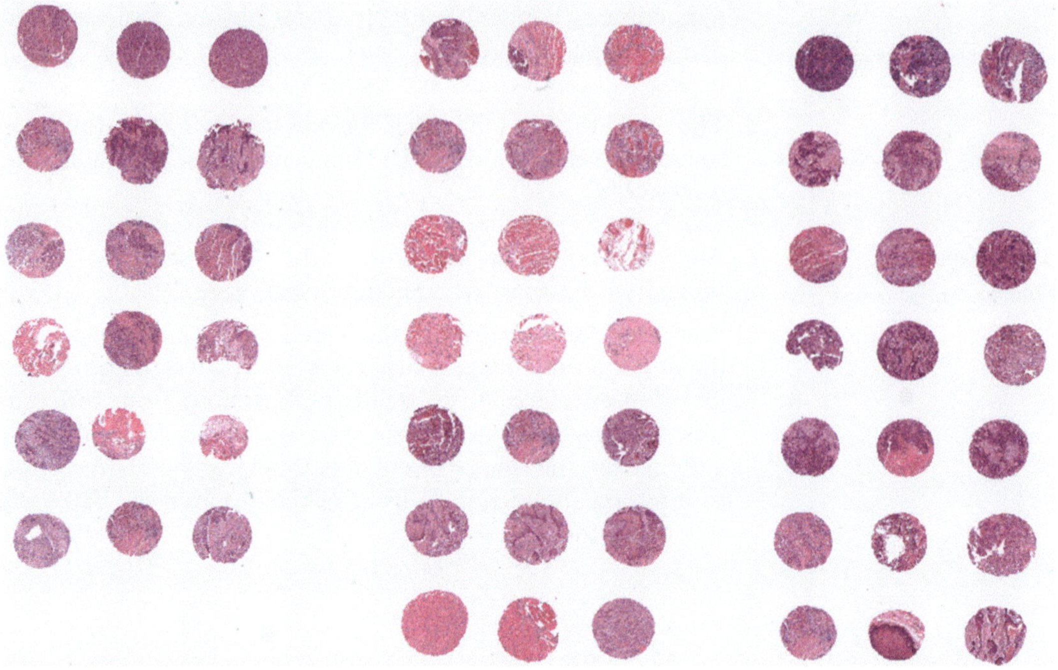

b

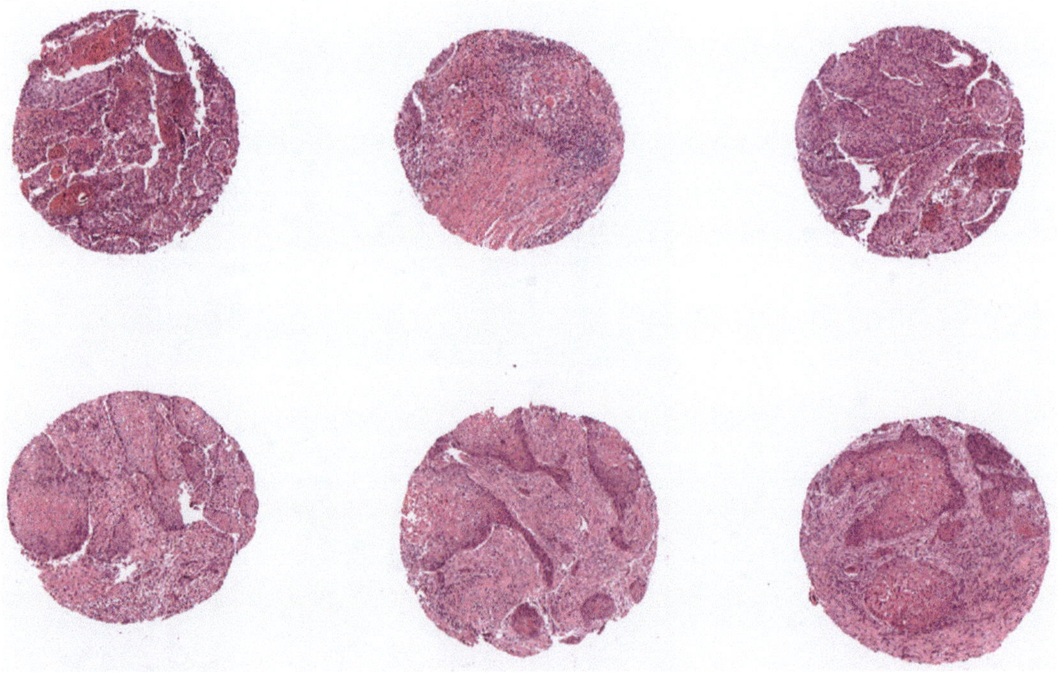

Fig. 9 (**a**) Whole-slide image of a TMA section captured. (**b**) High magnification of two rows (two cases) from the TMA section. (**c**) High magnification showing detailed morphology of esophageal squamous cell carcinoma. (**d**) Image of the TMA section showing expression of a protein marker stained by immunohistochemistry

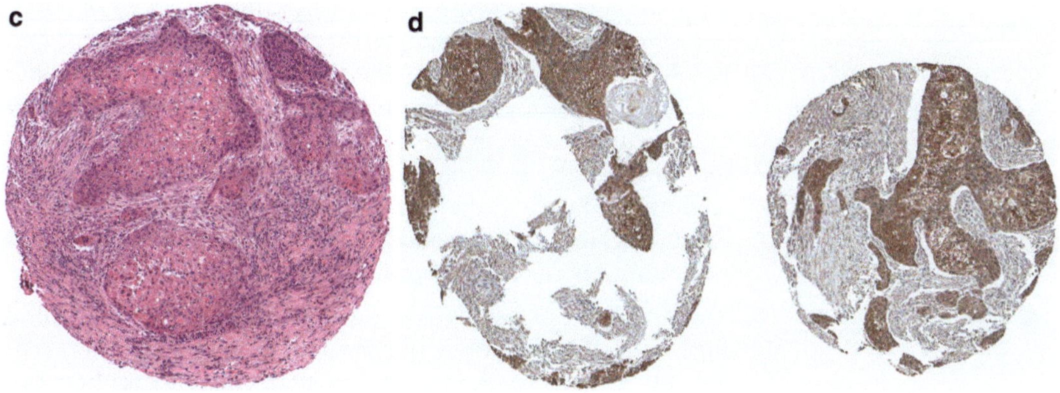

Fig. 9 (continued)

4 Notes

1. Paraffin with a lower melting point (50–54 °C) has better tissue infiltration. However, it is more brittle and may create holes larger than tissue cores during the punching. Based on our experience, mixing 30% of paraffin with a higher melting point (60 °C) can improve the circularity of the tissue cores while preserving the adhesion between tissue and wax.
2. One of the advantages of trimming the surface of "recipient" block is lowering the punching debris on the automatic method. Trimming can make sure the surface is parallel to the base of the cassette. This can also ensure all the tissues are inserted at the same surface height on the automatic method.
3. Some tissues may have compositions that can be difficult to punch out. For example, the calcification of the cancerous tissue may appear shrivelled and very hard. The process of decalcification can remove the mineral from the tissue but may destroy essential pathologic characteristics. Some particularly thin tissue of only 2–3 mm in thickness can also be difficult to punch out due to the lack of friction on the inner wall of the puncher. Re-processing may have to be considered.
4. To minimize the amount of damage to the "donor" blocks, some may prefer to use a smaller core size. However, one may concern that the tissue of 0.6 mm biopsies does not show enough characteristics to represent the carcinoma. One way to resolve the issue is by having multiple cores per "donor" block.
5. If we wish to construct TMA with more samples, the space between cores needs to be smaller. However, squeezing the cores in a tight space may cause crack or deformation among them. Based on our experience, the space between edges of two cores should be at least 0.5 mm, and the ideal space between

the centers of two cores should be 1.5 times the size of cores. For example, the ideal space between two cores of size 2.0 mm should be 3.0 mm, meaning that the space between their edges is 1.0 mm. Although the number of cores in an array depends on the surface area of "recipient" block, an adequate margin should be saved to avoid cracking during the punching and sectioning. Leaving the minimum of 2–5 mm margins can avoid cracking of the paraffin when punching the holes or sectioning for the TMA slides.

6. The drawback of having two punchers is that the mechanical alignment of having two punchers on the same position is very difficult to achieve. A slight offset may create a gap between them and can result in the core dropping off from the slide when sectioning the TMA blocks.
7. The fully automated TMA system must be able to adapt different conditions of the donor blocks retrieved from the laboratory. For example, the samples may come in different thickness, and the experienced technicians use the caliper to measure thickness, as shown in Fig. 1c. Such difference may cause the recipient block not having all the samples level up on the surface or even devastating when precious samples are thicker than the recipient blocks and the extra will need to be cut off. Some automated TMA systems are also equipped with the laser height sensor (Fig. 5b) to measure the "donor" blocks before the process.
8. Designing the layout for the TMA block, the technician needs to pay attention to the allocation of the array within the enclosed area on the "recipient" block. The vision of the process over the computer screen and overlaid schematic drawing can be used to guide the process. Users can center the pseudo-array on the paraffin blocks and to reserve enough margin on edge to avoid the crack due to the tension when punching the holes (Fig. 5d).
9. Another crucial step takes place in selecting the targeting positions of the core on the "donor" blocks. The histopathologist investigates the region of interest on the hematoxylin and eosin-stained section and marks them on the slide for each "donor" block. After the selection, the technician needs to find the corresponding positions on the "donor" blocks. The automated method can ease this procedure by selecting the positions on the screen.

References

1. Saremi N, Lam AK (2018) Application of tissue microarray in esophageal adenocarcinoma. Methods Mol Biol 1756:105–118
2. van Zwieten A (2013) Tissue microarray technology and findings for diagnostic immunohistochemistry. Pathology 45:71–79
3. Chan D, Tsoi MY, Liu CD, Chan SH, Law SY, Chan KW, Chan YP, Gopalan V, Lam AK, Tang JC (2013) Oncogene GAEC1 regulates CAPN10 expression which predicts survival in esophageal squamous cell carcinoma. World J Gastroenterol 19:2772–2780
4. Yu VZ, Wong VC, Dai W, Ko JM, Lam AK, Chan KW, Samant RS, Lung HL, Shuen WH, Law S, Chan YP, Lee NP, Tong DK, Law TT, Lee VH, Lung ML (2015) Nuclear localization of DNAJB6 is associated with survival of patients with esophageal cancer and reduces AKT signaling and proliferation of cancer cells. Gastroenterology 149:1825–1836.e5
5. Chai AW, Cheung AK, Dai W, Ko JM, Ip JC, Chan KW, Kwong DL, Ng WT, Lee AW, Ngan RK, Yau CC, Tung SY, Lee VH, Lam AK, Pillai S, Law S, Lung ML (2016) Metastasis-suppressing NID2, an epigenetically-silenced gene, in the pathogenesis of nasopharyngeal carcinoma and esophageal squamous cell carcinoma. Oncotarget 7:78859–78871
6. Li B, Xu WW, Lam AKY, Wang Y, Hu HF, Guan XY, Qin YR, Saremi N, Tsao SW, He QY, Cheung ALM (2017) Significance of PI3K/AKT signaling pathway in metastasis of esophageal squamous cell carcinoma and its potential as a target for anti-metastasis therapy. Oncotarget 8:38755–38766
7. Islam F, Gopalan V, Law S, Tang JC, Lam AK (2019) FAM134B promotes esophageal squamous cell carcinoma in vitro and its correlations with clinicopathologic features. Hum Pathol 87:1–10
8. Xu WW, Li B, Lam AK, Tsao SW, Law SY, Chan KW, Yuan QJ, Cheung AL (2015) Targeting VEGFR1- and VEGFR2-expressing non-tumor cells is essential for esophageal cancer therapy. Oncotarget 6:1790–1805
9. Ng HY, Li J, Tao L, Lam AK, Chan KW, Ko JMY, Yu VZ, Wong M, Li B, Lung ML (2018) Chemotherapeutic treatments increase PD-L1 expression in esophageal squamous cell carcinoma through EGFR/ERK activation. Transl Oncol 11:1323–1333
10. Rong L, Liu Y, Hui Z, Zhao Z, Zhang Y, Wang B, Yuan Y, Li W, Guo L, Ying J, Song Y, Wang L, Zhou Z, Xue L, Lu N (2019) PD-L1 expression and its clinicopathological correlation in advanced esophageal squamous cell carcinoma in a Chinese population. Diagn Pathol 14:6
11. Wei Q, Li X, Yu W, Zhao K, Qin G, Chen H, Gu Y, Ding F, Zhu Z, Fu X, Sun M (2019) microRNA-messenger RNA regulatory network of esophageal squamous cell carcinoma and the identification of miR-1 as a biomarker of patient survival. J Cell Biochem 120:12259–12272
12. Melling N, Norrenbrock S, Kluth M, Simon R, Hube-Magg C, Steurer S, Hinsch A, Burandt E, Jacobsen F, Wilczak W, Quaas A, Bockhorn M, Grupp K, Tachezy M, Izbicki J, Sauter G, Gebauer F (2019) p53 overexpression is a prognosticator of poor outcome in esophageal cancer. Oncol Lett 17:3826–3834

Chapter 11

Patient-Derived Xenograft and Mice Models in Esophageal Squamous Cell Carcinoma

Alfred K. Lam and Johnny C. Tang

Abstract

Mouse models are important in the study of pathogenesis, testing new treatment, and monitoring the progress of treatment in patients with esophageal squamous cell carcinoma (ESCC). The mice commonly used are immunosuppressed. The first category of models is for basic research and includes genetically engineered mouse models and carcinogen- or diet-induced mouse models. The second category of models involves either injection of cells with altered gene function related to pathogenesis of ESCC or ESCC cell lines. This method is commonly used and relatively inexpensive and simple to use. These cells commonly being subcutaneous injected in flank (subcutaneous xenograft model), tail vein, or peritoneum of immunodeficient mice. Direct implantation into the esophagus (orthotopic xenograft model) is also performed despite the cost and technical difficulties. The third category of mouse model is the patient-derived xenograft (PDX) model. In this model, ESCC tissues (instead of cell lines) removed from the patient are implanted into immunodeficient mice. This model appears promising for personalized medicine and of high resemblance to the nature of human ESCC, but there are many limitations for the use. It is likely to be used more in research in ESCC in the future. In this chapter, we detailed the preparation and experiments of PDX model from a patient with ESCC.

Key words ESCC, Esophageal, Squamous cell carcinoma, Patient-derived xenograft, Mice model

1 Introduction

Mouse models are important in the study of pathogenesis, testing new treatment, and monitoring the progress of treatment in patients with esophageal squamous cell carcinoma (ESCC). The mice used are immunosuppressed to allow the growth of the cancer. There are four different types of mice for making animal models of cancer [1]. They are athymic nude mice, SCID (severely compromised immunodeficient) mice, NOD/SCID (nonobese diabetic/SCID) mice, and NSG (NOD.Cg-*Prkdcscid Il2rgtm1Wjl*/SzJ) mice. Athymic nude and SCID mice are preferably used for implanting cancer cell lines. Athymic nude mice have no functional T cells. SCID mice have no functional T cells and B cells. NOD/SCID and NSG mice are often used for the transplantation of human

Alfred K. Lam (ed.), *Esophageal Squamous Cell Carcinoma: Methods and Protocols*, Methods in Molecular Biology, vol. 2129,
https://doi.org/10.1007/978-1-0716-0377-2_11,

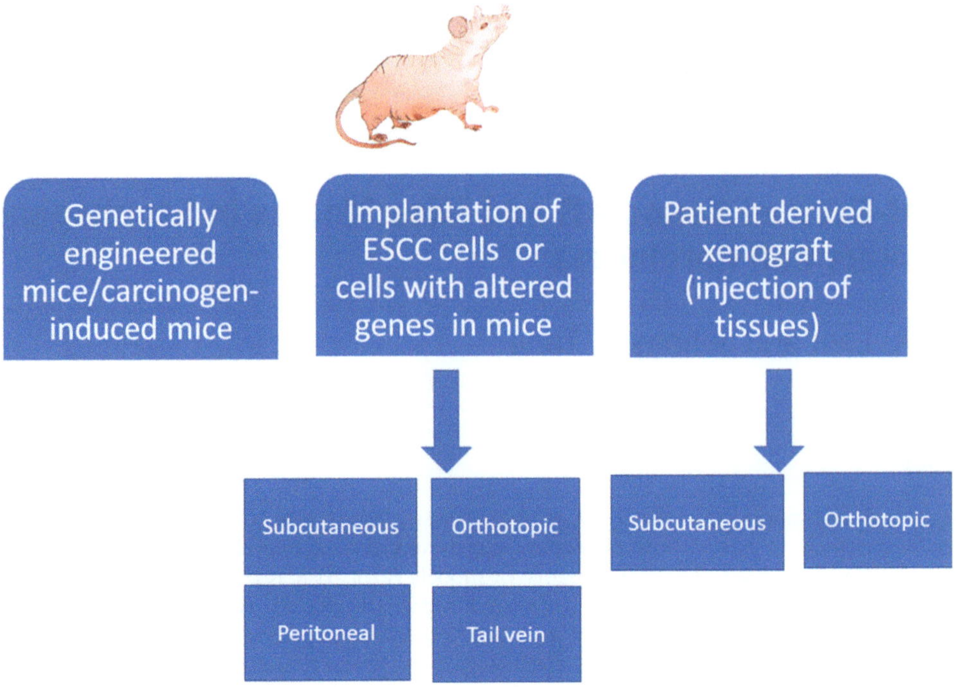

Fig. 1 The different mice models for investigation of esophageal squamous cell carcinoma

tumors. NOD/SCID mice have no functional T cells and B cells as well as impaired natural killer cells, whereas NSG mice have no functional T cells, B cells, or natural killer cells. Using these mice, there are three broad categories of mouse models for ESCC (Fig. 1).

The first category of mouse modules is mainly for basic research. These include genetically engineered mouse models (contain loss or gain of function of genes of interest in the esophageal cancer) and carcinogen- or diet-induced mouse models (treated by carcinogens or diet deficient in specific nutrients to induce esophageal cancer).

The second category involves the implantation of cells with transfected gene or ESCC cell lines into immunosuppressed mice. Using the first type of method, cells with altered gene function related to pathogenesis of ESCC could be put in athymic nude mice. This method is important in the confirmation of biological effects of cancer-related genes in ESCC. *GAEC1* (*gene amplified in esophageal cancer 1*) plays a crucial role in pathogenesis and was discovered in 2007 [2, 3]. Injection of GAEC1-transfected 3T3 cells into athymic nude mice formed undifferentiated sarcoma in vivo, indicating that GAEC1 is a transforming oncogene in ESCC [2, 3]. Similarly, other genes important in the pathogenesis of ESCC, *JK-1* (*FAM134B/RETREG1*) and *JS-1*, were identified in the same experiment as *GAEC1*. Subcutaneous sarcomas were formed in athymic nude mice after the National Cancer Institute (NIH) 3T3 cells overexpressing JK-1 were injected subcutaneously [4, 5].

The other method in this category is the injection of ESCC cell lines into immunosuppressed mice. This method is commonly used and relatively inexpensive and simple to use, and many ESCC cell lines are available [6–8]. The cells from the cell lines most commonly being subcutaneous injected into athymic nude mice (subcutaneous xenograft model). The in vivo anti-cancer effect of potential novel target therapies, such as quinoline derivate, could be studied by this model [9]. The other means of injection involve the injection of ESCC cells into the tail vein and injection into the peritoneum of immunodeficient mice. However, the cancer developed in this category of method lacks the resemblance of microenvironment of ESCC and could not adequately represent the behavior of the tumor in patient.

The other means of implantation of ESCC cell lines is engraftment into the esophagus of the mice (orthotopic xenograft model). It closely resembles the usual microenvironment of ESCC but needs high expertise to implant the tumor (*see* Chapter 12) [10]. The other disadvantage is the need of sophisticated imaging system to follow up the growth of the tumor as the tumor is situated internally. In ESCC, the orthotopic xenograft model has been used to study the effect of chemotherapy on the programmed cell death-1 (PD-L1) expression (important marker in immunotherapy) [11]. In addition, orthotopic xenograft model has been used to demonstrate the antiproliferative effect of mTOR inhibitor (temsirolimus) in ESCC [12].

The third category of mouse model is the patient-derived xenograft (PDX) model. In this model, ESCC tissues (instead of cell lines) removed from the patient are implanted into immunodeficient mice. As the tumor in the mouse is directly from the patient with ESCC, it represents best, when compared with using other patients' cell lines, the clinical pathological characteristics of the ESCC of the patient. Thus, PDX model is a personalized model to study the effects of different therapies on patients with ESCC. In the literature, PDX model has been used in preclinical drug testing (combination chemotherapy) in ESCC [13–15]. In addition, ESCC cell lines could be obtained from this method [6–8].

Although this model appears promising for personalized medicine and of high resemblance to the nature of human ESCC, there are many limitations for the use. First, the main challenge is the low tumor implantation rate. As a result, there is a high cost involved in making a successful mouse model. Also, the tumor needs more time to grow as compared with cell line implant. The time for tumor growth in mice may be too long as the patient's condition may change during the time. In addition, the mice could not be used to test vaccines or immunotherapy (checkpoint blocking antibodies).

The other aspect is the human resources needed for getting ethics for collection of human tissues (in addition to animal ethics) and coordination of transferring the tumor tissues after operative procedures to the mice as soon as possible after the operation.

Overall, PDX model is likely to be used more in research in ESCC in the future despite the limitations of this approach. Thus, technical advances are needed to get successful PDX model for clinical applications. In addition, the data obtained by personalized therapy could be fit into a database. The data could be used to planning optimal treatment of patients with similar genomic characteristics [16]. In this chapter, we detailed the preparation and experiments of PDX model from a patient with ESCC. The injection of the ESCC cell lines was also presented.

2 Materials

2.1 Implantation of ESCC into Mice

1. Fresh ESCC tissue.
2. ESCC cell lines.
3. Phosphate-buffered saline.
4. Dissection kits (forceps, scalpel, blade, surgical sutures, etc.).
5. Culture medium—Eagle's Minimum Essential Medium.
6. Animal housing facilities.
7. Athymic nude mice of 6–8 weeks old.
8. Well-ventilated cages for holding the mice.
9. Restrainer for mice (helps to hold the mice during anesthesia or tail injection).
10. 5% halothane with airtight container.
11. 70% ethanol for disinfection on mice skin.
12. Cotton swab.

2.2 Experimental Phase

1. A 25–27 gauge or smaller needle (for injection of experimental drug).
2. Safety cabinet and protective measures—gloves, mask, sharp bin, etc.
3. Electronic balance (weighing).
4. Caliper or ruler for measurement.
5. Small gauge syringe (1 mL) for tail vein injection.

2.3 Dissection of Mice

1. Dissection Table.
2. 5% carbon dioxide for euthanasia with airtight container.
3. Digital camera.
4. Histology cassette for tissue collection.

5. Foil paper for storage of frozen sample.
6. −80°C freezer.
7. EDTA (ethylenediaminetetraacetic acid) or heparin tube for blood collection.
8. 10% formaldehyde.
9. Reagents for decontamination after working with animals.
10. Embedding machine for paraffin blocks.
11. Hematoxylin and eosin staining stations (*see* Chapter 7) or autostainer.
12. Mounting medium and coverslips or automatic coverslip machine.
13. Light microscope.

3 Method

3.1 Implantation of ESCC into Mice

1. Obtain ethnics for working on projects with animals.
2. Induction of the operator into the procedures and safety measures in animal facilities as well as fulfilment of training requirements of handling mice including dissection and injection.
3. Collect the fresh ESCC tissues after surgical operation as soon as possible (*see* Chapter 8).
4. Put the ESCC tissues immediately into cell culture medium—Eagle's Minimum Essential Medium (MEM).
5. Cut the ESCC collected into small pieces—with each to less than 1 mm in diameter.
6. Prepare the athymic mice in ventilated cages. The mice should be restrained properly.
7. Anesthetize each of the athymic nude mice with appropriate concentration of halothane by inhalation (*see* **Note 1**).
8. Under sterilized condition (with disinfection of the skin with 70% ethanol wipes), cut open the skin in the flank region of the mouse with a maximum size of 2 mm. The preparation of cell line injection to mice is similar except for cutting open the skin (*see* **Note 2**).
9. Insert the tumor tissues into the subcutaneous region of the cut site of the mouse.
10. Close the wound with surgical suture.
11. Observe the mice. If mice show sign of distress, pain killer could be used (*see* **Note 3**).

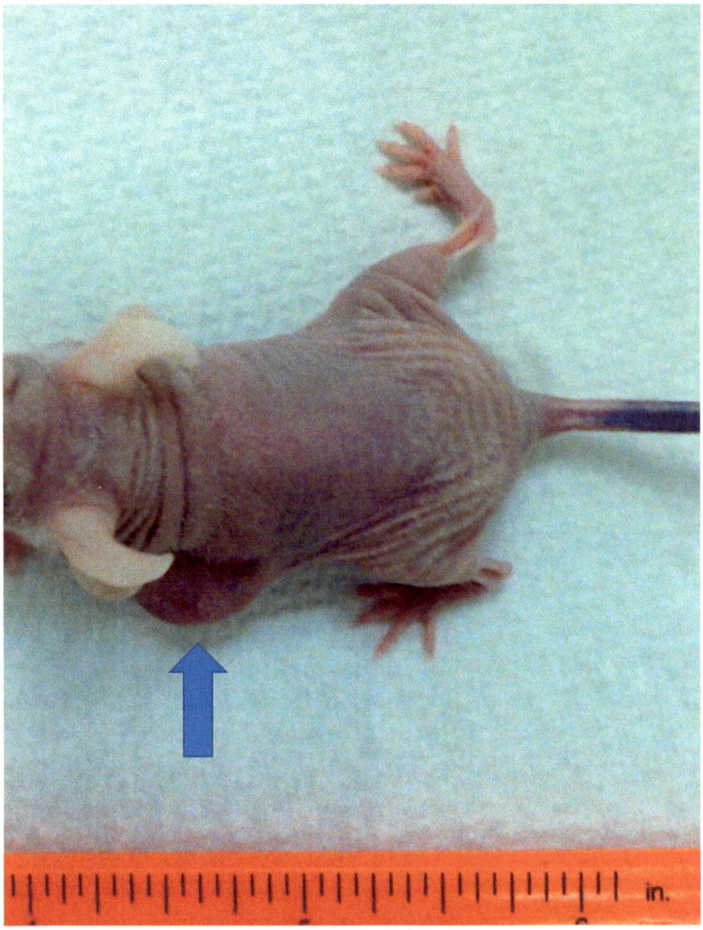

Fig. 2 The growth of the patient-derived xenograft of esophageal squamous cell carcinoma in the subcutaneous tissue of mice (arrow)

3.2 Experimental Phase

1. Weight the mice every day.
2. Observe the growth of the subcutaneous tumor daily (Fig. 2).
3. Record the tumor size with caliper. Calculate the volume of the tumor from the measurements (*see* **Note 4**).
4. Monitor the growth for approximately 1 month (4 weeks) to wait until the tumors reach a stable size of approximately 150 mm^3.
5. Select the mouse with the tumor that grows largest. Harvest the tumor, and perform re-transplantation to another batch of nude mice, and repeat the above procedures until the tumor reaches the similar size of approximately 150 mm^3.
6. Group some mice as experimental and some as controls.
7. Inject the experimental therapeutics into the mice (*see* **Note 5**) (Fig. 3).
8. Observe the mice daily with measurements as described above (*see* **Note 6**).

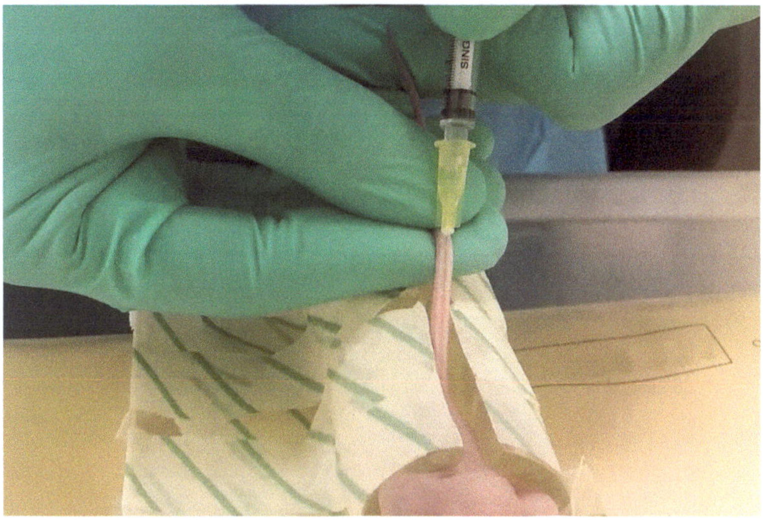

Fig. 3 Injection of therapeutic intervention through the vein

3.3 Dissection of Mice

1. Euthanasia will be performed at the predefined experimental endpoint (depending on the status of the mice and the type of experiment). Standard monitoring procedure determines an animal to be deteriorating.
2. At the experimental endpoint, the mice could be euthanized by 5% carbon dioxide and cervical dislocation.
3. Dissect out the tumor. The tumor of the mice should be dissected out completely including the skin and subcutaneous tissue (Fig. 4).
4. The size and weight of the tumor in the controls and subjects are recorded.
5. Postmortem of the mice (*see* **Note 7**).
6. Process of the collected tissues. Put half of the sampled tissues in cassette and process for paraffin blocks. The other half was stored in frozen at −80 °C (*see* Chapter X on biobanking). The frozen tissues are best for genomic studies, expression analysis, and Western blot for detection of proteins, etc.
7. Cut sections of the collected tissue from paraffin blocks for hematoxylin staining.
8. Examine under microscope (Fig. 5) (*see* **Note 8**).
9. Proper disposal of the mice and kits as well as decontamination.

4 Notes

1. The number of mice depends on the research project and the success rate of implants into the mice. At least one group needs

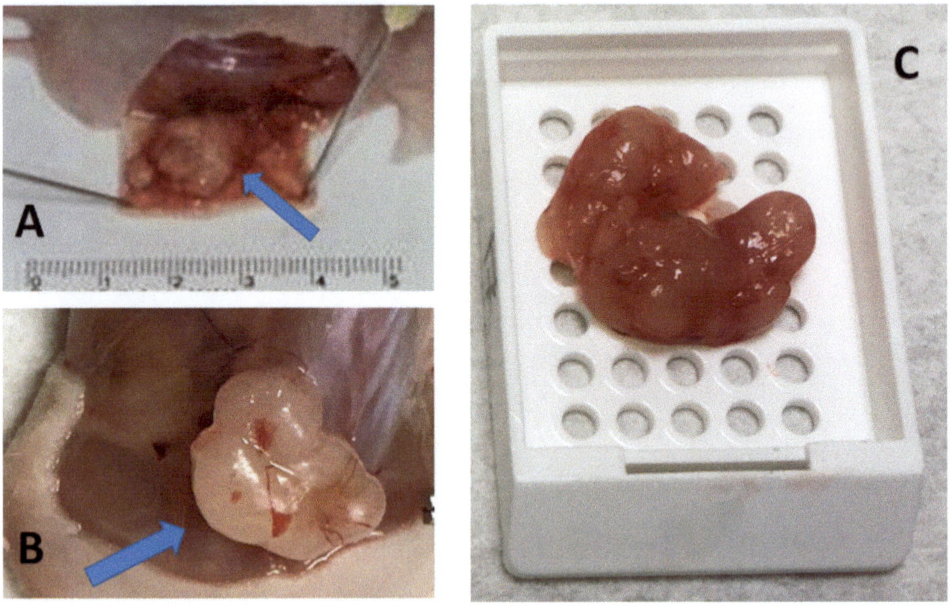

Fig. 4 (**a**) Dissection of the skin to expose the tumor (arrow). (**b**) Higher magnification showing removal of tissue around the tumor (arrow). (**c**) Half of the tumor was puts in the cassette for formalin fixation and then embeds in paraffin whereas half fresh frozen in −80 °C

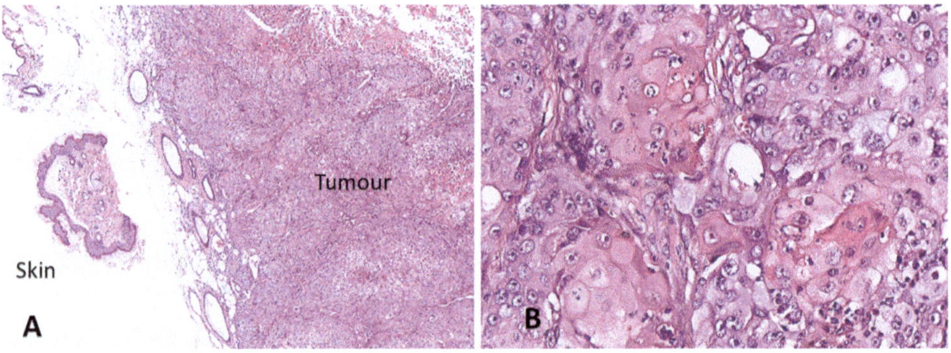

Fig. 5 Histological examination of the patient-derived xenograft. (**a**) There is a big tumor underneath the skin of the nude mouse (hematoxylin and eosin ×4). (**b**) Higher magnification shows that the tumor is a squamous cell carcinoma comprising of polygonal tumor cells with keratinization resembling the parent carcinoma in the esophagus of the patient

to be set as controls. Approximately five mice may be used in one run of the study. The success rate of implant varies and may be as low as 5%. Thus, more viable ESCC tissue should be obtained as well as more mice should be implanted per patient.

2. The loose skin in the flank is good for subcutaneous implantation. For ESCC cell line injection instead of tissue, prepare cell lines with approximately 3×10^6 cells in 0.1 mL phosphate-

buffered saline Then, a 25–27 gauge or smaller needle could be inserted through the skin into subcutaneous tissue. Make sure the needle tip not mistakenly entered into the muscle. After retraction of the needle, place sterilized cotton swab over the injection site for 30 s to prevent bleeding and spillage of tumor cells.

3. The clinical signs may involve the behavior signs (walking behavior) as well as bowel movement (solid or diarrhea). Buprenorphine could be used for pain killing. The dosage could be sustained-release formulation of buprenorphine (SB, 2.2 mg/kg) with a standard protocol of three injections of buprenorphine (Temgesic, 0.1 mg/kg/8 h) in mice [17].
4. There are many formulas for determining the volume of the tumor in athymic mice [18]. The most accurate way is to measure the three dimensions (length [L], width [W], and height [H]) of the tumor, but it may not always be possible to determine all these dimensions. The formulas are tumor volume $= \pi/6 \times L \times W \times H$ or $1/2 \times L \times W \times H$. For convenience, tumor volume $= L \times W \times W/2$.
5. The experimental agent could be injected into lateral tail veins or by intraperitoneal approach. Tail vein is small and sometimes difficult to deliver 100% with leakage of the dosage. Do not do more than four attempts on one mouse.
6. The mice should be monitored. Tumor size could not be more than 5% of the body weight.
7. A midline incision to open the skin from below the chin to above the pubic bone. Inspect for evidence of metastases under the subcutaneous tissue. Open the rib case and inspect the mediastinum and diaphragm. Cut open the rib cage and inspect the heart and lung surface. If necessary, take blood directly from the heart of the animal with a syringe, and store. Then, carefully detach the trachea and esophagus from the posterior mediastinal wall. By holding the trachea and esophagus, dissect along the posterior mediastinum and the posterior peritoneum. All the organs in the chest and abdomen could be removed to examine on the dissection table. Section the large organs to examine the internal aspects for cancer. Take blocks for any organs with cancer. Sample the large organs such as the lungs, spleen, liver, kidney, heart, etc.
8. The microscopic examination of internal organs serves three major purposes. The first is to examine the effect of tested therapeutic measures in terms of metastases. The other purpose is to examine any toxic effects to the organs by the drugs. Lastly, we could use the block to examine for parameters such as expression of protein makers of EMT (epithelial-mesenchymal transition), stem cell, proliferative index (Ki-67), vascularization (VEGF), etc. [19, 20].

References

1. Jung J, Seol HS, Chang S (2018) The generation and application of patient-derived xenograft model for cancer research. Cancer Res Treat 50:1–10
2. Tang JC, Lam KY, Law S, Wong J, Srivastava G (2001) Detection of genetic alterations in esophageal squamous cell carcinomas and adjacent normal epithelia by comparative DNA fingerprinting using inter-simple sequence repeat PCR. Clin Cancer Res 7:1539–1545
3. Law FB, Chen YW, Wong KY, Ying J, Tao Q, Langford C, Lee PY, Law S, Cheung RW, Chui CH, Tsao SW, Lam KY, Wong J, Srivastava G, Tang JC (2007) Identification of a novel tumor transforming gene GAEC1 at 7q22 which encodes a nuclear protein and is frequently amplified and overexpressed in esophageal squamous cell carcinoma. Oncogene 26:5877–5888
4. Tang WK, Chui CH, Fatima S, Kok SH, Pak KC, Ou TM, Hui KS, Wong MM, Wong J, Law S, Tsao SW, Lam KY, Beh PS, Srivastava G, Chan AS, Ho KP, Tang JC (2007) Oncogenic properties of a novel gene JK-1 located in chromosome 5p and its overexpression in human esophageal squamous cell carcinoma. Int J Mol Med 19:915–923
5. Fatima S, Chui CH, Tang WK, Hui KS, Au HW, Li WY, Wong MM, Cheung F, Tsao SW, Lam KY, Beh PS, Wong J, Law S, Srivastava G, Ho KP, Chan AS, Tang JC (2006) Transforming capacity of two novel genes JS-1 and JS-2 located in chromosome 5p and their overexpression in human esophageal squamous cell carcinoma. Int J Mol Med 17:159–170
6. Hu YC, Lam KY, Law SY, Wan TS, Ma ES, Kwong YL, Chan LC, Wong J, Srivastava G (2002) Establishment, characterization, karyotyping, and comparative genomic hybridization analysis of HKESC-2 and HKESC-3: two newly established human esophageal squamous cell carcinoma cell lines. Cancer Genet Cytogenet 135:120–127
7. Tang JC, Wan TS, Wong N, Pang E, Lam KY, Law SY, Chow LM, Ma ES, Chan LC, Wong J, Srivastava G (2001) Establishment and characterization of a new xenograft-derived human esophageal squamous cell carcinoma cell line SLMT-1 of Chinese origin. Cancer Genet Cytogenet 124:36–41
8. Hu Y, Lam KY, Wan TS, Fang W, Ma ES, Chan LC, Srivastava G (2000) Establishment and characterization of HKESC-1, a new cancer cell line from human esophageal squamous cell carcinoma. Cancer Genet Cytogenet 118:112–120
9. Pun IH, Chan D, Chan SH, Chung PY, Zhou YY, Law S, Lam AK, Chui CH, Chan AS, Lam KH, Tang JC (2017) Anti-cancer effects of a novel quinoline derivative 83b1 on human esophageal squamous cell carcinoma through down-regulation of COX-2 mRNA and PGE (2). Cancer Res Treat 49:219–229
10. Ip JC, Ko JM, Yu VZ, Chan KW, Lam AK, Law S, Tong DK, Lung ML (2015) A versatile orthotopic nude mouse model for study of esophageal squamous cell carcinoma. Biomed Res Int 2015:910715
11. Ng HY, Li J, Tao L, Lam AK, Chan KW, Ko JMY, Yu VZ, Wong M, Li B, Lung ML (2018) Chemotherapeutic treatments increase PD-L1 expression in esophageal squamous cell carcinoma through EGFR/ERK activation. Transl Oncol 11:1323–1333
12. Nishikawa T, Takaoka M, Ohara T, Tomono Y, Hao H, Bao X, Fukazawa T, Wang Z, Sakurama K, Fujiwara Y, Motoki T, Shirakawa Y, Yamatsuji T, Tanaka N, Fujiwara T, Naomoto Y (2013) Antiproliferative effect of a novel mTOR inhibitor temsirolimus contributes to the prolonged survival of orthotopic esophageal cancer-bearing mice. Cancer Biol Ther 14:230–236
13. Hou W, Qin X, Zhu X, Fei M, Liu P, Liu L, Moon H, Zhang P, Greshock J, Bachman KE, Ye BC, Wang H, Zang CY (2013) Lapatinib inhibits the growth of esophageal squamous cell carcinoma and synergistically interacts with 5-fluorouracil in patient-derived xenograft models. Oncol Rep 30:707–714
14. Zhang J, Jiang D, Li X, Lv J, Xie L, Zheng L, Gavine PR, Hu Q, Shi Y, Tan L, Ge D, Xu S, Li L, Zhu L, Hou Y, Wang Q (2014) Establishment and characterization of esophageal squamous cell carcinoma patient-derived xenograft mouse models for preclinical drug discovery. Lab Investig 94:917–926
15. Wu X, Zhang J, Zhen R, Lv J, Zheng L, Su X, Zhu G, Gavine PR, Xu S, Lu S, Hou J, Liu Y, Xu C, Tan Y, Xie L, Yin X, He D, Ji Q, Hou Y, Ge D (2012) Trastuzumab anti-tumor efficacy in patient-derived esophageal squamous cell carcinoma xenograft (PDECX) mouse models. J Transl Med 10:180
16. Xu C, Li X, Liu P, Li M, Luo F (2019) Patient-derived xenograft mouse models: a high fidelity tool for individualized medicine. Oncol Lett 17:3–10
17. Jirkof P, Tourvieille A, Cinelli P, Arras M (2015) Buprenorphine for pain relief in mice: repeated injections vs sustained-release depot formulation. Lab Anim 49:177–187

18. Tomayko MM, Reynolds CP (1989) Determination of subcutaneous tumor size in athymic (nude) mice. Cancer Chemother Pharmacol 24:148–154
19. Vosgha H, Ariana A, Smith RA, Lam AK (2018) miR-205 targets angiogenesis and EMT concurrently in anaplastic thyroid carcinoma. Endocr Relat Cancer 25:323–337
20. Maroof H, Islam F, Dong L, Ajjikuttira P, Gopalan V, McMillan NAJ, Lam AK (2018) Liposomal delivery of miR-34b-5p induced cancer cell death in thyroid carcinoma. Cell 7: E265

Chapter 12

Orthotopic Xenograft Mouse Model in Esophageal Squamous Cell Carcinoma

Valen Z. Yu, Joseph C. Y. Ip, Josephine M. Y. Ko, Lihua Tao, Alfred K. Lam, and Maria L. Lung

Abstract

Orthotopic xenograft model recapitulates the faithful organ-specific microenvironment and facilitates analyses involving tumor-stromal interactions that are crucial for developing new-generation cancer therapy. Herein, we describe the detailed rationales and protocols of a versatile orthotopic xenograft model for esophageal squamous cell carcinoma.

Key words Esophageal squamous cell carcinoma, Orthotopic model, Xenograft, Live animal imaging, Bioluminescence imaging

1 Introduction

Cancer cells have been the focus for cancer treatment. Other than the malignant epithelial components, the contribution of the tumor stroma, including immune cells, fibroblasts, and endothelial cells, to tumor development and therapeutic resistance has been gaining attention [1]. Compared to the routinely used subcutaneous model for cancer, the orthotopic xenograft model (establishment of the cancer in the usual site of occurrence) recapitulates the faithful organ-specific microenvironment and facilities the interactions between the cancer cells and the stromal compartment. Such interaction plays crucial roles in cancer development and drug responses. Hence, the establishment of orthotopic xenograft models for various cancer types has been the preferred choice for translational studies.

There are a few established orthotopic models in esophageal squamous cell carcinoma (ESCC). Furihata and colleagues introduced the first orthotopic model of esophageal squamous cell carcinoma (ESCC) in which they injected a single ESCC cell line into the submucosa of the lower esophagus [2]. Ohara and

Alfred K. Lam (ed.), *Esophageal Squamous Cell Carcinoma: Methods and Protocols*, Methods in Molecular Biology, vol. 2129, https://doi.org/10.1007/978-1-0716-0377-2_12,

colleagues injected ESCC cell lines through the cervicothoracic esophageal lumen from the mouth and monitored tumor progression by computed tomography imaging [3]. Song and colleagues implanted fragments of a pre-established subcutaneous ESCC cell line-derived tumor into the abdominal esophagus and monitored tumor growth by bioluminescent imaging [4]. Kuroda and colleagues injected a single ESCC cell line near the gastro-esophageal junction and observed local lymph node metastases and peritoneal disseminations [5]. Recently, Tung and colleagues described an orthotopic model in which cells were injected into the wall of the cervical esophagus through a surgical opening in the neck of the mouse [6].

Here we describe the detailed procedures for a versatile orthotopic ESCC xenograft model, as well as bioluminescence imaging in live animals [7]. Cells are injected into the intra-esophageal wall at the middle-lower esophagus of the mouse. We target the middle-lower portion for injection because more than 70% of human ESCC cases originate at the middle-lower esophagus [8]. We aim at introducing an orthotopic model with highly reproducible and well-controlled surgical procedures and maximal mouse recovery after surgery. In addition, the procedures can be easily modified for injection of other materials such as organoid cultures of ESCC.

2 Materials

2.1 Reagents and Consumables

1. Mice: inbred BALB/cAnN-nu athymic nude mice, female, 4–6 weeks old (*see* **Note 1**).
2. Cancer cell lines: human esophageal squamous cell carcinoma cell lines [9–11]: 81-T; SLMT-1; KYSE30; KYSE150 (*see* Table 1 and **Note 2**).
3. RPMI-based culture medium: plain RPMI-1640 medium, 10% fetal bovine serum (FBS), 1% penicillin-streptomycin solution (*see* **Note 3**).
4. Dulbecco's Modified Eagle's Medium (DMEM)-based culture medium: plain DMEM, 10% FBS, 1% penicillin-streptomycin solution.
5. Dulbecco's phosphate-buffered saline (DPBS) (*see* **Note 4**).
6. Trypsin-ethylenediaminetetraacetic acid (EDTA) (0.25%) (*see* **Note 5**).
7. Cell culture flasks with filter cap.
8. 1.5 mL Eppendorf microcentrifuge tube.
9. Polypropylene centrifuge tube.
10. 1 mL insulin syringe with 30 G needle (*see* **Note 6**).
11. 1 mL syringe with 25 G needle (*see* **Note 7**).

Table 1
Summary of the ESCC cell lines used

Cell line	ExPASy/ cellosaurus cell line identification	Cell line characteristics	Cell density (per cm^2)	Cell number used in orthotopic injection (in 10 μL)	Reference
81-T	CE81T/VGH (CVCL_Y011)	Well-differentiated ESCC; unknown anatomical location; Taiwan Chinese, male, age 57	$0.6–1 \times 10^5$	1×10^5	[9]
SLMT-1	SLMT-1 (CVCL_E305)	Well-differentiated ESCC in lower esophagus; Hong Kong Chinese, male, age 49	$0.6–1 \times 10^5$	1×10^5	[10]
KYSE30	KYSE-30 (CVCL_1351)	Well-differentiated ESCC in middle esophagus; Japanese, male, age 64	$0.8–1.2 \times 10^5$	5×10^4	[11]
KYSE150	KYSE-150 (CVCL_1348)	Poorly differentiated ESCC in upper esophagus; Japanese, female, age 49	$0.8–1.2 \times 10^5$	1×10^5	[11]

12. Meloxicam (*see* **Note 8**).
13. Anesthetic: ketamine (e.g., 10% ketamine hydrochloride) and xylazine (e.g., 2% xylazine hydrochloride) (*see* **Note 9**).
14. Ophthalmic ointment (*see* **Note 10**).
15. Iodophors (*see* **Note 11**).
16. Cotton swab for infant baby (*see* **Note 12**).
17. Vicryl absorbable sutures (*see* **Note 13**).
18. Reflex wound clips (*see* **Note 14**).
19. D-Luciferin, potassium salt (*see* **Note 15**).

2.2 Equipment

1. Biosafety level 2 cabinet (*see* **Note 16**).
2. Water-jacketed CO_2 incubator (*see* **Note 17**).
3. Bright-field microscope with phase contrast (*see* **Note 18**).
4. Benchtop centrifuge with swinging bucket (*see* **Note 19**).
5. Cell counter (*see* **Note 20**).
6. Small animal surgery system for mouse.
7. Laboratory animal warm water blankets and circulators (*see* **Note 21**).
8. Infrared heat lamp.

9. Sterile gauze pad (*see* **Note 22**).
10. Germinator 500 Glass Bead Sterilizer (*see* **Note 23**).
11. Dissecting microscope (*see* **Note 24**).
12. Auxiliary lighting device for dissecting microscope scientific digital scale (*see* **Note 25**).
13. Animal ear punch (*see* **Note 26**).

3 Methods

3.1 Preparation of ESCC Cells

1. Culture all ESCC cell lines in RPMI-based culture medium, except SLMT-1, which is cultured in DMEM-based culture medium. Cell cultures are maintained at 37 °C with 5% CO_2 in a humidified incubator.
2. Expand the cell culture according to your experimental design (*see* Table 1 and **Note 27**).
3. Harvest the cells by trypsinization. Wash the cells with adequate DPBS before trypsinization. Add 0.5 mL of trypsin-EDTA per 25 cm^2 culture surface, e.g., 3.5 mL for a T-175 flask. Incubate at 37 °C for 5 min or until cells detach (*see* **Note 28**).
4. Neutralize trypsin by adding at least two volumes of RPMI- or DMEM-based culture medium (*see* **Note 29**).
5. Transfer the solution to a centrifuge tube. Mix the solution well by pipetting. Aliquot 500 μL to a microcentrifuge tube and perform cell counting (*see* **Note 30**).
6. Pellet the cells by centrifugation at 200 × *g* for 5 min at room temperature.
7. Aspirate the supernatant without disturbing the pellet. Resuspend the pellet in at least 10 mL of DPBS. Pellet the cells.
8. Resuspend the cells in plain RPMI or DMEM medium without FBS or penicillin–streptomycin solution according to the cell count. Keep the cell on ice before injection (*see* **Note 31**).

3.2 Orthotopic Inoculation

1. Perform all mouse experiments in accordance with guidelines and roles of the relevant institutions and national regulations.
2. Administer the anti-inflammatory drug meloxicam to reduce pain or discomfort. Meloxicam is provided in the drinking water 2 days prior to surgery and 3 days after surgery (*see* **Note 32**).
3. Set up the working bench including the dissecting microscope with lighting device, the small animal surgery system with the warm blanket, and all the surgical instruments. Wipe the surface of the equipment with 70% ethanol, and sterilize the surgical instruments using the glass bead sterilizer.

4. Identify the individual mouse by ear punch and weigh all mice (*see* **Note 33**).
5. Restrain the mouse in a head-down position. Anesthetize the mouse by intraperitoneal injection of ketamine/xylazine solution using a syringe with 25 G or 27 G needle. Inject a final volume of 200 μL per 20 g mouse into the lower right quadrant of the abdomen at an angle of 30–45°. Before injecting, ensure negative pressure by pulling the plunger after inserting the needle intraperitoneally (*see* **Note 34**).
6. Keep the mouse in the cage until it is fully anesthetized (*see* **Note 35**).
7. Coat the eyes of the animal with ointment (*see* **Note 36**).
8. Place the mouse ventrally on the small animal surgery system, with a pre-heated warm blanket beneath the body. The intended operation area is below the left side of the rib cage and diaphragm near the stomach (*see* Fig. 1a). Disinfect that area with iodophors, followed by 70% ethanol.
9. Make a skin incision around 10 mm along the edge of the rib cage, followed by an aligned peritoneal dissection. Gently keep the wound open using the retractors on the surgery system to maximize visualization (*see* **Note 37**).
10. Locate the stomach and the esophagus. Carefully separate the connective tissues between the small left liver lobe and the esophagus.
11. Gently straighten the esophagus by pulling out the stomach caudally. Rest the gastroesophageal junction on a cotton swab (*see* Fig. 1b and **Note 38**).
12. Remove the plunger of an insulin syringe with 30G needle, and load 10 μL of plain medium containing desired number of cells

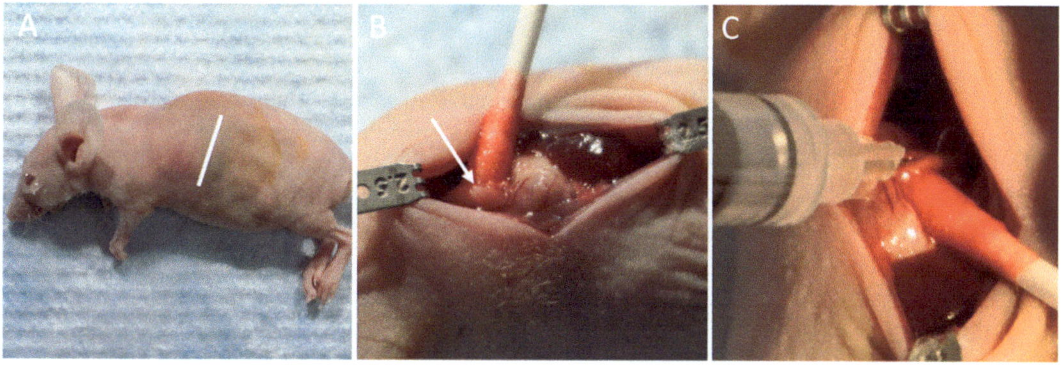

Fig. 1 Representative photos showing surgical procedures of the implantation of cancer cells in the mouse. (**a**) Ventral positioning of the mouse ready for surgery. The skin incision site is indicated by a white line. (**b**) Esophagus (arrow) resting on a cotton swap. The asterisk indicates the stomach of the mouse. (**c**) Insertion of needle into the esophageal wall for cell injection

into the syringe from the opening using a P10 or P20 pipetman. Re-insert the plunger gently avoiding any bubbles. Insert the whole needle horizontally with bevel facing outward along the esophageal wall. Expel the cells into the muscularis externa of the esophagus under the microscope. Edema should be observed at the inoculation site immediately (*see* Fig. 1c and **Note 39**).

13. After injection, press a cotton swab at the inoculation site while gently retracting the needle to minimize cell leakage to the peritoneum (*see* **Note 40**).
14. Release the retractors. Close the peritoneum wound using vicryl absorbable sutures; close the skin incision by reflex wound clips.
15. Remove the mouse from the surgery system, and place it near a heat lamp for recovery. Closely monitor the mouse until it regains full motility (*see* **Note 41**).
16. Mice are then housed and monitored daily. Clips are removed in 14 days. Body weight and activity status are routinely recorded.

3.3 Live Animal Imaging

1. Live animal imaging is performed weekly using in vivo imaging system. Luciferase-labelled cells can be monitored by the bioluminescent signals in the mouse body.
2. Anesthetize the mouse by intraperitoneal injection of ketamine/xylazine solution, and apply ointment to the eyes (*see* **Note 42**).
3. Inject the firefly luciferase substrate luciferin at 150 mg/kg (100 μL of stock solution for a 20 g mouse) by intraperitoneal injection (*see* **Notes 15** and **43**).
4. Mouse is then imaged in the prone position by the IVIS spectrum system 10–20 min after injection of luciferin. Image up to 6–12 mice each time (*see* Fig. 2 and **Note 44**).
5. Euthanize all mice at the end of study. Examine the orthotopic tumor growth. Collect and divide the tumors, and store in liquid nitrogen or fix in formalin followed by paraffin embedding for future analyses (*see* Fig. 3 for autopsy photos showing tumor formation and Fig. 4 for hematoxylin and eosin (H&E) staining of the tumors).

4 Notes

1. Choosing nude mice for human orthotopic xenograft experiments is preferable. Nude mice possess a more intact host immune microenvironment as compared to other commonly

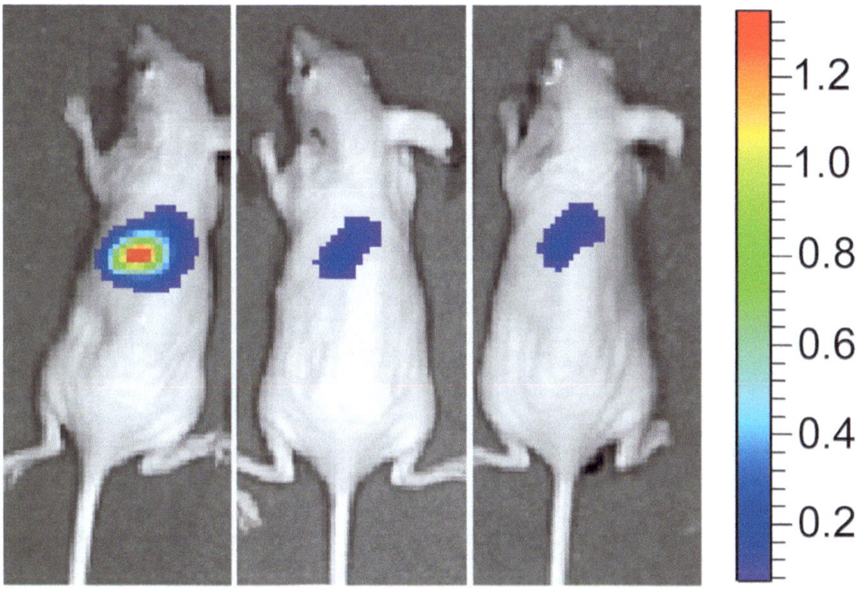

Fig. 2 Representative live animal images showing bioluminescent signals indicating tumor formation. Unit of signal intensity: million photons/second/square centimeter/steradian

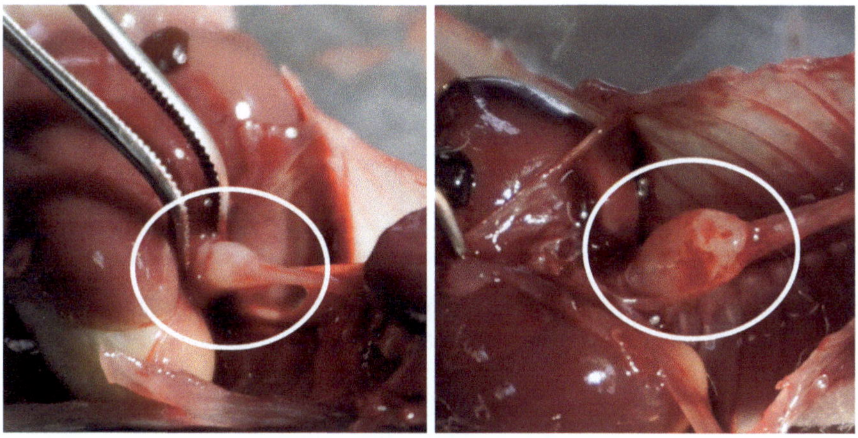

Fig. 3 Representative autopsy photos of the mouse showing esophageal tumor formation above the diaphragm (circled)

used immunodeficient mouse models, e.g., severe combined immunodeficient mice and NOD scid gamma (NSG) mice. Nude mouse model is also frequently used in other xenograft experiments, and the results from orthotopic xenograft experiments can be easily compared side by side with other xenograft experiments, e.g., subcutaneous xenograft and tail vein experimental metastasis experiments.

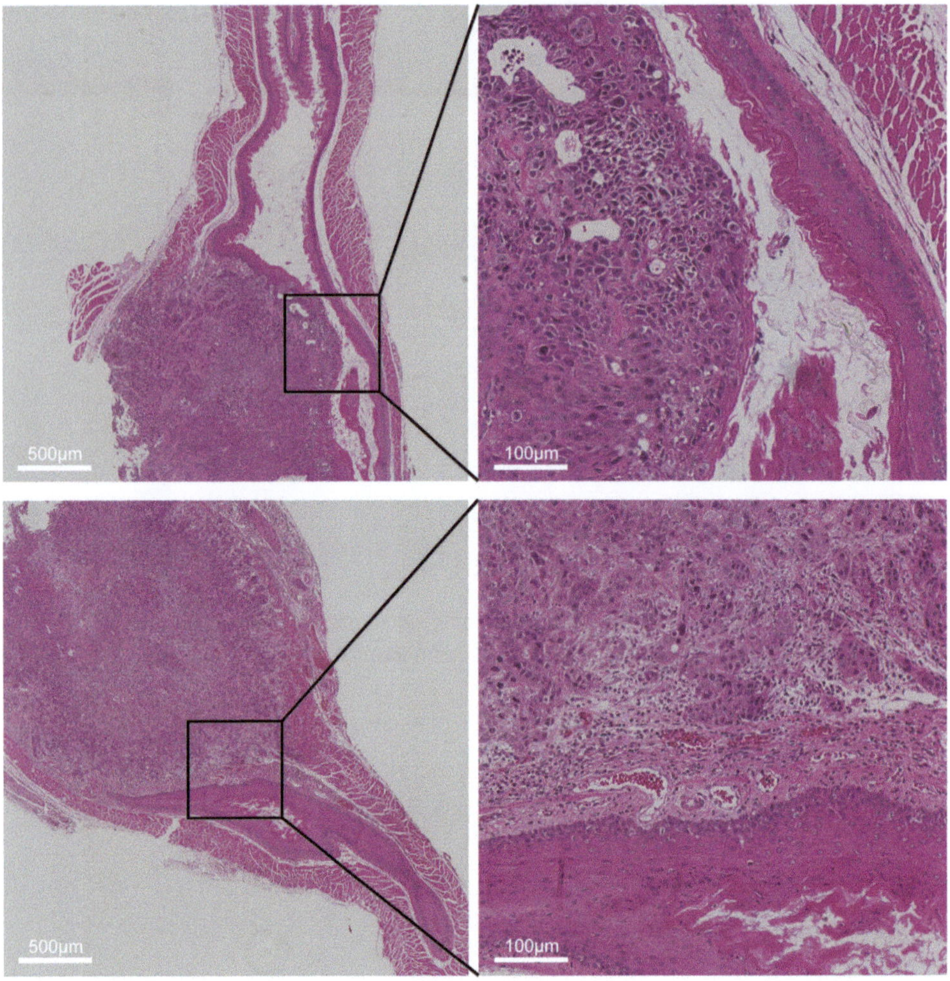

Fig. 4 Representative hematoxylin and eosin staining images of two orthotopic ESCC xenografts showing disrupted (upper panel) or intact (lower panel) epithelia

2. All cell lines used are labelled with bioluminescent firefly luciferase to facilitate live animal imaging of the orthotopic tumors [7].
3. Appropriate tissue culture practice done according to guidelines by the American Type Culture Collection and the European Collection of Cell Cultures. Tissue culture using biosafety level 2 cabinet should follow the National Institute of Health guidelines. FBS is heat-inactivated at 56 °C for 30 min to disable the complement system. Penicillin–streptomycin solution is used in tissue culture medium in a final concentration of 100 U/mL (1% v/v), as a broad-spectrum antibiotic to prevent bacterial contamination.
4. Dulbecco's phosphate-buffered saline is used to wash the cells before trypsinization to remove serum and before injection to

remove any residual trypsin and for drug/substrate preparation.

5. Trypsin-EDTA is used for cell dissociation from the culture surface.
6. The insulin syringe with 30G needle is used for orthotopic injection due to its minimal dead space and small needle size.
7. The 1 mL syringe with 25G needle is used to administer the anesthetic and luciferin through intraperitoneal injection.
8. Meloxicam is used to reduce pain or discomfort caused by the surgery.
9. The ketamine/xylazine combination is a reliable anesthetic for mouse surgery. The final working concentration for mouse is 100 mg/kg ketamine and 10 mg/kg xylazine. Dilute the stock in sterile water. Store the working solution at 4 °C for a maximum of 2 weeks.
10. Ophthalmic ointment is applied to the eyes of the animal to prevent desiccation; the eyes of animal under anesthesia remain open, which can lead to corneal drying and trauma.
11. Iodophors are used to disinfect skin of the mouse at the surgical site.
12. Cotton swab for infant baby has a smaller cotton bud than the usual type, which is suitable for the limited space near the mouse esophagus.
13. The absorbable suture is used to close the peritoneum wound.
14. The absorbable suture is used to close the skin incision.
15. Luciferin is the substrate for firefly luciferase. The stock solution is prepared in DPBS at a concentration of 30 mg/mL.
16. Appropriate tissue culture practice done according to guidelines by the American Type Culture Collection and the European Collection of Cell Cultures. Tissue culture using biosafety level 2 cabinet should follow the National Institute of Health guidelines.
17. Water-jacketed incubator is used for its better temperature stability compared to direct heat incubator. CO_2 level is maintained at 5%. High humidity is maintained using a pan of water in the incubator. The insides of the incubator, including shelves and water pan, are routinely cleaned and disinfected by ethanol and germicidal ultraviolet light.
18. Microscope is used for routine inspection of cell status.
19. Centrifuge is used to pellet cells after trypsinization and wash.
20. An automatic cell counter is used to accurately count the cell number in solution and to determine cell status by monitoring the size distribution pattern. Healthy cell populations display a

typical bell-shaped Gaussian distribution, while unhealthy populations display a left shift in the histogram. A 60 μm sensor, designed for particles/cells of a diameter between 6 μm and 36 μm, is used as the ESCC cells growing on culture surface have a diameter between 15 μm and 20 μm when detached.

21. The warm blanket is used to maintain body temperature during surgery. Alternatively, a microwave heat pack can be used.
22. The gauze pad is used to cover the mouse during recovery.
23. The glass bead sterilizer is used to sterilize surgical instruments. Turn on the sterilizer in advance to reach optimal working temperature. Gently insert and pull out the surgical instruments to avoid any damages to the blades.
24. The dissecting microscope is used for better visualization during mouse surgery.
25. The scale is used to weigh the mouse to accurately deliver the needed amount of anesthetic and bioluminescent substrate.
26. The ear punch is used to differentiate mice for subsequent experiment and future data recording.
27. It is crucial to maintain the culture under full confluency during subculture and for orthotopic injection to achieve consistency between batches.
28. Avoid over-trypsinization longer than 10 min to maintain best cell status. Cell surface proteins/structures will be damaged after prolonged trypsinization, and cell integrity will be compromised.
29. Serum contains protease inhibitors as α1-anti-trypsin that inhibit trypsin activity.
30. Automated cell counter shows top accuracy when the test cell concentration is between 5×10^4 and 5×10^5/mL. Results from solution outside the range may be faulty and should not be used in following analysis. Perform dilution to achieve the optimal range if necessary.
31. Keeping the cells on ice in serum-free medium slows down metabolic activity and minimizes cell death.
32. The stock of meloxicam is 5 mg/mL. Administrating meloxicam (1.5 mg/mL in drinking water) in advance allows the mice to accept the drug.
33. The weight of individual mouse is for estimation of the volume of anesthetic that will be needed.
34. Hold the mouse head-down, and perform intraperitoneal injection at the lower right abdomen to minimize damages to the internal organs. Negative pressure ensures that the needle is in the peritoneal cavity. Mouse will start to wake up in around

half an hour; therefore, do not anesthetize too many mice at the same time.

35. Apply pressure to the footpad of the mouse; absence of any reflex response indicates good anesthesia.
36. Avoid touching the eyes with the tip of the ointment dispenser.
37. Minimize the incision to facilitate better closure of the wound and better recovery. Minimize the force needed of the retractor to avoid unnecessary damage to the wound.
38. Perform this step with extreme care; the esophagus is fragile and may be damaged by excessive pulls, endangering the mouse. The cotton swab is used to hold the junction in position and to absorb any leaked cell solution during injection. Do not over-straighten the esophagus; cells may leak out from the inoculation site due to excessive pressure.
39. Well-mix the cell-containing solution before loading; avoid any bubbles. Keep the cell-containing syringe on ice until injection. To maximize accuracy of such a small volume, do not re-use syringe. Try to inject the cells in the upper region of the esophagus to better recapitulate the tumor growth site in human of ESCC.
40. Used syringe with needle should be discarded instantly into a biohazard sharp box.
41. Do not directly expose the mouse to the heat lamp as it may cause skin burns and dehydration. Cover the mouse with sterile gauze pad.
42. Do not anesthetize too many mice at the same time; the whole imaging process takes around 20 min. Image up to 6–12 mice each time.
43. Keep the mouse warm by heat lamp or heat pad before imaging.
44. Mouse can be imaged individually and sequentially or can be imaged in a group of up to 12 mice altogether. The luciferin injected is of excess amount; bioluminescent signal reaches maximum in 10 min and lasts for at least half an hour.

Acknowledgments

The Research Grants Council of Hong Kong Special Administrative Region, People's Republic of China (HKU 774413M to Maria Li Lung), supported this work. The DSMZ (German Collection of Microorganisms and Cell Culture) provided the KYSE series cell lines. The University of Hong Kong Li Ka Shing Faculty of Medicine Faculty Core Facility provided access to the live animal imaging system.

References

1. Turley SJ, Cremasco V, Astarita JL (2015) Immunological hallmarks of stromal cells in the tumour microenvironment. Nat Rev Immunol 15:669–682
2. Furihata T, Sakai T, Kawamata H et al (2001) A new in vivo model for studying invasion and metastasis of esophageal squamous cell carcinoma. Int J Oncol 19:903–907
3. Ohara T, Takaoka M, Sakurama K et al (2010) The establishment of a new mouse model with orthotopic esophageal cancer showing the esophageal stricture. Cancer Lett 293:207–212
4. Song S, Chang D, Cui Y et al (2014) New orthotopic implantation model of human esophageal squamous cell carcinoma in athymic nude mice. Thorac Cancer 5:417–424
5. Kuroda S, Kubota T, Aoyama K et al (2014) Establishment of a non-invasive semi-quantitative bioluminescent imaging method for monitoring of an Orthotopic esophageal cancer mouse model. PLoS One 9:e114562
6. Tung LN, Song S, Chan KT et al (2018) Preclinical study of novel curcumin analogue SSC-5 using orthotopic tumor xenograft model for esophageal squamous cell carcinoma. Cancer Res Treat 50:1362–1377
7. Ip JC, Ko JM, Yu VZ et al (2015) A versatile orthotopic nude mouse model for study of esophageal squamous cell carcinoma. Biomed Res Int 2015:910715
8. Daly JM, Fry WA, Little AG et al (2000) Esophageal cancer: results of an American College of Surgeons patient care evaluation study. J Am Coll Surg 190:562–572; discussion 572-563
9. Hu CP, Hsieh HG, Chien KY et al (1984) Biologic properties of three newly established human esophageal carcinoma cell lines. J Natl Cancer Inst 72:577–583
10. Tang JC, Wan TS, Wong N et al (2001) Establishment and characterization of a new xenograft-derived human esophageal squamous cell carcinoma cell line SLMT-1 of Chinese origin. Cancer Genet Cytogenet 124:36–41
11. Shimada Y, Imamura M, Wagata T et al (1992) Characterization of 21 newly established esophageal cancer cell lines. Cancer 69:277–284

Chapter 13

In Vitro Assays of Biological Aggressiveness of Esophageal Squamous Cell Carcinoma

Farhadul Islam, Vinod Gopalan, and Alfred K. Lam

Abstract

Researchers are developing new techniques and technologies to determine the characteristic features for cancer progression, thereby identifying potential targets and therapeutics to interfere these hallmark processes of cancer pathogenesis. The transformative researches using these in vitro methods have enable researchers to design precision treatments of patients with esophageal squamous cell carcinoma (ESCC). These in vitro methods mainly include analysis of cell proliferation, cytotoxicity, colony formation, invasion, and migration in ESCC cells for analyzing manipulations affecting the biological behavior of ESCC. Because of these studies, important information on molecular mechanisms of different genes and proteins as well as result of therapeutic interventions are confirmed in ESCC.

Key words Biological aggressiveness, Cell proliferation, Cytotoxicity, Invasion, Migration

1 Introduction

Carcinogenesis is a multi-step process in which normal cells progressively convert to malignant cells. During this transformation, key processes of cells, i.e., sustained proliferation, evading growth suppressors, resisting death, enabling replicative immortality, angiogenesis, invasion, and metastasis, which are regarded as cancer biological hallmarks are aberrantly activated [1, 2]. Genomic instability in cancer cells drives these fundamental processes of tumor development, while inflammation nurtures and accelerates tumor formation [3]. In addition, epigenetic changes, altered energy metabolism, and avoiding immune destruction emerged as crucial players in the initiation and progression of cancer [4, 5]. Furthermore, dynamic interaction of cancer cells and tumor microenvironment critically contributed in the development of cancer [2]. The significance of these cancer biological hallmarks and other contributing factors deregulation in particular cancer pathogenesis depends on the underlying molecular features of the cancer [2, 3].

Alfred K. Lam (ed.), *Esophageal Squamous Cell Carcinoma: Methods and Protocols*, Methods in Molecular Biology, vol. 2129, https://doi.org/10.1007/978-1-0716-0377-2_13, © Springer Science+Business Media, LLC, part of Springer Nature 2020

Abnormalities of growth and/or survival pathways or their component regulate the cancer biological hallmarks [2]. Functional assays especially in vitro assays are the best available options for examining the role of a given hallmark in a particular cancer pathogenesis [2, 6, 7]. However, selection of appropriate assays for investigating a particular hallmarks or concurrent analysis of multiple hallmarks in cancer cell is challenging. Assay combination provides better insight of cancer hallmarks, but factors such as multiplexing, sequential measurement, cost, time, quantitative real-time or end point analysis, etc. need to be considered [3]. The in vitro functional assays are being used to investigate biological hallmarks on cancer, to identify cancer-promoting or cancer-inhibiting genes, or to test new drugs summarized in Table 1.

In vitro assays play essential roles in research in esophageal squamous cell carcinoma (ESCC) [8–19]. They are important in understanding the roles of many genes and proteins and miRNA expressions in ESCC. In addition, they can be used to identify the function of novel genes and test therapeutic interventions in ESCC. Moreover, these in vitro assays guide the researchers for the development of new therapeutics; thereby transfer the information from laboratories to clinical settings for better management of patients with ESCC. Similarly, in other cancers, these assays are being used as the quick tools for discovery and developing new therapeutics against other cancers [20–24].

Understanding of pathogenesis and alterations in proliferation-related factors (nuclear proteins), apoptotic factors (pro−/anti-apoptotic proteins), metastatic factors (cell adhesion molecules and enzyme related to degradation of extracellular matrix), and angiogenic factors continue to evolve in ESCC [25]. To acheive advancement in the field of molecular biology in ESCC, we need to apply many in vitro assays for analyzing hallmarks of ESCC and discovering potential drugs for ESCC. These assays include cell proliferation assays, colony formation assays, wound healing assays, as well as invasion and migration assays performed with proper controls.

2 Materials

Use all the chemicals and reagents of analytical grade. Prepare required solutions using ultrapure water, and store all the reagents and solutions at room temperature unless otherwise indicated. Follow the guidelines and regulations of waste disposal during disposing waste materials, and use the appropriate personal protective equipment during experiments to minimize the laboratory hazards.

Table 1
In vitro assays used to evaluate biological aggressiveness and drug development in cancer

Cancer processes	Biochemical/ cellular event	Assays	Principle	References
Sustained proliferation and evading growth suppressors	Metabolic activity	MTT, XTT, MTS, WST-1, WST-8	Redox reaction—colorless compounds are reduced by living cells to brightly colored metabolites	[26–30]
	Protein content	Sulforhodamine B staining	Binds amino acid residues in living cell proteins through its sulfonic group and gives an estimation of total protein mass	[31]
	Membrane integrity	Trypan blue Propidium iodide SYTOX Yo-PRO-1 Lactate dehydrogenase	Dead cells or substances released from a cell take up the dye	[31–34]
	DNA synthesis	BrdU $3H$-thymidine	Substances are incorporated into new strands during de novo DNA synthesis	[35, 36]
	Colony formation	Colony counting	Cells grown in culture	[16]
Resisting cell death	Morphological changes	Microscopic imaging	Cell staining	[37]
	Genome fragmentation	DNA laddering	DNA staining	[38]
		DNA content analysis	DNA staining: PI, acridine orange, ethidium bromide, Hoechst 33,342, etc.	[32]
		TUNEL	Labeling DNA breaks by terminal transferase with fluorescently marked dUT	[39]
	Plasma membrane changes	Annexin binding	PS-binding Annexin V-labeled FITC or phycoerythrin	[40]
		LDH activity	LDH enzyme reaction linked to NADH reduction leads to absorbance changes of specific probes	[41]
	Caspase activity	Direct detection	Using specific mAbs for active or inactive form of the proteins	[42]
		PARP assay	Using specific mAbs for cleaved or uncleaved caspase target protein PARP	[43]

(continued)

Table 1
(continued)

Cancer processes	Biochemical/ cellular event	Assays	Principle	References
Replicative immortality	Length of telomeres	TRF analysis	Identification of telomeres through Southern blotting or in-gel hybridization using a probe specific for telomeric DNA	[44]
	Telomerase activity	TRAP analysis	Using substrate specificity of telomerase	[45]
Inducing angiogenesis	Blood vessel formation	Tube formation	Endothelial cells rapidly form capillary-like structures when plated on top of a basement membrane extracellular matrix	[46]
	Angiogenesis activators	Direct detection	Using mAbs for angiogenesis activators, i.e., VEGF, FGF, EGF, etc. by immunoblot or ELISA	[47]
Activating invasion and metastasis	Transwell migration and invasion	Boyden chamber	Cell counting based on fluorescent staining	[48]
	Wound healing	Scratch healing	Cell counting with time-lapse microscopy	[49]

MTT 3-(4,5-dimethylthiazol-2-yl)-2,5-diphenyltetrazolium bromide, *XTT* (2,3-bis-(2-methoxy-4-nitro-5-sulfophenyl)-2*H*-tetrazolium-5-carboxanilide), *MTS* (3-(4,5-dimethylthiazol-2-yl)-5-(3-carboxymethoxyphenyl)-2-(4-sulfophenyl)-2*H*-tetrazolium), *WST-1* water-soluble tetrazolium salt 1, *WST-8* water-soluble tetrazolium salt 8, *BrdU* 5-bromo-2′-deoxyuridine, *TUNEL* terminal deoxynucleotidyl transferase dUTP nick end labeling, *PS* phosphatidylserine, *FITC* fluorescein isothiocyanate, *LDH* lactate dehydrogenase, *NADH* nicotinamide adenine dinucleotide hydrogen, *PARP* poly(ADP-ribose) polymerase, *TRF* terminal restriction fragments, *TRAP* telomeric repeat amplification protocol, *VEGF* vascular endothelial growth factor, *FGF* fibroblast growth factor, *EGF* epidermal growth factor, *ELISA* enzyme-linked immunosorbent assay

2.1 Cell Culture

1. Esophageal squamous cell carcinoma cells.
2. Cell culture media: Roswell Park Memorial Institute (RPMI) 1640, L-glutamine, pH 7.2. Add 900 mL water to a glass beaker and stir gently. Add 10.4 g RPMI 1640 powder media to the water (*see* **Note 1**). Stir to dissolve completely the powder. Do not heat the media (*see* **Note 2**). Then, weigh 2.0 g of sodium bicarbonate and pour to the media. Stir for complete dissolving. Then adjust the pH with 1 N HCl (hydrogen chloride) and NaOH (sodium hydroxide). Add water up to mark 1 L, sterilize with 0.22 micron membrane filter, and aseptically transfer media into sterile container. Store at 4 °C.
3. 10% fetal bovine serum (FBS) in sterile media (*see* **Note 3**). Store at 4 °C.
4. 1% mixture of penicillin and streptomycin antibiotic in sterile media. Store at 4 °C (*see* **Note 4**).

5. Cell washing buffer: phosphate-buffered saline (PBS), pH 7.4. Add 8.0 g NaCl, 0.2 g KCl, 1.42 g Na_2HPO_4, and 0.24 g KH_2PO_4 in glass beaker. Dissolve all the salts in 800 mL water, and adjust the pH with 1 N HCl. Add water to a total volume of 1 L. Sterilize and store 4 °C.
6. Cell dissociation solution: 0.25% trypsin-ethylenediaminetetraacetic acid (EDTA), pH 7.2–8. Stored at −20 °C (*see* **Note 5**).
7. Cell culture flasks: polystyrene 25 cm^2 and 75 cm^2 flasks.
8. Falcon 15 mL and 50 mL conical centrifuge tubes.
9. Microscope.
10. Centrifuge machines.
11. 80% ethanol in water (v/v).
12. CO2 incubator.
13. 1.5 mL and 10 mL serological pipettes.
14. Gloves.

2.2 Cell Proliferation

1. Cell proliferation assay kit.
2. Cell culture plates: 6-wells, 12-wells, 48-wells, and 96-wells.
3. Plate reader with 450 nm filter.
4. 10 μL, 100–200 μL pipettes.
5. Multi-channel pipettes.
6. 10 μL, 100–200 μL, 1 mL tips.
7. 0.4% trypan blue or equivalent viability stain.
8. Automated cell counter or hemocytometer.

2.3 Cytotoxicity Assay

1. Tested drugs/compounds.
2. Positive controls.
3. Negative control or solvent control.

2.4 Colony Formation Assay

1. 0.5% crystal violet in water (w/v).
2. Methanol.
3. Glacial acetic acid.
4. Fixation solution: acetic acid/methanol 1:7 (v/v).
5. Stereomicroscope.
6. ImageJ software.

2.5 Wound Healing Assay

1. 200 μL tips.
2. 6-well plates.
3. Stereomicroscope.
4. ImageJ software.

2.6 Invasion and Migration Assays

1. Low-speed centrifuge.
2. Cell invasion and migration assay kit.
3. 50 and 500 mL graduated cylinders.
4. −80 °C, −20 °C, and 4 °C storage facility.
5. Ice bucket.
6. Standard light microscope (or inverted).
7. Timer.
8. Vortex mixer.
9. Fluorescent 96-well plate reader, top reader (485 nm excitation, 520 nm emission).
10. Black 96-well plate (for standard curve).
11. Serum-free media: tissue culture growth media without serum.
12. Drugs or pharmacological agents to be tested.
13. Distilled deionized water.

3 Methods

3.1 Cell Culture

1. Take the cryovial containing ESCC cells from liquid nitrogen facility, and transfer them into a 37 °C water bath.
2. Quickly thaw the cells by gently swirling the vial in water bath at 37 °C (*see* **Note 6**).
3. Carefully transfer the vial into a biosafety cabinet, and wipe out the sides of the vial with 80% ethanol.
4. Add pre-warmed complete growth media (2 mL) in a 15 mL centrifuge tube.
5. Add the thawed cells drop-wise into the tube.
6. Centrifuge the cell suspension at approximately 400 × *g* for 3–5 min.
7. Check the cell pellet after centrifugation, and aseptically decant the supernatant without disrupting the cell pellet.
8. Add 2 mL PBS and resuspend the cell pellet with slow pipetting.
9. Centrifuge the suspension at 400 × *g* for 3–5 min and discard the supernatant.
10. Resuspend the cell pellets in complete growth media (containing FBS), and transfer them into an appropriate cell culture flask containing recommended growth media.
11. Incubate in the CO_2 incubator at appropriate conditions (*see* **Note 7**).

3.2 Cell Proliferation Assay

1. Grow the ESCC cells up to 70–80% confluency.
2. Collect cells after trypsinization followed by resuspension in growth media.
3. Inoculate cell suspension (100 μL/well) in a 96-well plate (*see* **Note 8**). Pre-incubate the plate in a humidified incubator (37 °C, 5% CO_2).
4. Thaw the cell proliferation assay kit on the bench top or in a water bath at 37 °C, if it is frozen (*see* **Note 9**).
5. Add 10 μL (or suggested by the kit manufacturer) of the cell proliferation assay solution to each well of the plate (*see* **Note 10**).
6. Incubate the plate for 1–4 h in the incubator to develop color.
7. Take the reading at 450 nm using a microplate reader at the end of intended time point (Fig. 1).
8. Prepare a calibration curve using the data obtained from the wells that contain known numbers of viable cells (*see* **Note 11**) (Fig. 2a).

3.3 Cytotoxicity Assay

1. Grow and collect ESCC cells as described in previous sections (Subheadings 3.1 and 3.2).
2. Dispense 100 μL of cell suspension (5000 cells/well) in a 96-well plate.

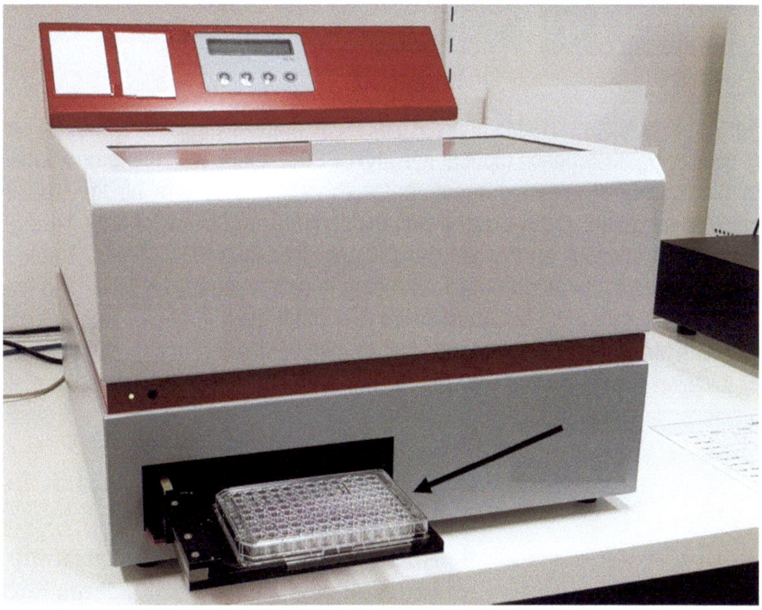

Fig. 1 Microplate reader with 96-well plate. The 96-well plate (arrow) with experimental samples being inserted into the reader to measure the absorbance

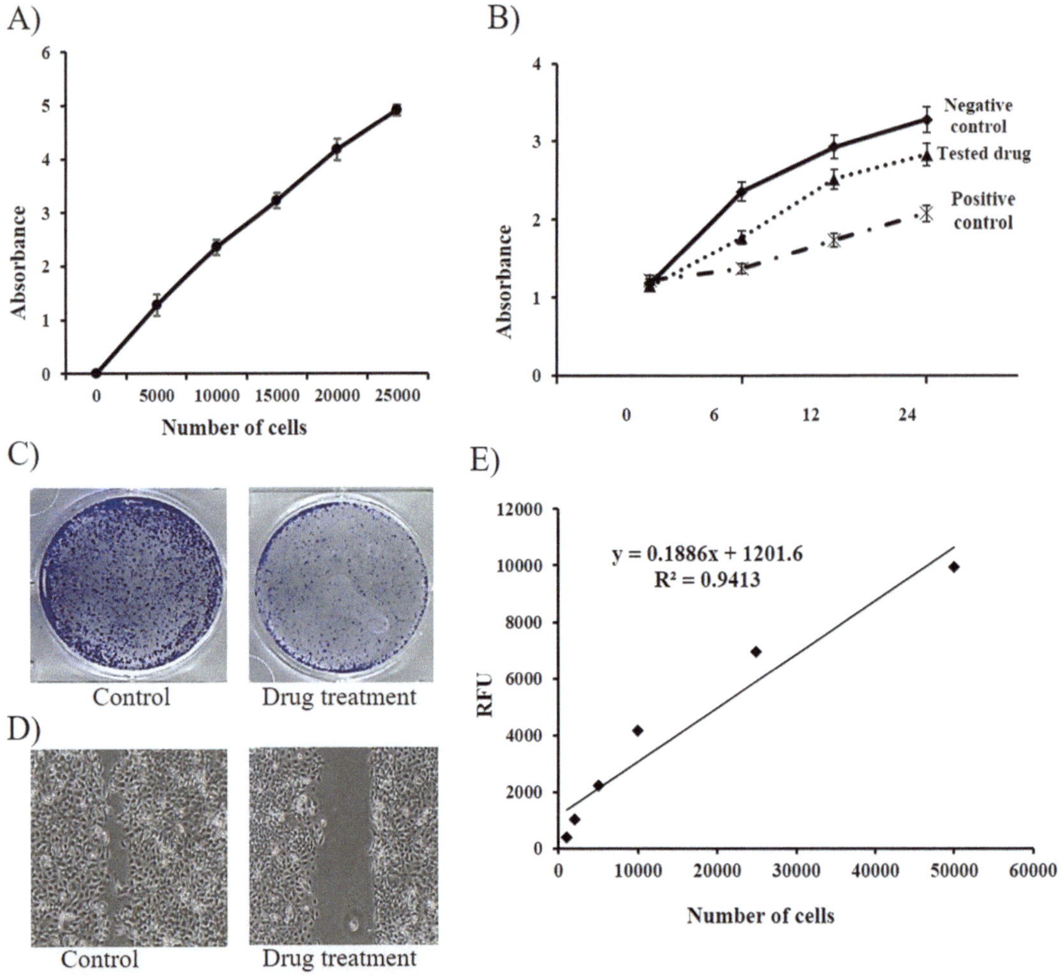

Fig. 2 In vitro assays used to analyze biological aggressiveness of ESCC. (**a**) Cell proliferation was determined by measuring absorbance (optical density) of ESCC cells, which is proportional to the number of viable cells. (**b**) Cytotoxicity of potential agents/drugs examined by observing the viability of ESCC cells (absorbance) following treatment and compared with the controls. (**c**) Colony formation assay used to examine the effects of chemical compounds on the biological aggressiveness of ESCC cells. Treatment of ESCC cells with drug or agent induces death of ESCC cells, resulting in decreased colony formation when compared to that of control cells. (**d**) Wound healing assay employed to monitor the migration properties of ESCC cells. Treatment of ESCC cells with biological active compound or drug induces reduced migration in comparison to that of control cells. (**e**) Invasion assay used to investigate the invasion and migration properties of ESCC cells. RFU (relative fluorescence units)

3. Pre-incubate the plate for 24 h in a humidified incubator (37 °C, 5% CO_2).
4. Add 10 μL of various concentrations of interested toxicant or drugs or pharmacological agents into the culture media in the plate.

5. Incubate the plate for an appropriate length of time such as 6, 12, 24, or 48 h in the incubator.
6. Thaw the assay kit on the bench top or in a water bath at 37 °C, if it is frozen.
7. Add 10 μL or amount suggested by kit manufacturer of assay solution to each well of the plate.
8. Incubate the plate for 1–4 h in the incubator.
9. Measure the absorbance at 450 nm using a microplate reader.
10. Calculate the growth inhibition in comparison to that of negative or solvent control, and compare with positive control (Fig. 2b).

3.4 Colony Formation Assay

1. Culture the cells up to 70–80% confluency in polystyrene 25 cm^2 flask.
2. Remove medium and rinse the ESCC cells with 5 mL 1× PBS.
3. Add 4 mL 0.25% trypsin to the cells, and incubate at 37 °C for 2–5 min until the cells appear round, and tap the flask gently to detach the cells quickly.
4. Add 4 mL medium with 10% FBS and detach the cells by pipetting.
5. Count the cells using a hemocytometer or automated cell counter as appropriate.
6. Prepare desired seeding concentration and seed cells into dishes or 6-well plates in triplicates (at least duplicates). Plate the cells either before or after the treatment (*see* **Note 12**).
7. For plating the cells before treatment, incubate cells for a few hours in a CO_2 incubator at 37 °C, and allow them to attach the plate/dish.
8. Treat the cells with chemicals at various concentrations (1–100 μM), radiation (2–10 Gy), or a combination of both.
9. Incubate the cells in a CO_2 incubator at 37 °C for 1–3 weeks until cells in control plates have formed colonies of a substantially good size (50 cells per colony is the minimum for scoring).
10. For plating the cells after treatment, harvest cells after treatment. Approximately, 50×10^4 cells can be plated.
11. Prepare serial dilutions with different numbers of cells. For radiation treatment, the cells can be plated immediately after treatment, and keep the cells on ice before re-plating.
12. Follow **step 9** to incubate the cells.
13. Remove medium and then rinse cells with 5 mL 1× PBS twice.
14. Remove PBS, and add 2–3 mL of fixation solution, and leave the dishes/plates at room temperature for 15 min.

15. Remove fixation solution.
16. Add 0.5% crystal violet solution and incubate at room temperature for 2 h.
17. After the incubation, add 10 mL medium with 10% FBS, and detach the stain by pipetting.
18. Carefully remove crystal violet by immersing the dishes/plates in tap water gently to rinse off crystal violet.
19. Air-dry the dishes/plates on a tablecloth at room temperature for up to a few days.
20. Count the number of colonies with a stereomicroscope (Fig. 2c).
21. Analyze the data, and calculate plating efficiency (PE) and surviving fraction (SF) (*see* **Note 13**).

3.5 Wound Healing Assay

1. Grow cells in media supplemented with 10% FBS.
2. Seed cells into 6-well tissue culture plates, and grow them until they reach ~70–80% confluence as a monolayer.
3. Do not change the medium; gently and slowly scratch the monolayer with a new 1 mL pipette tip across the center of the well (*see* **Note 14**).
4. Scratch another straight line perpendicular to the first line to create a cross in each well.
5. Then gently wash the well twice with medium to remove the detached cells.
6. Replenish the well with fresh medium (*see* **Note 15**).
7. Grow cells for additional 48 h (or the time required to heal the wound).
8. Wash the cells twice with 1× PBS, and fix the cells with 3.7% paraformaldehyde for 30 min.
9. Then stain the fixed cells with 1% crystal violet in 2% ethanol for 30 min.
10. Take photos for the stained monolayer using a microscope (Fig. 2d).
11. Set the same configurations of the microscope when taking pictures for different views of the stained monolayer. Measure the gap distance using software ImageJ.

3.6 Invasion and Migration Assays

Day 0

1. Culture cells per manufacturer's recommendation: adherent cells should be cultured to no more than 80% confluence, and each well requires at least 50,000 cells, so plan accordingly.

2. Twenty-four hours prior to beginning assay, starve cells in a serum-free medium (0.5% FBS may be used if needed) to allow expression of free receptors.
3. Coat membrane of top invasion chamber (leave three chambers uncoated for a migration control) with 50 μL of 0.1× to 1× basement membrane extract (BME) solution, and incubate for 4 h or overnight at 37 °C in a CO_2 incubator.

Day 1

4. After 24 h of serum starvation (optional), harvest and count cells.
5. Centrifuge cells at 250 × *g* for 10 min, remove supernatant, and wash with 1× wash buffer.
6. Count and resuspend at 1 × 10^6 cells/mL in a serum-free medium.
7. Aspirate top chamber of cell invasion device, and do not allow top or bottom chambers to dry.
8. Add 50 μL of cells per well to top chamber (with or without drugs/chemical agents).
9. Add 150 μL of medium per well to bottom chamber using access port (with or without drugs/agents).
10. Incubate chamber at 37 °C in CO_2 incubator for 24 h.
11. Put different known number of cells in the remaining assay wells for standard curve generation (Fig. 2d).

Day 2

12. Aspirate top chamber carefully and do not puncture membrane.
13. Wash each well with 100 μL of 1× wash buffer.
14. Aspirate the bottom chamber, and wash each well twice with 200 μL 1× wash buffer.
15. Transfer top chambers to assay chamber plate (usually black or other format supplied by manufacturer).
16. Add 12 μL of Calcein-AM solution to 10 mL of cell dissociation solution.
17. Put 100 μL of cell dissociation solution/Calcein-AM to bottom chamber.
18. Assemble cell invasion device, and incubate at 37 °C in CO_2 incubator for 1 h.
19. After the incubation time, remove top chamber, and read plate at 485 nm excitation and 520 nm emission using a fluorescent 96-well plate reader.

20. Using standard curve, convert relative fluorescence units to cell number.
21. Determine the percent of invasion.

4 Notes

1. Powdered media are highly hygroscopic. Therefore, they should be protected from atmospheric moistures. In addition, preparing a concentrated media solution may form precipitation.
2. pH needs to be reduced to 4.0 with 1 N HCl to dissolve the media completely, and the pH can be raised up to 7.2 with 1 N NaOH prior to adding sodium bicarbonate.
3. We noted that 10% FBS is good for the growth and maintenance of the ESCC cells. You may need to optimize the appropriate concentration for your cells.
4. The combined antibiotics penicillin and streptomycin were used to prevent the bacterial contamination of cultured ESCC cells. We found that this concentration is enough to maintain and keep the cells free from bacterial contaminations.
5. Avoid repeated freeze thawing and warm-up of trypsin, and multiple freezing, thawing, and warming may cause the reduced enzymatic activity of trypsin.
6. Thawing procedures is stressful for the frozen cells, and using the good techniques and fast thawing at 37 °C ensure high proportion of the cells survive the procedures. Dilute the frozen cells with pre-warmed complete media, and mix with slow pipette up and down.
7. Flask size depends on the number of frozen cells present in the cryovial, and culture conditions vary based on cell type and media used. Generally, cells seeded at 10,000 cells/cm^2 in 5% CO_2 at 37 °C are used for routine culture and passages.
8. Prepare wells that contain known numbers of viable cells for generation of calibration curve.
9. It takes about 30 min on the bench top at 25 °C or 5 min in a water bath at 37 °C.
10. Be careful not to introduce bubbles to the wells, since they interfere with the OD reading.
11. To measure the absorbance later, add 10 μL of 1% w/v SDS to each well, cover the plate, and store it with protection from light at room temperature. No absorbance change should be observed for 48 h.

12. It is critical to get a relatively accurate number for the cells for equal plating. The number of cells for seeding should be determined by the aggressiveness of the treatment.
13. PE = no. of colonies formed divided by no. of cells seeded × 100%
    SF = no. of colonies formed after treatment divided by no. of cells seeded × PE.
14. While scratching across the surface of the well, the long axial of the tip should always be perpendicular to the bottom of the well. The resulting gap distance therefore equals to the outer diameter of the end of the tip. The gap distance can be adjusted by using different types of tips. Scratch a straight line in one direction.
15. Medium may contain ingredients of interest that you want to test, e.g., chemicals that inhibit/promote cell motility and/or proliferation.

References

1. Chang JC (2016) Cancer stem cells: role in tumor growth, recurrence, metastasis, and treatment resistance. Medicine (Baltimore) 95:S20–S25
2. Hanahan D, Weinberg RA (2011) Hallmarks of cancer: the next generation. Cell 144:646–674
3. Menyhárt O, Harami-Papp H, Sukumar S, Schäfer R, Magnani L, Barrios d et al (2016) Guidelines for the selection of functional assays to evaluate the hallmarks of cancer. Biochim Biophys Acta 1866:300–319
4. Weisenberger DJ, Liang G, Lenz HJ (2018) DNA methylation aberrancies delineate clinically distinct subsets of colorectal cancer and provide novel targets for epigenetic therapies. Oncogene 37:566–577
5. Islam F, Gopalan F, Lam AKY (2019) Cancer stem cells: role in tumor progression and treatment resistance. In: Dammacco F, Silvestris F (eds) Oncogenomics: from basic research to precision medicine. Academic Press, Cambridge, pp 77–87
6. Grillet F, Bayet E, Villeronce O, Zappia L, Lagerqvist EL, Lunke S et al (2017) Circulating tumour cells from patients with colorectal cancer have cancer stem cell hallmarks in ex vivo culture. Gut 66:1802–1810
7. Vinci M, Gowan S, Boxall F, Patterson L, Zimmermann M, Court W et al (2012) Advances in establishment and analysis of three-dimensional tumor spheroid-based functional assays for target validation and drug evaluation. BMC Biol 10:29
8. Chan D, Zhou Y, Chui CH, Lam KH, Law S, Chan AS, Li X, Lam AK, Tang JCO (2018) Expression of insulin-like growth factor binding protein-5 (IGFBP5) reverses cisplatin-resistance in esophageal carcinoma. Cell 7: E143
9. Li B, Xu WW, Lam AKY, Wang Y, Hu HF, Guan XY, Qin YR, Saremi N, Tsao SW, He QY, Cheung ALM (2017) Significance of PI3K/AKT signaling pathway in metastasis of esophageal squamous cell carcinoma and its potential as a target for anti-metastasis therapy. Oncotarget 8:38755–38766
10. Pun IH, Chan D, Chan SH, Chung PY, Zhou YY, Law S, Lam AK, Chui CH, Chan AS, Lam KH, Tang JC (2017) Anti-cancer effects of a novel quinoline derivative 83b1 on human esophageal squamous cell carcinoma through down-regulation of COX-2 mRNA and PGE (2). Cancer Res Treat 49:219–229
11. Islam F, Gopalan V, Law S, Tang JC, Chan KW, Lam AK (2017) MiR-498 in esophageal squamous cell carcinoma: clinicopathological impacts and functional interactions. Hum Pathol 62:141–151
12. Chai AW, Cheung AK, Dai W, Ko JM, Ip JC, Chan KW, Kwong DL, Ng WT, Lee AW, Ngan RK, Yau CC, Tung SY, Lee VH, Lam AK, Pillai S, Law S, Lung ML (2016) Metastasis-suppressing NID2, an epigenetically-silenced gene, in the pathogenesis of nasopharyngeal

carcinoma and esophageal squamous cell carcinoma. Oncotarget 7:78859–78871
13. Gopalan V, Islam F, Pillai S, Tang JC, Tong DK, Law S, Chan KW, Lam AK (2016) Overexpression of microRNA-1288 in oesophageal squamous cell carcinoma. Exp Cell Res 348:146–154
14. Yu VZ, Wong VC, Dai W, Ko JM, Lam AK, Chan KW, Samant RS, Lung HL, Shuen WH, Law S, Chan YP, Lee NP, Tong DK, Law TT, Lee VH, Lung ML (2015) Nuclear localization of dnajb6 is associated with survival of patients with esophageal cancer and reduces AKT signaling and proliferation of cancer cells. Gastroenterology 149:1825–1836
15. Xu WW, Li B, Lam AK, Tsao SW, Law SY, Chan KW, Yuan QJ, Cheung AL (2015) Targeting VEGFR1- and VEGFR2-expressing non-tumor cells is essential for esophageal cancer therapy. Oncotarget 6:1790–1805
16. Chan D, Tsoi MY, Liu CD, Chan SH, Law SY, Chan KW, Chan YP, Gopalan V, Lam AK, Tang JC (2013) Oncogene GAEC1 regulates CAPN10 expression which predicts survival in esophageal squamous cell carcinoma. World J Gastroenterol 19:2772–2780
17. Pak KC, Lam KY, Law S, Tang JC (2009) The inhibitory effect of Gleditsia sinensis on cyclooxygenase-2 expression in human esophageal squamous cell carcinoma. Int J Mol Med 23:121–129
18. Law FB, Chen YW, Wong KY, Ying J, Tao Q, Langford C, Lee PY, Law S, Cheung RW, Chui CH, Tsao SW, Lam KY, Wong J, Srivastava G, Tang JC (2007) Identification of a novel tumor transforming gene GAEC1 at 7q22 which encodes a nuclear protein and is frequently amplified and overexpressed in esophageal squamous cell carcinoma. Oncogene 26:5877–5888
19. Tang WK, Chui CH, Fatima S, Kok SH, Pak KC, Ou TM, Hui KS, Wong MM, Wong J, Law S, Tsao SW, Lam KY, Beh PS, Srivastava G, Ho KP, Chan AS, Tang JC (2007) Inhibitory effects of *Gleditsia sinensis* fruit extract on telomerase activity and oncogenic expression in human esophageal squamous cell carcinoma. Int J Mol Med 19:953–960
20. Islam F, Gopalan V, Lam AK, Kabir SR (2018) Pea lectin inhibits cell growth by inducing apoptosis in SW480 and SW48 cell lines. Int J Biol Macromol 117:1050–1057
21. Islam F, Gopalan V, Lam AK (2018) RNA interference-mediated gene silencing in esophageal adenocarcinoma. Methods Mol Biol 1756:269–279
22. Islam F, Khatun H, Khatun M, Ali SM, Khanam JA (2014) Growth inhibition and apoptosis of Ehrlich ascites carcinoma cells by the methanol extract of Eucalyptus camaldulensis. Pharm Biol 52:281–290
23. Islam F, Raihan O, Chowdhury D, Khatun M, Zuberi N, Khatun L et al (2015) Apoptotic and antioxidant activities of methanol extract of Mussaenda roxburghii leaves. Pak J Pharm Sci 28:2027–2034
24. Islam F, Khanam JA, Khatun M, Zuberi N, Khatun L, Kabir SR et al (2015) A p-menth-1-ene-4,7-diol (EC-1) from Eucalyptus camaldulensis Dhnh. Triggers apoptosis and cell cycle changes in Ehrlich ascites carcinoma cells. Phytother Res 29:573–581
25. Lam AK (2000) Molecular biology of esophageal squamous cell carcinoma. Crit Rev Oncol Hematol 33:71–90
26. Berridge MV, Herst PM, Tan AS (2005) Tetrazolium dyes as tools in cell biology: new insights into their cellular reduction. Biotechnol Annu Rev 11:127–152
27. Mosmann T (1983) Rapid colorimetric assay for cellular growth and survival: application to proliferation and cytotoxicity assays. J Immunol Methods 65:55–63
28. Scudiero DA, Shoemaker RH, Paull KD, Monks A, Tierney S, Nofziger TH et al (1988) Evaluation of a soluble tetrazolium/formazan assay for cell growth and drug sensitivity in culture using human and other tumor cell lines. Cancer Res 48:4827–4833
29. Cory AH, Owen TC, Barltrop JA, Cory JG (1991) Use of an aqueous soluble tetrazolium/formazan assay for cell growth assays in culture. Cancer Commun 3:207–212
30. Maekawa Y, Yagi K, Nonomura A, Kuraoku R, Nishiura E, Uchibori E et al (2003) A tetrazolium-based colorimetric assay for metabolic activity of stored blood platelets. Thromb Res 109:307–314
31. Skehan P, Storeng R, Scudiero D, Monks A, McMahon J, Vistica D (1990) New colorimetric cytotoxicity assay for anticancer-drug screening. J Natl Cancer Inst 82:1107–1112
32. Riccardi C, Nicoletti I (2006) Analysis of apoptosis by propidium iodide staining and flow cytometry. Nat Protoc 1:1458–1461
33. Roth BL, Poot M, Yue ST, Millard PJ (1997) Bacterial viability and antibiotic susceptibility testing with SYTOX green nucleic acid stain. Appl Environ Microbiol 63:2421–2431
34. Cho MH, Niles A, Huang R, Inglese J, Austin CP, Riss T et al (2008) A bioluminescent cytotoxicity assay for assessment of membrane

integrity using a proteolytic biomarker. Toxicol In Vitro 22:1099–10106

35. Sidman RL, Miale IL, Feder N (1959) Cell proliferation and migration in the primitive ependymal zone: an autoradiographic study of histogenesis in the nervous system. Exp Neurol 1:322–333
36. Duque A, Rakic P (2011) Different effects of BrdU and (3) H-thymidine incorporation into DNA on cell proliferation, position and fate. J Neurosci 31:15205–15217
37. Artymovich K, Appledorn DM (2015) A multiplexed method for kinetic measurements of apoptosis and proliferation using live-content imaging. Methods Mol Biol 1219:35–42
38. Oberhammer F, Wilson JW, Dive C, Morris ID, Hickman JA, Wakeling AE et al (1993) Apoptotic death in epithelial cells: cleavage of DNA to 300 and/or 50 kb fragments prior to or in the absence of internucleosomal fragmentation. EMBO J 12:3679–3684
39. Ehemann V, Sykora J, Vera-Delgado J, Lange A, Otto HF (2003) Flow cytometric detection of spontaneous apoptosis in human breast cancer using the TUNEL-technique. Cancer Lett 194:125–131
40. van Engeland M, Ramaekers FC, Schutte B, Reutelingsperger CP (1996) A novel assay to measure loss of plasma membrane asymmetry during apoptosis of adherent cells in culture. Cytometry 24:131–139
41. Decker T, Lohmann-Matthes ML (1988) A quick and simple method for the quantitation of lactate dehydrogenase release in measurements of cellular cytotoxicity and tumor necrosis factor (TNF) activity. J Immunol Methods 115:61–69
42. Smolewski P, Bedner E, Du L, Hsieh TC, Wu JM, Phelps DJ et al (2001) Detection of caspases activation by fluorochrome-labeled inhibitors: multiparameter analysis by laser scanning cytometry. Cytometry 44:73–82
43. Soldani C, Lazzè MC, Bottone MG, Tognon G, Biggiogera M, Pellicciari CE et al (2001) Poly(ADP-ribose) polymerase cleavage during apoptosis: when and where? Exp Cell Res 269:193–201
44. Kimura M, Stone RC, Hunt SC, Skurnick J, Lu X, Cao X et al (2010) Measurement of telomere length by the southern blot analysis of terminal restriction fragment lengths. Nat Protoc 5:1596–1607
45. Skvortsov DA, Zvereva ME, Shpanchenko OV, Dontsova OA (2011) Assays for detection of telomerase activity. Acta Nat 3:48–68
46. Gagnon E, Cattaruzzi P, Griffith M, Muzakare L, LeFlao K, Faure R et al (2002) Human vascular endothelial cells with extended life spans: in vitro cell response, protein expression, and angiogenesis. Angiogenesis 5:21–33
47. Fan F, Wey JS, McCarty MF, Belcheva A, Liu W, Bauer TW et al (2005) Expression and function of vascular endothelial growth factor receptor-1 on human colorectal cancer cells. Oncogene 24:2647–2653
48. Boyden S (1962) The chemotactic effect of mixtures of antibody and antigen on polymorphonuclear leucocytes. J Exp Med 115:453–466
49. Liang CC, Park AY, Guan JL (2007) In vitro scratch assay: a convenient and inexpensive method for analysis of cell migration in vitro. Nat Protoc 2:329–333

Chapter 14

Detention and Identification of Cancer Stem Cells in Esophageal Squamous Cell Carcinoma

Farhadul Islam, Vinod Gopalan, and Alfred K. Lam

Abstract

Cancer stem cells (CSCs) are a small subpopulation of cells associated with cancer initiation, progression, metastasis, therapy resistant, and recurrence. In esophageal squamous cell carcinoma (ESCC), several cell surface and intracellular markers, for example, CD44, ALDH, Pygo2, MAML1, Twist1, Musashi1, side population (SP), CD271, and CD90, have been proposed to identify CSCs. In addition, stem cell markers such as ALDH1, HIWI, Oct3/4, ABCG2, SOX2, SALL4, BMI-1, NANOG, CD133, and podoplanin were associated with pathological stages of cancer, cancer recurrence, prognosis, and therapy resistance of patients with ESCC. Identification and isolation of CSCs could play an important part of improved cancer management regime in ESCC. Furthermore, CSCs may be used as the predictive tool for chemoradiotherapy response in ESCC. Different methods such as in vitro functional assays, cell sorting using various intracellular, and cell surface markers and xenotransplantation techniques are frequently used for the identification and isolation of CSCs in different cancers, including ESCC. However, none of these methods solely can guarantee complete isolation of CSC population. Therefore, a combination of methods is used for reliable detection and isolation of CSCs. Herein, we describe the identification and isolation of CSCs from ESCC cells by cell sorting after Hoechst 33342 staining followed by in vitro functional assays and in vivo mouse xenotransplantation techniques.

Key words Cancer stem cell, Esophageal squamous cell carcinoma, In vitro assays, CSC identification, CSC isolation

1 Introduction

Cancer stem cells (CSCs) are the cells that have the capacity of self-renewal and undergo asymmetric divisions to produce more CSCs and differentiated cells of various lineage resulting in forming a tumor [1–7]. In this aspect, identification and isolation of CSCs in ESCC might have potential to improve the therapeutic management of patients with ESCC [6]. Nonneoplastic stem cells and CSCs share some functional characteristics such as membrane transport, DNA repair, self-renewal, and multi-lineage differentiation. Therefore, there are challenges to identify CSCs in different cancers, including in ESCC [6]. Accordingly, identification and

Alfred K. Lam (ed.), *Esophageal Squamous Cell Carcinoma: Methods and Protocols*, Methods in Molecular Biology, vol. 2129, https://doi.org/10.1007/978-1-0716-0377-2_14,

isolation of CSCs from non-CSCs with specific single method have not been reported yet. A combination of methods, for example, cell sorting based on cell surface and intracellular protein marker, in vitro functional assays, and xenograft, are commonly in use to identify CSCs in different cancers including ESCC.

Importantly, the translational definition of CSCs and the gold standard for exhibiting "stemness" of CSCs is the ability to regenerate primary tumor in immunocompromised xenograft mice. This xenotransplantation demonstrates the capacity of CSCs to reproduce the variety of differentiated cells present in original primary cancer [1]. Several biomolecules, including cell surface and intracellular markers, could be used to detect and isolate CSCs in different cancers. A well-defined panel of markers for CSC in ESCC has not been identified and characterized, but many tentative molecules are being used to functionally identify the CSC in ESCC. Table 1 presents the markers used to identify CSCs in ESCC.

1.1 Implications of CSC Markers in ESCC Prognosis

Local invasion and metastases are the major causes of cancer-related deaths in patients with ESCC. Studies have indicated that CSCs are responsible for cell invasion and metastasis in many cancers, including ESCC [8, 9]. Biomarkers such as CD44, ALDH, Pygo2, MAML1, HIWI, Twist1, Musashi1, side population (SP), CD271, and CD90 are used to identify CSCs in ESCC. They could help in the assessment of prognosis of patients with ESCC. For example, expression of ALDH1 (ALDH1A1), an isoform of ALDH, was reported to be positively correlated with the advanced pathological stages of ESCC [10, 11]. In addition, overexpression of ALDH1A1 protein was associated with shorter survival of patients with ESCC. Another study reported that significant cancer regression correlated with the expression of ALDH1 after chemoradiotherapy [12]. It was demonstrated that overexpression of HIWI protein in ESCC cell lines and in cancer tissues was significantly associated with high histological grade, higher T stage, and poorer survival of patients with ESCC [13].

Oct3/4 is a transcription factor which regulates the stemness and development of stem cells. The expression of Oct3/4 in ESCC significantly correlated with high histological grade and poor survival of patients with ESCC [14]. Another study found that ESCC with $Oct4^+$ had increased capacity of tumor-sphere formation in culture and xenograft model when compared to differentiated cells [15]. SOX2 is another transcription factor, which can regulate the stemness and development of stem cells. Expression of SOX2 protein in ESCC was associated with lymphatic metastasis, vascular invasion, high histological grade, and poorer patient's survival [14, 16, 17]. In addition, NANOG is a transcription factor involved in self-renewal of embryonic stem cells, and expression of NANOG in ESCC can be used as a prognostic marker.

Table 1
Markers used to identify cancer stem cells in esophageal squamous cell carcinoma

Name of marker	Source of CSCs in ESCC	Assay method	References
Cripto-1	ESCC cell lines (EC109, TE1)	Colony formation, tumor-sphere formation, and xenotransplantation assays	[24]
EZH2	KYSE30 cells	Gene expression analysis	[25]
CD47, CD133	ESCC tissues	Spheres formation assay and immunohistochemistry	[26]
CD44	Primary ESCC cell lines (ESC1 and ESC2)	Colony formation assay, therapy-resistant assay, and xenotransplantation assay in immune-deficient mice	[27]
ALDH	ESCC cell lines (KY-5, KY-10, TE-1, TE-8, YES-1, YES-2)	Flow cytometry (attached-cell Aldefluor assay), immunocytochemistry, tumor-sphere formation assay, and therapy-resistant assay	[28]
CD271	ESCC cell lines (KYSEs) and tissues	Colony formation assay, flow cytometry, immunocytochemistry, and TUNEL assay	[29]
CD90	ESCC clinical specimen (tissues) and cell lines (EC18, EC109, HKESC1, KYSE520, YSE30, KYSE140, KYSE180, KYSE410, and KYSE510)	Flow cytometry, sphere formation assay, differentiation assay, chemoresistance assay, tumorigenicity and serial transplantation assay in NOD/SCID mice, cell invasion and motility assays, and experimental metastasis assay in NOD/SCID mice	[8]
Side population (Hoechst 33342 dye exclusion)	ESCC cell lines EC9706 and EC109 cells	Clone formation assay, xenotransplantation into nonobese diabetic/severe combined immunodeficiency mice	[30, 31]

ABCG2, an isoform of ATP-binding cassette transporter (ABC-transporter), mediates the translocation of various substances across cell membrane. Expression of ABCG2 correlated with presence of lymph node metastasis and poorer prognosis of patients with ESCC [18, 19]. Patients with ESCC having ABCG2 expression require more intensive or targeted therapy.

BMI1 is an oncoprotein which regulates cell cycle events in cancer cells. Expression of BMI1 protein correlated with tumor

Table 2
Putative *cancer stem cell* (CSC) markers in esophageal squamous cell carcinoma

Name of marker	Expression in nonneoplastic stem cells	Function	Role in ESCC	References
Cripto-1	Bone marrow and immune tissues	An extracellular, membrane-bound protein; plays an essential role in embryonic development and tumor growth	Overexpression correlated with pathological stage (depth and lymph node metastasis) of ESCC	[24]
EZH2	Bone marrow and immune tissues, reproductive system, and lung tissues	This protein associates with the embryonic ectoderm development and may play a role in the hematopoietic and central nervous systems	Deregulation of the protein associated with tumor cell invasiveness, metastasis, and the patients' poor survival	[25]
CD47	Embryonic cells and neuronal cells in the stomach	Membrane protein and play a role in membrane transport and signal transduction	Patients with ESCC having high CD47 or CD133 expression exhibited poor overall survival and progression-free survival rate	[18, 26]
SOX-2	Embryonic cells and neuronal cells in the stomach and central nervous system	Transcription factor and regulates self-renewal or pluripotency of undifferentiated embryonic stem cells	Elevated expression associated with high tumor grade, metastasis, and poorer patient's survival	[14, 32]
ABCG2	Placenta, hematopoietic stem cells, and other stem cells	ATP-binding cassette transporter (membrane transporter)	Overexpression correlated with lymph node metastasis and poor patient's prognosis	[18, 19]
SALL4	Epithelial cells and stem cells of various organs	Transcription factors and maintenance of pluripotency, self-renewal, and cell fate decision	Overexpression associated with invasion and metastasis	[35]
NANOG	Embryonic stem cells and epithelial cells	Transcriptional regulator and self-renewal	Expression linked with lower tumor regression after chemoradiotherapy	[33]
BMI1	Hematopoietic stem cell	Cell cycle regulator	Expression associated with early relapse, poor prognosis, and chemotherapy resistance	[34]

(continued)

Table 2 (continued)

Name of marker	Expression in nonneoplastic stem cells	Function	Role in ESCC	References
Oct3/4	Stem cell in different organs	Regulate stemness and development	Upregulation of this factor linked to poorer survival and advanced tumor stages	[12, 14]
Podoplanin	Various vascular endothelium in different organs	Regulates invasion	Positive expression associated with cancer recurrence, poorer prognosis, and metastasis	[22]
CD133	Stem cell in different organs	Regulates stemness	Cytoplasmic expression correlated with overall patient's survival	[18, 21]
HIWI	Stem cell in different organs	Regulate stemness of nonneoplastic stem cells	Overexpression correlated with high grade and poorer patient's survival	[13]

ESCC Esophageal squamous cell carcinoma

regression grade and could predict early relapse of cancer and poor prognosis in patients with ESCC after chemoradiotherapy [12, 20].

CD133, also known as prominin-1, is a transmembrane glycoprotein, which has been used as cancer stem cell marker in ESCC. The cytoplasmic expression of CD133 was significantly correlated with overall survival of patients with ESCC [21]. Podoplanin is another small mucin-like transmembrane protein that is involved in cancer progression. Cancer recurrence, presence of lymph node metastasis, and poorer prognosis of patients with ESCC were correlated with podoplanin-positive expression [22]. Another study found that high expression of podoplanin in ESCC was associated with lymphovascular invasion and shorter survival times of patients with ESCC [23].

Table 2 summarizes the potential role of some putative CSCs markers in ESCC prognosis.

1.2 Therapeutic Applications of CSCs in ESCC

CSCs are the only cells in cancer with the ability to expand and promote cancer growth and more importantly with the capacity of distant metastasis. Thus, therapeutics strategies and modalities could target these special CSC populations in ESCC. As CSCs are relatively resistant to the currently available chemoradiotherapy, new treatment options to target these cells directly would be of immense benefit. Therefore, the main objective in CSC research is to devise new strategies that will selectively kill CSCs. Accordingly, much of the research in the field focused either on searches for targets expressed in CSCs, but not in nonneoplastic stem cells, or on screening for selective drugs or RNA interference (RNAi) molecules that specifically kill CSCs over nonneoplastic stem cells.

Overall, CSCs are primarily responsible to drive and maintain cancer. Markers of these cells have prognostic implications, and developing drugs targeting this subpopulation of ESCC cells could have provide better clinical outcome of patients with ESCC. Therefore, herein, we describe the identification of CSCs from ESCC cells using a combination of multiple techniques including (1) isolating CSC from ESCC cells by fluorescence-activated cell sorting (FACS) followed by Hoechst 33342 staining (2) functional assays such as in vitro spheres formation assay and in vivo mouse xenotransplantation. For this, firstly, SP (side population) fraction of cells from ESCC cells will be sorted out with FACS using Hoechst 33342 dye staining. This step is based on differential efflux of fluorescent DNA-binding dye Hoechst 33342 in ESCC stem cells relative to the non-stem cells and poorly stained cells, which are called side population with CSCs properties [1–3]. Secondly, the sorted SP cells will then be tested for tumor spheres formation capacity in vitro and tumorigenic properties in xenograft mouse.

2 Materials

Remember to use ultrapure water to prepare all the reagents and solutions and store at room temperature unless otherwise indicated. Also, use appropriate personal protective equipment during experiments, and follow the rules and regulations of waste disposal during disposing the waste materials.

2.1 Cell Culture

1. Esophageal squamous cell carcinoma cells.
2. Cell culture media: Roswell Park Memorial Institute (RPMI) 1640, L-glutamine, pH 7.2. Take 900 mL water to a glass beaker, and add 10.4 g of RPMI1640 powder media to the water with gentle stir (*see* **Note 1**). Dissolve the powder completely and do not heat the media (*see* **Note 2**). Add 2.0 g of sodium bicarbonate to the media and stir for complete dissolving. Adjust the pH with 1 N HCl (hydrogen chloride) and NaOH (sodium hydroxide). Finally, add water up to mark 1 L, sterilize with 0.22 μm membrane filter, and aseptically transfer media into sterile container. Store at 4 °C.
3. 10% fetal bovine serum (FBS) in sterile media (*see* **Note 3**). Store at 4 °C.
4. 1% penicillin and streptomycin. Store at 4 °C (*see* **Note 4**).

5. Cell washing buffer: Phosphate buffer saline (PBS), pH 7.4. Take 8.0 g sodium chloride (NaCl), 0.2 g potassium chloride (KCl), 1.42 g disodium hydrogen phosphate (Na_2HPO_4), and 0.24 g potassium dihydrogen phosphate (KH_2PO_4) in a glass beaker and dissolve all the salts in 800 mL water. Adjust the pH with 1 N HCl and add water to a total volume of 1 L. Sterilize by autoclaving at 121 °C for 30 min. Cool it down and store at 4 °C.
6. Cell dissociation solution: 0.25% trypsin-ethylenediaminetetraacetic acid (EDTA), pH 7.2–8. Stored at −20 °C (*see* **Note 5**).
7. Cell culture flasks: Polystyrene 25 cm^2 and 75 cm^2 flasks.
8. Falcon 15 mL and 50 mL conical centrifuge tubes.
9. Microscope and benchtop centrifuge machines.
10. 80% ethanol in water (v/v).

2.2 Cell Staining and Sorting

1. Cell staining dye: 5 μg/mL Hoechst 33342 in water (*see* **Note 6**).
2. Dead cell dye: 10 μg/mL propidium iodide (PI) in water (*see* **Note 7**).
3. Wash buffer: Cold phosphate-buffered saline (PBS), pH 7.2.
4. ATP-binding cassette (ABC)-transporters inhibitor: 50 μM verapamil or 10 μM fumitremorgin C.
5. Centrifuge tubes: 1.5 mL.
6. Vortex mixer.
7. Flow cytometer.
   (a) Excitation wavelength 325 nm or 351–364 nm.
   (b) Detection filters: 450/20 nm band-pass (BP) filter, 675 nm longpass (LP) filter, and 610 nm shortpass dichroic mirror.
8. Cell counter/hemocytometer.
9. 0.4% trypan blue solution in PBS, pH 7.2–7.3.
10. Polystyrene tubes: 5 mL.
11. Collection tube: 15 mL falcon tube.

2.3 In Vitro Functional Assay

1. Cell culture plates: 6-well plates, 96-well ultralow attachment plates.
2. Cell culture media: RPMI1640 (*see* Subheading 2.1).
3. Tumor spheres formation media: RPMI1640, 50× B27, 20 ng/mL epidermal growth factor (EGF), 10 ng/mL basic fibroblast growth factor (FGF), 5 μg/mL insulin. Take 10 μg EGF, 5 μg FGF, 2.5 μg insulin, and 0.5 mL B27 supplement to 500 mL of RPMI1640 media (*see* **Note 8**). Store at 4 °C.

2.4 In Vivo Xenotransplantation

1. Cell culture media: RPMI1640 (*see* Subheading 2.1).
2. Cancer cells: SP-positive, SP-negative.
3. Animal: Nonobese diabetic/severe combined immunodeficiency (NOD/SCID) (*see* **Note 9**).
4. Anesthetic agents: 1–3% isoflurane, 80–100 mg/kg ketamine (intraperitoneal) (*see* **Note 10**).
5. Syringe: 1 mL with 27- or 30-gauge needle.
6. Digital caliper.

3 Methods

3.1 Cell Culture

1. Bring the cryovial containing ESCC cells from liquid nitrogen facility, and transfer them into a 37 °C water bath.
2. Thaw the cells quickly by gently swirling the vial in water bath at 37 °C (*see* **Note 11**).
3. Aseptically take the vial containing ESCC into a biosafety cabinet, and wipe out site of the vial with 80% ethanol.
4. Add pre-warmed complete growth media (2 mL) in a 15 mL centrifuge tube, take the cells from the vial with a pipette, and add dropwise into the tube.
5. Centrifuge the cell suspension at approximately 400 × *g* for 3–5 min.
6. Check the cell pellet after centrifugation, and aseptically decant the supernatant without disrupting the cells pellet.
7. Add 2 mL PBS and resuspend the cells pellet by slow pipetting.
8. Centrifuge the suspension at 400 × *g* for 3–5 min and discard the supernatant.
9. Resuspend the cell pellets in complete growth media.
10. Transfer the cells into an appropriate cell culture flask/plate containing recommended growth media, and incubate in the CO_2 incubator at appropriate conditions (*see* **Note 12**).

3.2 Cell Staining and Sorting

1. Grow the ESCC cells up to 70–80% confluency and harvest them by trypsinization.
2. Take the flask (s) inside the biosafety cabinet, discard the media, and rinse with 1× warm PBS.
3. Vacuum off the PBS, add 0.25% trypsin-EDTA to the flask/plate, and incubate for 5–10 min or until disassociation of cells (*see* **Note 13**).
4. After completing the detachment of cells from the flask/plate, add growth media to neutralize the EDTA.

5. Rinse the flask/plate and pipette off cells to ensure maximum collection of cells.
6. Centrifuge for 3–5 min at 400 × *g*, discard the media, and wash the cells with PBS.
7. Resuspend the cells in cold PBS, and count the cells with a cell counter or hemocytometer using trypan blue (*see* **Note 14**).
8. Readjust the ESCC cell number to 1×10^7 cells/mL in cold PBS (*see* **Note 15**).
9. Label tubes as “Inhibitor,” “SP-stained,” and “Unstained” (*see* **Note 16**).
10. Take 100 μL of prepared cell suspension (equal to one million cells) to each tube.
11. Add 10 μL of Verapamil to the “Inhibitor” tube.
12. Add 10 μL of Hoechst 33342 satin to the “SP-stained” and “Inhibitor” label tubes.
13. Vortex gently for a few seconds and incubate for 15–30 min in a covered ice bucket.
14. Add 1–2 mL cold PBS to wash off excess staining, and centrifuge for 5 min at 800 × *g*.
15. Aspirate the supernatant without disturbing the cells pellet.
16. Resuspend the cells in 500 μL cold PBS, and add 5 μL propidium iodide stock solution to “SP-stained” and “Inhibitor” label tubes.
17. Incubate for 15–30 min on ice and keep in the dark.
18. Wash off excess propidium iodide with cold PBS, and resuspend cells in 500 μL cold PBS with 1% bovine serum albumin (BSA) (*see* **Note 17**).
19. Mix the cell suspension with pipette up and down several times, and transfer to the FACS tube for analysis and sorting.
20. Set up and optimize the cell sorter (*see* **Note 18**).
21. Perform compensation, and set gates for controls and stained samples (*see* **Note 19**).
22. Select the gates for sorting into external collection tubes (*see* **Note 20**).
23. Run the experimental sample tubes at 4 °C (*see* **Note 21**).
24. Stop the sorting when desired number of cells were obtained in the collection tubes, and perform the post-sort analysis.
25. Collect the sorted cells in complete growth media for subsequent in vitro and in vivo experiments.

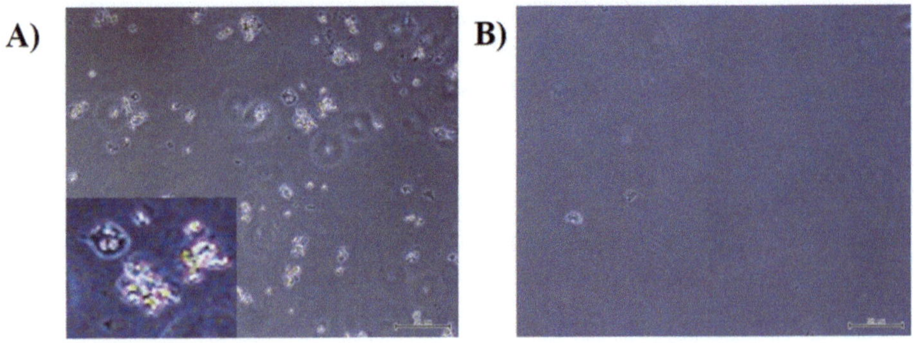

Spheres generated by CSCs

No spheres generated by non-CSC cells

Fig. 1 Tumor spheres formation by CSCs derived from ESCC cells. (**a**) Tumor spheres under phase-contrast microscope at 40× magnifications by CSCs cells. Inset showing the spheres at 100×. (**b**) No tumor spheres generated by non-CSCs cells. Scale bar 20 μm

3.3 In Vitro Tumor Spheres Formation Assay

1. Count the FACS-isolated SP-positive cells. Adjust the cells number as 1000 cells/mL in growth media.
2. Take 100 μL of PBS to the first and last columns (column 1 and 12) of the 96-well ultralow attachment plate to minimize the evaporation of tumor spheres formation media.
3. Put 100 μL of tumor spheres formation media into the rest of the wells.
4. Place the SP-positive cells in columns 2–11 at 200, 100, 50, 10, 5, and 1 cell into each well (*see* **Note 22**).
5. Seal the edges of the plate with lab film to avoid media evaporation.
6. Incubate the plate for 1–3 weeks at 37 °C with 5% CO_2 until spheres formed (Fig. 1).
7. Count the number of tumor spheres under phase-contrast microscope using 40× magnifications.
8. Finally, calculate the percentages of spheres formation capacity of the SP-positive cells.

3.4 Xenotrans-spi1; plantation

1. Readjust the freshly FACS-sorted SP-positive and SP-negative cells to a concentration of 1.0×10^7 cells/mL in cold PBS. Keep the cells always on ice.
2. Slowly pull up 100 μL of cells using 1 mL syringe fitted with 27- or 30-gauge needle.
3. Carefully anesthetize the mice using isoflurane (*see* **Note 10**).
4. Inject 1.0×10^6 cells into the flank of NOD/SCID mice. Pinch the skin of the mouse between the index finger and the thumb. Pull the skin away from the body of the mouse.
5. Inject the cells slowly and evenly into the created pouch.

6. Monitor the tumor growth by palpation regularly.
7. Sacrifice the animals when largest subcutaneous tumors reach ~50–60 mm^3 in diameter.
8. Measure tumor diameter with digital caliper, and calculate the tumor volume in mm^3 using the formula: $\text{Volume} = (\text{Width})^2 \times \text{Length}/2$.

4 Notes

1. Powdered media are highly hygroscopic and need to be protected from atmospheric moistures. In addition, preparing a concentrated media solution may form precipitation.
2. Reduce pH to 4.0 with 1 N HCl to dissolve the media completely. After that, adjust the pH up to 7.2 with 1 N NaOH prior to add sodium bicarbonate.
3. 10% FBS is good for the growth and maintenance of the ESCC cells. It is necessary to optimize the amount of the cells of interest.
4. Penicillin and streptomycin, the mixture of antibiotics, need to be used to prevent the bacterial contamination of cultured ESCC cells. One percent concentration is enough to maintain and keep the cells free from bacterial contaminations.
5. It is better to avoid repeated freeze thawing and warm up of trypsin as multiple freezing, thawing, and warming may cause the reduced enzymatic activity of trypsin.
6. Avoid re-solubilization of Hoechst 33342 dye in PBS. However, dilute solutions of the dye may be used with PBS or other phosphate-containing buffers. Water solution of the dye stored at 4 °C can be used at least for 6 months. Thus, the Hoechst 33342 dye solution should be stored at 2–6 °C and protected from light. The dye is a potential mutagen and should be handled with care. Disposal of the dye should be carried out safely in accordance to the proper regulations.
7. Prepare a stock of propidium iodide (PI) solution at 1 mg/mL (1.5 mM) in sterile distilled water, and store at 2–6 °C. Protect the solution from light, and it can be used at least for 6 months. PI is a potential mutagen; therefore, use with care and dispose in accordance to the proper regulations.
8. B27, a growth supplement, increased the spheres formation of sorted cells and attributed passages of spheres culture.
9. Consider the animals between ages 4–6 weeks old, and allow enough time, at least 5 days acclimation period of mice arrival. Obtain the animal ethics from the proper authority, and follow standard operating procedures in accordance to the approved guidelines.

10. Isoflurane, an inhaled anesthesia, or ketamine, a local anesthesia, makes the implantation of cells to mice easier and less stressful. Anesthesia with isoflurane is easier to preform by placing the mouse in a closed chamber/box with appropriate gas scavenging attached. Once writhing reflex is lost, remove the animal from the induction chamber and maintain on gas delivered via a fitted nose cone or endotracheal tube. Do not over anesthetize as the mice will succumb to respiratory depression.

11. Thawing procedures is stressful for the frozen cells. Using good techniques and fast thawing at 37 °C ensure high proportion of the cells to survive the procedures. For better survival of cells, dilute the frozen cells with pre-warmed complete media and mix by slow pipette up and down.

12. Culture flask/plate size depends on the number of frozen cells present in the cryovial and culture conditions. In addition, it may vary based on cell type and media used. In general, cells seeded at 10,000 cells/cm^2, in 5% CO_2 at 37 °C, are used for routine culture and passages.

13. Put 2 mL and 5 mL 0.25% trypsin-EDTA in 25 cm^2 and 75 cm^2 flask, respectively. Examine the cells every 2 min to ensure that they are being disassociated. Tap gently the flask to get maximum disassociation and recovery of cells as soon as possible. Keeping cells long time in trypsin may cause reduced viability of the cells.

14. Put 0.4% trypan blue stock solution and cell suspension in a 1.5 mL centrifuge tube (1:1). For example, add 100 μL trypan blue in 100 μL cells and mix by pipetting. Then, load 10 μL of this cell on a hemocytometer and examine and count the viable cells under microscope with low magnification. Count the blue or dead cells (dead cells take up trypan blue and become stained) and total number of cells. Finally, calculate the viability of cells using the formula: % of viable cells = [1 − (Number dead cells/Number of total cells)] × 100. Number of cells per mL of culture can be determined using the following formula: Number of viable cells × 10^4 × Dilution factor = Cells/mL of culture. At least 95% cell viability would be good for healthy log phase culture of cells.

15. Low cells counts need prolonged sorting time, which might affect the viability of cells. On the other hand, too many cells can reduce the purity and may cause blockages. A 1×10^6 to 2×10^7 cells/mL should be good for better sorting outcome. In addition, ensure that cells are in single-cell suspension and no cells clumps or aggregates are present. Use Ca-/Mg^{2+}-free PBS to avoid the formation of cells clumps. Add anti-clump agents such EDTA (1–5 mM) to the buffer to prevent formation of aggregates, if the cells have higher tendency to

aggregate. Also, add 20–50 μg/mL DNAse I and 5 mM magnesium chloride hexahydrate ($MgCl_2 \cdot 6H_2O$) to avoid cell clumping due to cell death.

16. For accurate SP fraction identification, control groups are required in which the ATP-binding cassette transporters responsible for Hoechst 33342 dye exclusion are blocked with inhibitor treatment. Commonly used ATP-binding cassette-transporters inhibitors are verapamil and fumitremorgin C. Use these cells to set gate, therefore discriminating SP population from non-SP cells. Unstained cell group will be used for initial gate setting of the cell-type analyte.
17. Prepared cells can be kept in refrigerator up to 1 week for analysis with flow cytometer. Use sorting buffer (PBS with 1% FBS) to avoid autofluorescence. Using high pressure during cell sorting can cause sorting buffer to become basic, and add 4-(2-hydroxyethyl)-1-piperazineethanesulfonic acid) (HEPES) (25 mM) to maintain the stable pH at 7.0–8.0.
18. Setup of flow cytometer is varied depending on the manufacturer and should be performed by trained personnel. In the process of setting up, first select the nozzle and sterilize the instrument. Then, perform the quality control with beads to check the lasers and functionality of the instrument. After that, install the 450/20 BP filter for Hoechst Blue, the 675 LP filter for Hoechst Red detection, and the 610 shortpass dichroic mirror for separation of blue and red signals. Propidium iodide (PI) fluorescence generated from ultraviolet excitation will also be captured by the 675 LP filter. High-fluorescence signals produced by PI-positive dead cells need to be discriminated from Hoechst Red-positive signals produced by live cells.
19. Set the compensation because it is essential to remove the spectral overlap between the detectors. However, according to the current literature, it is not absolute. As it is affected by intensity of signals produced by certain markers and by the signals of cells that have low autofluorescence, which led to poor resolution between dim and negative populations. Thus, to create appropriate gating for the isolation of SP cells, first plot Forward Scatter (FSC, related to cell size) and Side Scatter (SSC, related to cell granularity) to discriminate cells from debris. A dot plot of Hoechst Blue versus height is created to differentiate single cells from cell aggregates and doublets. Finally, Hoechst Blue versus Hoechst Red plot is created for SP fraction isolation. ABC-transporter inhibitor verapamil-treated cells are used to establish the SP gate. Run the sample, and adjust the FSC versus SSC plot by changing voltages of both parameters until all cells are captured on the dot plot. Adjust the voltages of Hoechst Blue and Red parameters until the cells stained brightly for Hoechst 33342 are visible on the

dot plot. If needed, increase the voltages until the cells stained weakly for Hoechst 33342 are visible on the lower left side of the plot. The SP subpopulation cells constitute a discrete cells population on the left side of the plot.

20. Use 15 mL falcon tube for two sorting (SP-positive and SP-negative) cells. Coat the tubes with BSA to prevent sorting cells sticking to the side of the tube. Add 10% BSA and incubate at 4 °C for overnight.
21. Always keep the sorted cells on ice, and protect from light exposure during analysis for further functional studies.
22. Seed the ESCC cells at different concentrations in a 12-well plate at each concentration; these can give you more reliable and comprehensive results of the spheres for the SP-positive.

References

1. Clarke MF, Dick JE, Dirks PB, Eaves CJ, Jamieson CH, Jones DL, Visvader J, Weissman IL, Wahl GM (2006) Cancer stem cells-perspectives on current status and future directions: AACR workshop on cancer stem cells. Cancer Res 66:9339–9344
2. Islam F, Gopalan V, Lam AK (2018) Identification of cancer stem cells in esophageal adenocarcinoma. Methods Mol Biol 1756:165–176
3. Gopalan V, Islam F, Lam AK (2018) Surface markers for the identification of cancer stem cells. Methods Mol Biol 1692:17–29
4. Wahab SMR, Islam F, Gopalan V, Lam AK (2017) The identifications and clinical implications of cancer stem cells in colorectal cancer. Clin Colorectal Cancer 16:93–102
5. Islam F, Gopalan V, Smith RA, Lam AK (2015) Translational potential of cancer stem cells: a review of the detection of cancer stem cells and their roles in cancer recurrence and cancer treatment. Exp Cell Res 335:135–147
6. Islam F, Gopalan V, Wahab R, Smith RA, Lam AK (2015) Cancer stem cells in oesophageal squamous cell carcinoma: identification, prognostic and treatment perspectives. Crit Rev Oncol Hematol 96:9–19
7. Islam F, Qiao B, Smith RA, Gopalan V, Lam AK (2015) Cancer stem cell: fundamental experimental pathological concepts and updates. Exp Mol Pathol 98:184–191
8. Tang KH, Dai YD, Tong M, Chan YP, Kwan PS, Fu L, Qin YR, Tsao SW, Lung HL, Lung ML, Tong DK, Law S, Chan KW, Ma S, Guan XY (2013) A CD90 tumor-initiating cell population with an aggressive signature and metastatic capacity in esophageal cancer. Cancer Res 73:2322–2332
9. Yang L, Ping YF, Yu X, Qian F, Guo ZJ, Qian C, Cui YH, Bian XW (2011) Gastric cancer stem-like cells possess higher capability of invasion and metastasis in association with a mesenchymal transition phenotype. Cancer Lett 310:46–52
10. Yang L, Ren Y, Yu X, Qian F, Bian BS, Xiao HL, Wang WG, Xu SL, Yang J, Cui W, Liu Q, Wang Z, Guo W, Xiong G, Yang K, Qian C, Zhang X, Zhang P, Cui YH, Bian XW (2014) ALDH1A1 defines invasive cancer stem-like cells and predicts poor prognosis in patients with esophageal squamous cell carcinoma. Mod Pathol 27:775–783
11. Wang Y, Zhe H, Gao P, Zhang N, Li G, Qin J (2012) Cancer stem cell marker ALDH1 expression is associated with lymph node metastasis and poor survival in esophageal squamous cell carcinoma: a study from high incidence area of northern China. Dis Esophagus 25:560–565
12. Hwang CC, Nieh S, Lai CH, Tsai CS, Chang LC, Hua CC, Chi WY, Chien HP, Wang CW, Chan SC, Hsieh TY, Chen JR (2014) Quantitative expression of Oct-3/4 defines differentiation, dedifferentiation or self-renewal of ES cells. PLoS One 9:e105676
13. He W, Wang Z, Wang Q, Fan Q, Shou C, Wang J, Giercksky KE, Nesland JM, Suo Z (2009) Expression of HIWI in human esophageal squamous cell carcinoma is significantly associated with poorer prognosis. BMC Cancer 9:426
14. Wang Q, He W, Lu C, Wang Z, Wang J, Giercksky KE, Nesland JM, Suo Z (2009) Oct3/4 and Sox2 are significantly associated with an unfavorable clinical outcome in human esophageal squamous cell carcinoma. Anticancer Res 29:1233–1241

15. Zhou X, Huang GR, Hu P (2011) Overexpression of Oct4 in human esophageal squamous cell carcinoma. Mol Cells 32:39–45
16. Saigusa S, Mohri Y, Ohi M, Toiyama Y, Ishino Y, Okugawa Y, Tanaka K, Inoue Y, Kusunoki M (2011) Podoplanin and SOX2 expression in esophageal squamous cell carcinoma after neoadjuvant chemo-radiotherapy. Oncol Rep 26:1069–1074
17. Gen Y, Yasui K, Zen Y, Zen K, Dohi O, Endo M, Tsuji K, Wakabayashi N, Itoh Y, Naito Y, Taniwaki M, Nakanuma Y, Okanoue T, Yoshikawa T (2010) SOX2 identified as a target gene for the amplification at 3q26 that is frequently detected in esophageal squamous cell carcinoma. Cancer Genet Cytogenet 202:82–93
18. Hang D, Dong HC, Ning T, Dong B, Hou DL, Xu WG (2012) Prognostic value of the stem cell markers CD133 and ABCG2 expression in esophageal squamous cell carcinoma. Dis Esophagus 25:638–644
19. Tsunoda S, Okumura T, Ito T, Kondo K, Ortiz C, Tanaka E, Watanabe G, Itami A, Sakai Y, Shimada Y (2006) ABCG2 expression is an independent unfavorable prognostic factor in esophageal squamous cell carcinoma. Oncology 71:251–258
20. Yoshikawa R, Tsujimura T, Tao L, Kamikonya N, Fujiwara Y (2012) The oncoprotein and stem cell renewal factor BMI1 associates with poor clinical outcome in oesophageal cancer patients undergoing preoperative chemoradiotherapy. BMC Cancer 12:461
21. Okamoto H, Fujishima F, Nakamura Y, Zuguchi M, Ozawa Y, Takahashi Y, Miyata G, Kamei T, Nakano T, Taniyama Y, Teshima J, Watanabe M, Sato A, Ohuchi N, Sasano H (2013) Significance of CD133 expression in esophageal squamous cell carcinoma. World J Surg Oncol 11:51
22. Ma W, Wang K, Yang S, Wang J, Tan B, Bai B, Wang N, Jia Y, Jia M, Cheng Y (2014) Clinicopathology significance of podoplanin immunoreactivity in esophageal squamous cell carcinoma. Int J Clin Exp Pathol 7:2361–2371
23. Chao YK, Chuang WY, Yeh CJ, Wu YC, Liu YH, Hsieh MJ, Cheng AJ, Hsueh C, Liu HP (2012) Prognostic significance of high podoplanin expression after chemoradiotherapy in esophageal squamous cell carcinoma patients. J Surg Oncol 105:183–188
24. Liu Q, Cui X, Yu X, Bian BS, Qian F, Hu XG, Ji CD, Yang L, Ren Y, Cui W, Zhang X, Zhang P, Wang JM, Cui YH, Bian XW (2017) Cripto-1 acts as a functional marker of cancer stem-like cells and predicts prognosis of the patients in esophageal squamous cell carcinoma. Mol Cancer 16:81
25. Karami Madani G, Rad A, Molavi M, Ardalan Khales S, Abbaszadegan MR, Forghanifard MM (2018) Predicting the correlation of EZH2 and cancer stem cell markers in esophageal squamous cell carcinoma. J Gastrointest Cancer 49:437–441
26. Wang JH, Huang ST, Zhang L, Liu ZG, Liang RX, Jiang SW, Jiang YN, Yu XJ, Jiang YC, Li XZ, Zhang PF, Wen ZS, Zheng M (2019) Combined prognostic value of the cancer stem cell markers CD47 and CD133 in esophageal squamous cell carcinoma. Cancer Med 8:1315–1325
27. Zhao JS, Li WJ, Ge D, Zhang PJ, Li JJ, Lu CL, Ji XD, Guan DX, Gao H, Xu LY, Li EM, Soukiasian H, Koeffler HP, Wang XF, Xie D (2011) Tumor initiating cells in esophageal squamous cell carcinomas express high levels of CD44. PLoS One 6:e21419
28. Almanaa TN, Geusz ME, Jamasbi RJ (2013) A new method for identifying stem-like cells in esophageal cancer cell lines. J Cancer 4:536–548
29. Okumura T, Tsunoda S, Mori Y, Ito T, Kikuchi K, Wang TC, Yasumoto S, Shimada Y (2006) The biological role of the low-affinity p75 neurotrophin receptor in esophageal squamous cell carcinoma. Clin Cancer Res 12:5096–50103
30. Wu C, Alman BA (2008) Side population cells in human cancers. Cancer Lett 268:1–9
31. Huang D, Gao Q, Guo L, Zhang C, Jiang W, Li H, Wang J, Han X, Shi Y, Lu SH (2009) Isolation and identification of cancer stem-like cells in esophageal carcinoma cell lines. Stem Cells Dev 18:465–473
32. Rizzino A (2009) Sox2 and Oct-3/4: a versatile pair of master regulators that orchestrate the self-renewal and pluripotency of embryonic stem cells. Wiley Interdiscip Rev Syst Biol Med 1:228–236
33. Mitsui K, Tokuzawa Y, Itoh H, Segawa K, Murakami M, Takahashi K, Maruyama M, Maeda M, Yamanaka S (2003) The homeoprotein Nanog is required for maintenance of pluripotency in mouse epiblast and ES cells. Cell 113:631–642
34. Hwang CC, Nieh S, Lai CH, Tsai CS, Chang LC, Hua CC, Chi WY, Chien HP, Wang CW, Chan SC, Hsieh TY, Chen JR (2014) A retrospective review of the prognostic value of ALDH-1, Bmi-1 and Nanog stem cell markers in esophageal squamous cell carcinoma. PLoS One 9:e105676
35. Tatetsu H, Kong NR, Chong G, Amabile G, Tenen DG, Chai L (2016) SALL4, the missing link between stem cells, development and cancer. Gene 584:111–119

Chapter 15

Liquid Biopsy: Detection of Circulating Tumor Cells in Esophageal Squamous Cell Carcinoma

Alfred K. Lam, Faysal Bin Hamid, and Vinod Gopalan

Abstract

Circulating tumor cells (CTC) harvested in the blood of patients with esophageal squamous cell carcinoma (ESCC) are associated with certain clinical pathological parameters as well as patients' prognosis and response to chemoradiation. They are the source of distant metastases and their mechanisms of pathogenesis is complex. In recent years, advance in technologies has allowed scientists to detect, enumerate, and isolate these cells for further analysis and monitor the diseases progression in patients with cancer. There are a few methods available for the identification of individual CTC and clusters of CTCs (circulating tumor microemboli). The most commonly used is detection by immunomagnetic method. Although all these methods have limitations, they are helpful for understanding the pathogenesis of CTCs with potential applications in clinical managements in patients with ESCC.

Key words Esophagus, Circulating tumor cell, CTC, CTM, Squamous carcinoma

1 Introduction

The ability of the cancer to go into lymphatics or blood vessels is the way for cancer metastases and cancer recurrence, which contributes to the mortality of patients with cancer. These cancer cells are termed circulating tumor cells (CTCs). This concept is not new as Thomas Ashworth identified CTCs in the blood of a man with metastatic cancer in 1869 [1]. In addition, pathologists often reported the presence of cancer cells in the lumina of small blood vessels or lymphatics in the surgical specimen even when there is an absence of metastatic cancer in the lymph node or distant organs (Fig. 1). This is especially true for esophageal squamous cell carcinoma (ESCC) as there are rich lymphatic networks in the esophagus [2].

Distant metastases and local recurrence are the two important factors contributing to high mortality in patients with ESCC [3]. Thus, the dynamics of CTCs are important factors to consider for improving the management of patients with ESCC. The

Alfred K. Lam (ed.), *Esophageal Squamous Cell Carcinoma: Methods and Protocols*, Methods in Molecular Biology, vol. 2129, https://doi.org/10.1007/978-1-0716-0377-2_15,

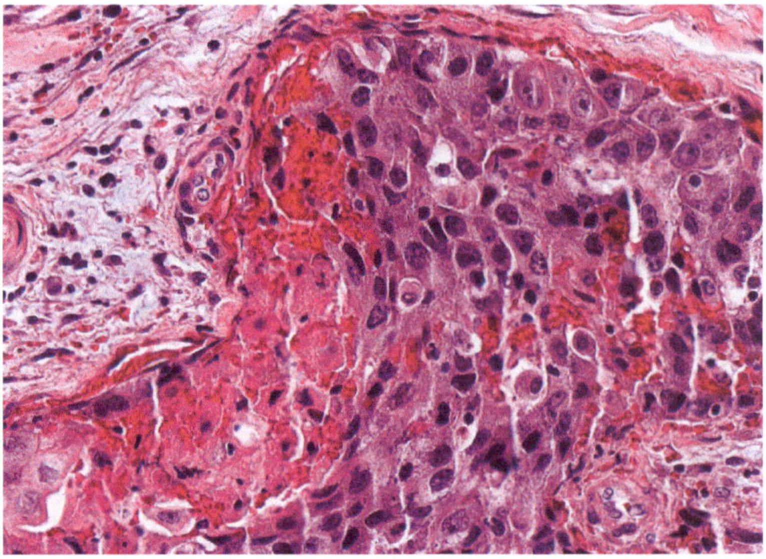

Fig. 1 Vascular invasion by esophageal squamous cell carcinoma. The blood vessel in the sub-adventitia of the esophagus shows sheets of carcinoma cells with eosinophilic cytoplasm, hyperchromatic nuclei, and mitotic figures. There are also red blood cells and fibrin in the vessel (hematoxylin and eosin ×25)

attractive aspect and potential application of CTC is the relative noninvasive nature of the procedure to obtain blood (termed liquid biopsy) when compared with tissue(s) biopsies in the serial assessment of patients with ESCC. When compared with looking at the mutation or mi-RNA expression in liquid biopsy, the assessment of CTCs has the advantage of being able to be directly visualized under the microscope.

Clinically, potential applications of detection, counting, and isolation of CTC may involve monitoring of minimal residual disease in terms of risk of relapse or progression, real-time monitoring of therapies, and identification of therapeutic targets and resistances [4]. The mechanism of CTC in the pathogenesis of cancer metastases is complex and needs continuous research [5]. The presence of CTCs in the blood is not enough for cancer metastases as the cells may die and interact with numerous factors in the human body. There are suppressor cells and promotor cells in the blood for CTCs. The forming of CTCs in clusters (circulating tumor microemboli [CTM]), shear stress, proliferation, property changes in CTC, size and blood flow of local blood vessels, as well as the nature of the host tissue affect the chance of forming distant metastases [6–8].

Table 1 showed the summary of studies on cytometric analysis of CTC in ESCC. Overall, the detection of CTC was noted in 8–100% of the patients with ESCC [9–23]. By pooling up the data in the literature, 55% (319 of 583) of these ESCC tested

Table 1
Circulating tumor cell detection by cytometric detection in esophageal squamous cell carcinoma

Author/year/ country	Subjects	Method	Positive	Correlations
Hiraiwa/2008/ Japan	33	PS	–	Distant metastases
Bobek/2014/ Czech	23	Size based	12/23 (52%)	–
Qiao/ 2015/China	1 with serial follow-up	NS	–	Cancer progression
Matsushita/ 2015/Japan	90 received adjuvant therapy	PS	25/90 (28%)	Patients' survival and cancer stage & progression
Reeh/2015/ Germany	29	PS	3/29 (10%)	Cancer metastatic stage and patients' survival
Tanaka/2015/ Japan	28	PS	19/38 (50%)	Patients' survival and treatment response
Li/2015/China	61	PS + size based	30/61 (32%)	Cancer stage, platelet count
Li/2016/China	140	NS	62/140 (44%)	Cancer stage and patients' survival
Su/2016/Taiwan	57 advanced cancers	NS + FC	57/57 (100%)	Patients' survival received adjuvant therapy
Qiao/ 2017/China	59	NS	47/59 (80%)	Cancer stage, grade, and patients' survival
Chen/ 2018/China	71	Size based	–	Cancer stage, size, adjuvant chemotherapy (mesenchymal type)
Choi/2018/ Korea	73	Size based	63/73 (86%)	Cancer stage
Han/2018/China	21	Size based	–	Cancer stage
Woestemeier/ 2018/Germany	13 resectable cancers	PS	1/13 (8%)	Patients' survival

PS positive selection, *NS* negative selection, *FC* flow cytometry

showed CTC. The presence of CTC correlated with pathological markers (grade, size, and stage of ESCC), response to adjuvant chemotherapy, and patients' survival. Epithelial-mesenchymal transition (EMT) occurred in CTC from patients with ESCC [19, 21]. CTC with EMT correlated with tumor size, cancer stage, and response to adjuvant chemotherapy in ESCC [19]. From the limited data, monitoring of CTC appears to be promising for the management of patients with ESCC.

Researches involving CTC often involve identification, counting, and extraction of CTC from patients with cancer. The isolated CTCs could be used to study mutations and protein expressions, cell cultures, and animal studies [7, 23, 24]. Nevertheless, the number of CTC in a patient with cancer is usually small [25]. A standardized protocol is ideal for the enrichment of CTCs (before detection) and use for downstream researches and clinical applications. The problems lie in the lack of recognized best procedure for pre-analytical workflows and methods of detection of CTCs. The pre-analytic problem centralizes on the collection of consistent quality blood specimens. Degeneration of CTC could occur in the waiting period before processing. CTC isolation methods can cause cellular damages or isolation of the cell cluster of CTCs into single cells.

In the processes of CTC detection, there are many methods and each of them has its own limitations. Among these, there are a few main mechanisms, which depend on the functional, physical properties (size, density, and other properties), immunological properties of CTCs, as well as the use of micro devices [24]. None of the methods of detection is perfect for workings on CTCs. Thus, there are continue search of new tools such as use of nanotechnology-based strategies as well as other capture agents like aptamers (screened oligonucleotide ligands with specific affinity for their target) which have potential to improve the detection of CTCs [24, 26].

The most commonly used type of method primarily relies on the expression of proteins (immunological properties) in CTC not found in other blood components [24]. In the settings of carcinoma, the proteins used are epithelial markers, used to identify carcinoma not easily to be confirmed by histopathological examination. There are basally two approaches in immunological-based methods, namely, positive selection and negative selection. The positive selection is to isolate the CTCs by tumor markers. The most common marker to epithelial cell is epithelial cell adhesion molecular (EpCAM). This is the principle employed by CELLSEARCH (Menarini Silicon Biosystems Inc., Huntingoton Valley, PA, USA). Currently, it is the only US FDA (Food and Drug Administration) approved method and most commonly employed to enumerate CTC. However, it may have challenges when targeting cancer cells with reduced expression of cancer-associated markers. On the other hand, negative selection is the removal of normal blood cells by anti-bodies. The method uses a magnet to remove the magnet beads coated with these antibodies to remove the unwanted hematopoietic cells. It is a promising technique. However, some of the CTCs associated with leukocytes may be removed in the process. In this chapter, a negative selection technique is used to demonstrate the extraction of CTC from blood samples of ESCC.

2 Materials

The material used is for working on the negative selection method.

1. Heparin containing collection tube for blood samples.
2. Magnet, magnetic beads in solution, and enrichment cocktail (buffer) (commercial kit).
3. 14 mL polystyrene round-bottom tube (to fit with the hole in magnet).
4. 50 mL of stock solution by mixing phosphate-buffered saline (PBS), fetal bovine serum (FBS), and 1 mM ethylenediamine-tetraacetic acid (EDTA), which can be stored up and use for multiple times (49 mL PBS mix with 1 mL FBS and 100 μL of EDTA resulting in 2% FBS).
5. Centrifuge.
6. Roswell Park Memorial Institute (RPMI) medium for cell culture.
7. 96-well plates.
8. Incubator.
9. Ice-cold 100% methanol.
10. 0.1% Triton X-100 containing PBS.
11. Bovine serum albumin (BSA).
12. Anti-EPCAM antibody (type for immunofluorescence).
13. Anti-CK-18 antibody (type for immunofluorescence).
14. Anti-CD45 antibody (type for immunofluorescence).
15. Secondary antibody (type for immunofluorescence)—must match the host species of primary antibody.
16. Humidified chamber in dark room.
17. 4′,6-diamidino-2-phenylindole (DAPI) (a blue-fluorescent DNA stain) or Hoechst (a blue-fluorescent DNA stain).
18. Fluorescence microscopy linked with computer in dark room.

3 Method

3.1 Extraction of CTC

1. Collect 5 mL of fresh blood in heparin containing collection tube.
2. Add the collected blood in 14 mL polystyrene round-bottom tube.
3. Add enrichment cocktail (buffer) to sample (50 μL/mL of sample, i.e., 250 μL).
4. Mix and incubate at room temperature for 5 min.

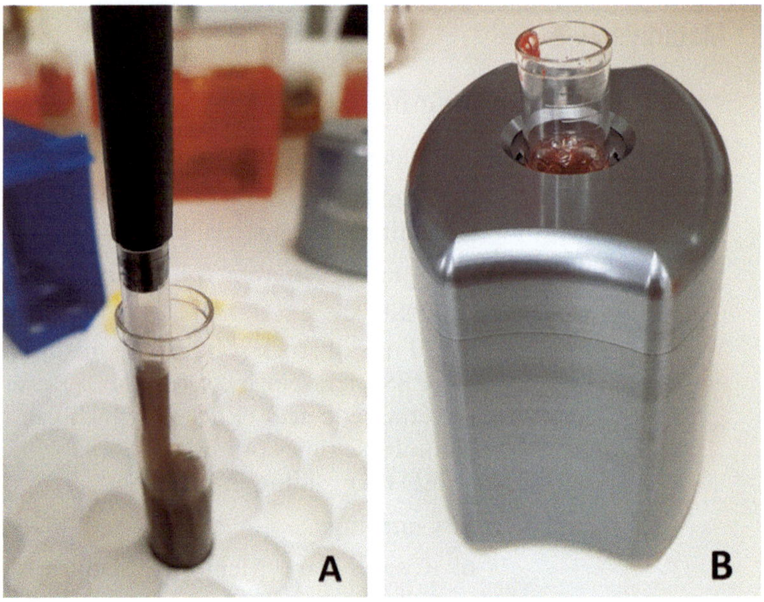

Fig. 2 (**a**) Add the solution with magnet beads to the blood sample in the tube. (**b**) Put the sample in (**a**) inside the hole in the magnet

5. Vortex magnet beads in solution for 30 s (contain antibodies to remove the unwanted cells such as white blood cells, red blood cells, platelets, and macrophages) (*see* **Note 1**).
6. Add magnetic beads in solution to sample (50 μL/mL of sample, i.e., 250 μL).
7. Add the 4.5 mL of stock solution (PBS, FBS, and EDTA) to the blood (5 mL), buffer, and magnetic beads (0.5 mL in total), which amount to 10 mL. Mix gently by pipetting up and down 2–3 times.
8. Place the tube (without lid) into the magnet and incubate at room temperature for 10 min (Fig. 2).
9. After incubation, pick up the magnet, and in one continuous motion invert the magnet and tube for 2–3 s to pour off the enriched cells suspension into a new 14 mL tube. Do not shake or blot off any drops (Fig. 3).
10. Repeat the separation procedure by adding magnet beads in solution to the new tube containing the enriched cells at **step 6** and mix.
11. Place the tube (without lid) into the magnet and incubate at room temperature for 10 min.
12. After incubation, pick up the magnet, and in one continuous motion invert the magnet and tube for 2–3 s to pour off the enriched cells suspension into a new 14 mL tube. Do not shake

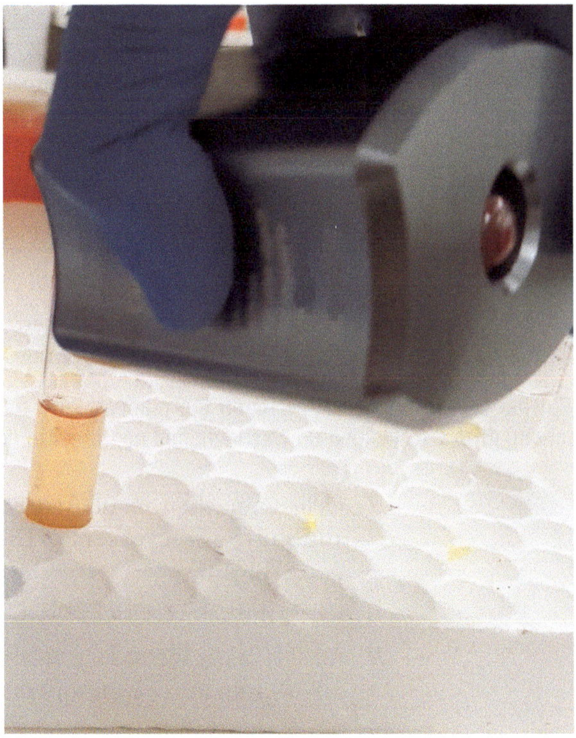

Fig. 3 Pour off the enriched cells suspension into a new 14 mL tube. Hematopoietic cells and platelets will stay in the previous tube with the magnet beads held in the magnet. Note that the collected sample is a clear fluid with the CTCs

or blot off any drops. This is the solution with isolated cells (CTC) ready for downstream use.

13. Spin down enriched cells suspension at 34 relative centrifugal force (RCF)/g for 7 min.
14. Discard supernatant and proceed for downstream application.

3.2 Detection Protocol

1. Add 400 μL RPMI medium to the tube in **step 14**.
2. Put the resulting mixture (RPMI medium and CTC extracted in **step 14**) in four wells in 96-well plates (approximately 100 μL in each well), maintained at in incubator at 37 °C with 5% CO_2 for 24 h (*see* **Note 2**).
3. The cells were fixed with ice-cold 100 μL 100% methanol (both fix and permeabilized) in −20 °C for 10 min.
4. Then, the cells were in 100 μL 0.1% Triton X-100 containing PBS for 10 min (permeabilization).
5. Wash with 100 μL PBS.
6. Block with 100 μL 1% BSA (avoid unwanted nonspecific protein binding).

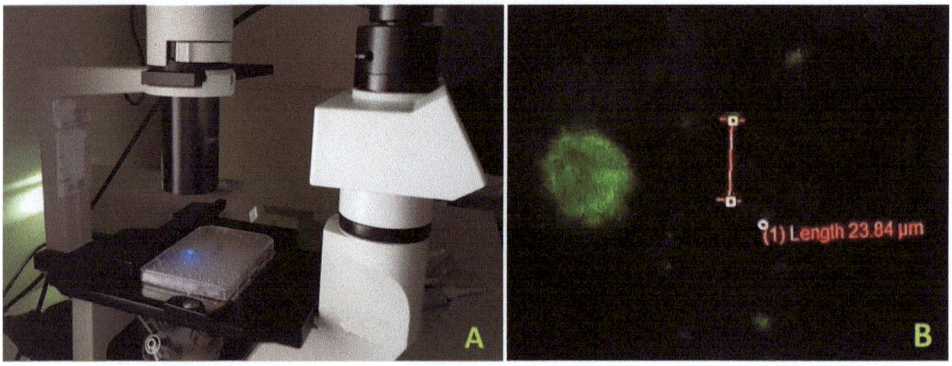

Fig. 4 (**a**) Put the culture plates with CTC on the platform of a fluorescence microscope attached to the computer screen. (**b**) A CTC stained up was identified and the size (length) of the CTC was noted

7. Cells were then incubated with 100 µL each of anti-EPCAM antibody, anti-cytokerain-18 antibody, and anti-CD45 antibody for 2 h.
8. Wash the samples twice with 100 µL PBS for 10 min each.
9. Add 100 µL secondary antibody (1:100) in 1% BSA/PBS for 30–60 min at room temperature (*see* **Note 3**).
10. Wash the samples twice with PBS for 10 min each.
11. Counter staining: stain the nuclei of cells with 100 µL DAPI or Hoechst for 5 min.
12. Wash the samples twice with 100 µL PBS for 10 min each.
13. Visualize and analyze the CTCs by fluorescent microscopy immediately or later (store at 4 °C in dark before use) (*see* **Note 4**) (Fig. 4).

4 Notes

1. Removal of hematopoietic cells by a cocktail of antibody-labelled immunomagnetic beads targeting CD2, CD14, CD16, CD19, CD45, CD61, CD66b, and glycophorin A. These hematopoietic cells after binding to the magnet beads with remain in the tube because of attractive force of the magnet. The cells in the fluid poured out from the tube will be mainly CTCs if present.
2. Culturing the CTCs overnight allows time for them to attach to the bottom of the plates. In addition, capturing CTCs at this stage under microscope is good for downstream experiments such as culture, implantation into mice, and mutation profiles.
3. The use of secondary antibody is to amply the signal of the antigen-antibody reaction to be visualized. Secondary antibody must match the host species of primary antibody used. In this

situation, the secondary antibody should conjugate to a dye in immunofluorescence. From this point onward, slides should be kept in the dark. Florescence antibodies are sensitive to light. The staining will fade when exposed to ambient light. The tube holding the antibodies should be wrapped in foils to keep in the dark and in a humidified chamber.

4. Study the number, dimension, and other properties (e.g., staining profiles) of the CTCs at this step.

References

1. Ashworth TR (1869) A case of cancer in which cells similar to those in the tumours were seen in the blood after death. Australas Med J 14:146–147
2. Lam KY, Ma LT, Wong J (1996) Measurement of extent of spread of oesophageal squamous carcinoma by serial sectioning. J Clin Pathol 49:124–129
3. Lam KY, Law S, Wong J (2003) Low prevalence of incidentally discovered and early-stage esophageal cancers in a 30-year autopsy study. Dis Esophagus 16:1–3
4. Alix-Panabieres C, Pantel K (2014) Challenges in circulating tumour cell research. Nat Rev Cancer 14:623–631
5. Zhang WW, Rong Y, Liu Q, Luo CL, Zhang Y, Wang FB (2019) Integrative diagnosis of cancer by combining CTCs and associated peripheral blood cells in liquid biopsy. Clin Transl Oncol 21:828–835
6. Lambert AW, Pattabiraman DR, Weinberg RA (2017) Emerging biological principles of metastasis. Cell 168:670–691
7. Lu Y, Lian S, Cheng Y, Ye Y, Xie X, Fu C, Zhang C, Zhu Y, Iqbal Parker M, Jia L (2019) Circulation patterns and seed-soil compatibility factors cooperate to cause cancer organ-specific metastasis. Exp Cell Res 375:62–72
8. Umer M, Vaidyanathan R, Nguyen NT, Shiddiky MJA (2018) Circulating tumor microemboli: Progress in molecular understanding and enrichment technologies. Biotechnol Adv 36:1367–1389
9. Hiraiwa K, Takeuchi H, Hasegawa H, Saikawa Y, Suda K, Ando T, Kumagai K, Irino T, Yoshikawa T, Matsuda S, Kitajima M, Kitagawa Y (2008) Clinical significance of circulating tumor cells in blood from patients with gastrointestinal cancers. Ann Surg Oncol 15:3092–3100
10. Bobek V, Matkowski R, Gürlich R, Grabowski K, Szelachowska J, Lischke R, Schützner J, Harustiak T, Pazdro A, Rzechonek A, Kolostova K (2014) Cultivation of circulating tumor cells in esophageal cancer. Folia Histochem Cytobiol 52:171–177
11. Qiao YY, Lin KX, Zhang Z, Zhang DJ, Shi CH, Xiong M, Qu XH, Zhao XH (2015) Monitoring disease progression and treatment efficacy with circulating tumor cells in esophageal squamous cell carcinoma: a case report. World J Gastroenterol 21:7921–7928
12. Matsushita D, Uenosono Y, Arigami T, Yanagita S, Nishizono Y, Hagihara T, Hirata M, Haraguchi N, Arima H, Kijima Y, Kurahara H, Maemura K, Okumura H, Ishigami S, Natsugoe S (2015) Clinical significance of circulating tumor cells in peripheral blood of patients with esophageal squamous cell carcinoma. Ann Surg Oncol 22:3674–3680
13. Reeh M, Effenberger KE, Koenig AM, Riethdorf S, Eichstädt D, Vettorazzi E, Uzunoglu FG, Vashist YK, Izbicki JR, Pantel K, Bockhorn M (2015) Circulating tumor cells as a biomarker for preoperative prognostic staging in patients with esophageal cancer. Ann Surg 261:1124–1130
14. Tanaka M, Takeuchi H, Osaki Y, Hiraiwa K, Nakamura R, Oyama T, Takahashi T, Wada N, Kawakubo H, Saikawa Y, Omori T, Kitagawa Y (2015) Prognostic significance of circulating tumor cells in patients with advanced esophageal cancer. Esophagus 12:352–359
15. Li H, Song P, Zou B, Liu M, Cui K, Zhou P, Li S, Zhang B (2015) Circulating tumor cell analyses in patients with esophageal squamous cell carcinoma using epithelial marker-dependent and -independent approaches. Medicine (Baltimore) 94:e1565
16. Li SP, Guan QL, Zhao D, Pei GJ, Su HX, Du LN, He JX, Liu ZC (2016) Detection of circulating tumor cells by fluorescent immunohistochemistry in patients with esophageal squamous cell carcinoma: potential clinical applications. Med Sci Monit 22:1654–1662

17. Su PJ, Wu MH, Wang HM, Lee CL, Huang WK, Wu CE, Chang HK, Chao YK, Tseng CK, Chiu TK, Lin NM, Ye SR, Lee JY, Hsieh CH (2016) Circulating tumour cells as an independent prognostic factor in patients with advanced oesophageal squamous cell carcinoma undergoing chemoradiotherapy. Sci Rep 6:31423
18. Qiao Y, Li J, Shi C, Wang W, Qu X, Xiong M, Sun Y, Li D, Zhao X, Zhang D (2017) Prognostic value of circulating tumor cells in the peripheral blood of patients with esophageal squamous cell carcinoma. Onco Targets Ther 10:1363–1373
19. Chen W, Li Y, Yuan D, Peng Y, Qin J (2018) Practical value of identifying circulating tumor cells to evaluate esophageal squamous cell carcinoma staging and treatment efficacy. Thorac Cancer 9:956–966
20. Choi MK, Kim GH, I H, Park SJ, Lee MW, Lee BE, Park DY, Cho YK (2019) Circulating tumor cells detected using fluid-assisted separation technique in esophageal squamous cell carcinoma. J Gastroenterol Hepatol 34:552–560
21. Han D, Chen K, Che J, Hang J, Li H (2018) Detection of epithelial-mesenchymal transition status of circulating tumor cells in patients with esophageal squamous carcinoma. Biomed Res Int 2018:7610154
22. Woestemeier A, Ghadban T, Riethdorf S, Harms-Effenberger K, Konczalla L, Uzunoglu FG, Izbicki JR, Pantel K, Bockhorn M, Reeh M (2018) Absence of HER2 expression of circulating tumor cells in patients with non-metastatic esophageal cancer. Anticancer Res 38:5665–5669
23. Tellez-Gabriel M, Cochonneau D, Cadé M, Jubellin C, Heymann MF, Heymann D (2018) Circulating tumor cell-derived pre-clinical models for personalized medicine. Cancers (Basel) 11:E19
24. Sharma S, Zhuang R, Long M, Pavlovic M, Kang Y, Ilyas A, Asghar W (2018) Circulating tumor cell isolation, culture, and downstream molecular analysis. Biotechnol Adv 36:1063–1078
25. Au SH, Edd J, Haber DA, Maheswaran S, Stott SL, Toner M (2017) Clusters of circulating tumor cells: a biophysical and technological perspective. Curr Opin Biomed Eng 3:13–19
26. Huang Q, Wang Y, Chen X, Wang Y, Li Z, Du S, Wang L, Chen S (2018) Nanotechnology-based strategies for early cancer diagnosis using circulating tumor cells as a liquid biopsy. Nano 2:21–41

Chapter 16

Liquid Biopsy for Investigation of Cancer DNA in Esophageal Squamous Cell Carcinoma

Robert A. Smith and Alfred K. Lam

Abstract

Early detection of cancer and the monitoring of cancer recurrence in treated patients are significant challenges in esophageal squamous cell carcinoma (ESCC). Liquid biopsy is the identification of tumor biomarkers from minimally invasive samples of biological fluids, including urine, blood, stool, saliva, or cerebrospinal fluid. Liquid biopsy offers a potential solution to the problems of detection and surveillance as DNA shed from cancer cells as cell-free DNA or in exosomes can be detected in body fluids. By detecting these DNAs, we can identify the presence of cancer-associated mutations for basic detection, as well as to obtain information on the recurrence and evolution of disease following initial treatment. These sources of information have the potential to significantly improve the management of patients with ESCC. In this chapter, we detail a method for the isolation of cell-free DNA from blood plasma and DNA associated with exosomes in blood from patients with esophageal squamous cell carcinomas.

Key words Liquid biopsy, Cell-free DNA, Exosome-associated DNA, Cancer surveillance, Cancer detection, Cancer management, Mutations

1 Introduction

Improved methods of early detection of esophageal squamous cell carcinoma are needed because of the high prevalence and high mortality of the cancer [1, 2]. Liquid biopsy offers a potential fulfillment of these requirements, thanks to its ability to detect signs of cancer presence in easily accessible tissues or bodily fluids rather than relying on direct biopsy of the less accessible esophageal tissue. An additional advantage of using liquid biopsies is that they provide material across the complete suite of cancer cells present in the body rather than the single localized population information provided by a traditional biopsy [3]. This has the potential to improve patient outcomes by detecting molecular signatures of increased tumor aggression in small, unnoticed tumor pockets not noticed or sampled in initial scans. Liquid biopsy can detect DNA, RNA, or protein derived from cancers in a variety of ways.

Alfred K. Lam (ed.), *Esophageal Squamous Cell Carcinoma: Methods and Protocols*, Methods in Molecular Biology, vol. 2129, https://doi.org/10.1007/978-1-0716-0377-2_16,

Biomarkers can be detected from actual circulating tumor cells, shed from apoptotic or necrotic cancer cells, or released by living cancer cells in the form of exosomes. Each of these different sources of biomarker has advantages and limitations, and the choice of which to use may depend on the intended treatment modality.

Circulating tumor cells are rare and difficult to obtain. There are methods to detect these circulating tumor cells in esophageal squamous cell carcinoma (*see* Chapter 15). The detection of these cells offers the ability to probe the behaviors of living members of the tumor population, and their survival in the bloodstream fundamentally biases them toward the more robust and aggressive subclones [4].

DNA shed from apoptotic or necrotic cancer cells necessarily reflects dead rather than active members of the tumor clonal population, but it is a relatively abundant source of material, and it enables the detection of common, cancer-specific mutations and can be used for prognostic testing and surveillance of recurrence [5, 6]. Exosomes may not contain all common mutations carried by the full tumor population, but analysis of their contents can provide insight into tumor effects on the microenvironment. As we come to know more about their composition and function, they may offer options for diagnosis, prognosis, and treatment [7].

Due to its relative ease of extraction and the known potential to detect tumor-specific DNA markers and profiles, cell-free DNA (cfDNA) shed from dead cancer cells has become a favored source of data for liquid biopsies. One of the advantages offered by cfDNA is its relatively short half-life, which has a few consequences [8–10]. The first of these is that cfDNA shed from dead or dying benign tissues exists at a roughly constant level, and so increases in the total amount of cfDNA can be a sign of the existence of cancer as a population of rapidly growing (and dying) cells, and increased cfDNA levels have been used to distinguish patients with non-small cell lung carcinoma from controls with reported sensitivities ranging from 69% to 79% and specificities of 83–89% [8]. The second consequence is that it can be used as a measure of both treatment success and disease recurrence, as levels drop sharply during effective treatment and rise detectably weeks to months before recurrence can be identified radiologically, potentially outperforming protein-based markers [9]. Third, it can be used to direct patient-specific risk profiling and surveillance. For instance, patients with no known tumor but who have detection of cancer-associated mutations in the blood have an increased risk of developing a detectable bladder carcinoma within 6 years [10]. Fourth, while cfDNA does measure dead cells, it measures the full breadth of the carious tumor clonal populations that exist at the time of sampling and can be used for effectively real-time tailoring of cancer treatment to resistance markers as soon as they appear.

The short half-life of cfDNA does provide a challenge for clinicians attempting to use it for liquid biopsy in that it continues to decay when removed from the body. This is in part due to its relatively small size, in multiples of ~166 bp as the leftover fragments of DNA bound to histone proteins, which makes it more vulnerable to larger DNA fragments to chemical attack [8]. Additionally, liquid biopsy samples left too long will begin to be contaminated by DNA shed from lysing benign cells collected along with the fluid medium, which can make it more difficult to detect cancer-specific mutations among the increased signal from benign DNA. As a result, cfDNA should be extracted as soon as possible after biopsy collection, and recommendations of between 2 and 24 h as the limit for extraction have been published [10]. The short survival time of cfDNA and the potential for increased benign DNA contamination have led to the development of specialist collection tubes with preservative reagents from companies such as Streck, Roche, and Qiagen. While preservative tubes do not seem to provide superior performance to nonspecialized tubes if extractions are performed within 6 h, preservative tubes do offer relatively unchanged detection abilities for between 5 and 7 days [10, 11].

Several studies have shown the potential value of liquid biopsy in esophageal squamous cell carcinoma, using markers including total cfDNA levels, detection of specific mutations or variants, and identification of aberrant methylation patterns in DNA. One of the earliest, conducted in 2003 by Eisenberger et al., examined plasma samples matched with tumor and normal tissue from 28 patients with ESCC and identified altered microsatellite lengths in at least one of twelve selected microsatellites in 96.4% (27/28) of their population's plasma samples [12]. Their results did not show complete matching of the detected changes in the tumor samples compared to the plasma samples, including one instance of detected instability in plasma where none was evident in the primary tumor, showing the capacity of liquid biopsy to identify a different range of mutations compared to sampling from primary or secondary tumors.

In 2007, Ijoma and colleagues compared the ability of *CEA* qPCR and a methylation-specific assay for *p16*, *E-cadherin*, and *RARβ* genes compared to detection of protein-based serum markers to detect the presence of cancer in the blood of patients with ESCC. They determined that the molecular-based tests were able to detect the presence of cancer in 53% of the 44 patients in their research population, while serum protein-based tests were only able to detect cancer in 32% of patients [13]. Detection by molecular mechanisms was not consistent. Different methods detected different patients with detection in six (14%), four (9%), and four patients (9%) for the p16, E-cadherin, and RARβ genes, respectively, while CEA qPCR was able to detect cancer in a further nine patients (20%). Their results indicate that while liquid biopsy and use of molecular methods may have high-detection rates, a variety of markers is more useful than a single marker for detection. A similar study in 2012 by Ling et al. examined methylation of *MSH2* in plasma and tumor samples of 209 patients with ESCC. They identified *MSH2* methylation in 77/209 patients, showing complete correlation between the primary tumor and plasma results [14]. Their results also indicated that continued detection of *MSH2* hypermethylation 1–3 months post-surgery was associated with worse prognosis, showing potential value for this marker and liquid biopsies in patient prognosis and surveillance. A similar study on hypermethylation of the *MGMT* gene in an Indian population by Das et al. detected promoter hypermethylation in 70/100 patients with ESCC [15]. The study also detected increased risk of *MGMT* hypermethylation for betel-quid and tobacco users, both cases and controls, with a combination of the methylation status and use of betel-quid or tobacco showing the highest risk for development of ESCC. Most interestingly, this study used whole-blood DNA extraction, indicating that hypermethylation was detectable as a biomarker with effects on nonmalignant DNA, though its presence in control subjects indicates that this biomarker is more useful for risk assessment and not for diagnosis.

Other studies in patients with ESCC looked at simple detection of total DNA levels using various means as a method for diagnosis or monitoring. In 2007, Tomita et al. examined the DNA levels and DNA integrity in 24 patients with ESCC having a mix of pathological characteristics and 21 healthy controls using qPCR of the *beta actin* gene with different-sized amplicons [16]. Their results indicated that patients with ESCC had on average higher concentrations of cell-free DNA in their plasma than controls and suggested a DNA concentration cutoff of 0.96 ng/mL of DNA, providing a 92% sensitivity and 95% specificity for detection of cancer in their data. A similar study conducted in 2016 by Hsieh and colleagues compared 81 patients with ESCC and 95 healthy controls who had no diagnosis of cancer within 2 years of blood collection [5]. Hsieh's study involved qPCR of the *cyclophilin* gene and DNA concentration as assessed as gene copies per milliliter. Like Tomita et al. before them, Hsieh and colleagues also found a significantly higher DNA copy number in patients with ESCC, with 96.3% sensitivity and 94.1% specificity with a cutoff value of 2447.26 copies/mL. In addition, they found a significant correlation between copy number and lymphovascular invasion, and a significant reduction in disease-free survival for high-cfDNA copy number patients, indicating the potential use for cfDNA levels as a prognostic marker in ESCC [5]. Interestingly, the samples for Hsieh et al.'s study came from a prospectively collected biobank, and there was no information provided in their publication about the time lag between collection of blood and spin-down for plasma, so it is possible that better diagnostic and prognostic capabilities might be available from plasma obtained as soon as possible after blood collection.

Finally, studies have also investigated the detection of cancer-specific mutations in patients with ESCC for diagnostic and prognostic purposes. In 2016, Luo et al. developed a custom sequencing panel following meta-analysis of 532 ESCC genomes and used this panel in eight patients with ESCC having whole exome sequencing in plasma derived from blood collected at 1-day pre-surgery and 7-day post-surgery [2]. Illumina TruSight Cancer sequencing was performed on the samples from three patients to assess this method. All samples were subject to sequencing not only in plasma but in tumor, tumor adjacent, and macroscopically normal tissues obtained during surgery. This study was successfully able to detect mutations from the primary cancer in cfDNA extracted from plasma, and the frequency of mutant alleles was reduced in postsurgical cfDNA, indicating a potential use for monitoring of recurrence. The Illumina TruSight system was also able to detect cancer-specific mutations, but Luo and colleagues observed that Illumina panel did not cover approximately 11% of the mutations in their meta-analysis of 532 samples, implying that tissue- or cancer-specific panels may have greater detection and monitoring capabilities than generally designed panels for sequencing-based surveillance [2].

In 2016, Ueda et al. utilized a panel of 53 genes and undertook next-generation sequencing in a cohort of 13 patients, utilizing tumor tissue as well as pre- and postsurgically collected cfDNA [6]. They were able to find 51.7% of the mutations detected in the primary tumor in the cfDNA from patients, and 81.3% of patients had more than one mutation detected using their panel. They detected some decrease in allele frequency of mutations post-surgery but did not find a significant difference between pre- and postsurgical samples. Interestingly, however, they did detect an increase in mutation allele frequencies approximately 9 months before recurrence was detected by imaging in two patients, which provides some useful information regarding the ability of liquid biopsy base sequencing as a surveillance mechanism for recurrence [6].

Most recently, Xu et al. utilized a qPCR-based approach in 66 patients with ESCC and esophageal adenocarcinoma treated with the EGFR tyrosine kinase inhibitor, gefitinib, to detect *EGFR* mutations [17]. Their study showed a higher EGFR mutation rate in patients with ESCC and indicated that patients with EGFR mutations detected in cfDNA samples had higher levels of overall response to gefitinib, showing the potential for liquid biopsies to be used in treatment targeting and other precision medicine approaches.

Most of the ESCC-based studies discussed here have used cfDNA extracted from plasma as the source for assays, and this choice is likely dictated by the ease of obtaining plasma as compared to live tumor cells, or even just exosomes, which require additional steps to isolate and prepare. Similarly, PCR-based approaches are popular and with high sensitivity for detection of either general DNA levels or specific mutations. On the other hand, next-generation sequencing is a useful alternative, especially because some studies have shown that relying on an individual mutation as marker may provide a false determination of overall tumor burden if it is restricted to the primary tumor and is no longer detectable following surgery, even if recurrence is later detected.

The protocol in this chapter is primarily concerned with isolation of nucleic acids from plasma but also includes provision for collection of exosomes if desired. Extraction of cfDNA from serum is also possible, but this has become less popular due to the potential for contamination from lysing normal cells during clotting. In general, spinning down rapidly after collection is advisable, though some studies have allowed for a several hours of gravity separation before centrifugation and still obtained useful results, such as the study by Xu et al. [17]. Fig. 1 shows a breakdown of different liquid biopsy targets and some suggested applications.

2 Materials

Prior to commencing the method, you will need the following:

1. EDTA vacutainer or similar anticoagulant-coated collection tube for blood samples.
2. Refrigerated centrifuge capable of at least 14,000 × *g*.
3. [For exosomes] Refrigerated ultracentrifuge capable of at least 105,000 × *g*.
4. [For exosomes] 0.22 μm filter and syringe to drive filtration.
5. Pipettes.
6. Centrifuge tubes, ranging from 10 mL to 1 mL, depending on volumes needed.
7. [For exosomes] Chromatographic separation column (e.g., Tricorn 5/20 Column).
8. [For exosomes] Sepharose 2B beads.
9. Spectrophotometer.
10. Agitating water bath.
11. Phosphate-buffered saline.

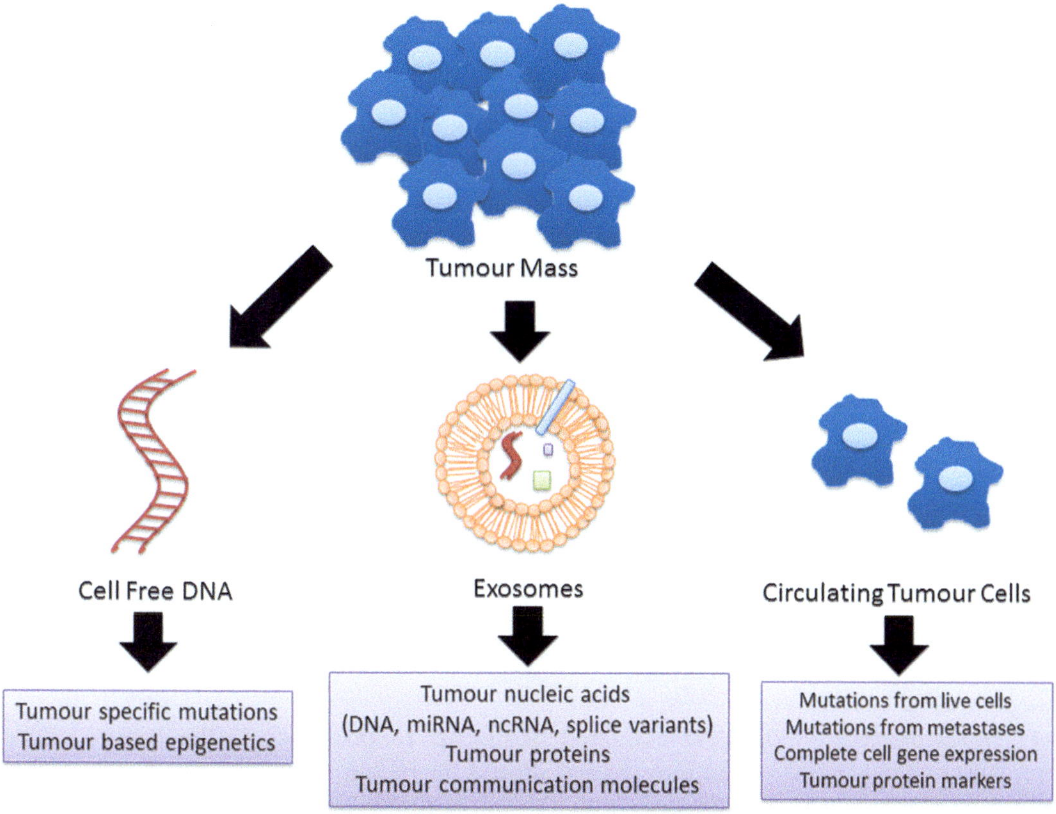

Fig. 1 Uses for different liquid biopsy targets. This figure shows the different uses to which categories of liquid biopsy targets can be put. Cell-free DNA enables the detection of tumor-based mutations and tumor-based epigenetic variants which can be used for diagnosis and surveillance. Exosomes contain a variety of molecules including a subset of various kinds of nucleic acids and tumor proteins, all tuned for manipulation of the surrounding microenvironment. Circulating tumor cells will provide the full range of tumor-associated molecules, slanted to live clonal subtypes and more aggressive clonal subtypes able to survive in the circulation before collection

12. Extraction buffer for plasma: 10 mM Tris–HCl (pH 8), 10 mM ethylenediaminetetraacetic acid (EDTA), 30 mM NaCl, 1 mM $CaCl_2$, 0.5% sodium dodecyl sulfate.
13. Extraction buffer for exosomes: 10 mM Tris–HCl (pH 8), 10 mM EDTA, 30 mM NaCl, 1 mM $CaCl_2$, 1% sodium dodecyl sulfate.
14. [Optional] Liquid nitrogen.

3 Method

3.1 Isolation of Cell-Free DNA from Plasma

3.1.1 Isolation of Plasma

1. Collect blood in a vacutainer or equivalent vessel containing EDTA, lithium heparin, or other anticoagulant (*see* **Note 1**).
2. Enough blood should be collected to maximize plasma yield and hence overall DNA produced. You may need to balance this with concerns over the amount of blood removed for other patient collection needs (*see* **Note 2**).
3. At the time of collection, gently invert collection tube 5–10 times to mix blood. Do not shake the blood or subject it to shocks that may cause cell lysis.
4. Centrifuge blood at 2000 × *g* for 15–20 min, until plasma separates.
5. [Alternative] Centrifuge blood at 250 × *g* for 30 min, followed by centrifugation at 1000 × *g* for 5 min, followed again by centrifugation at 2000 × *g* for 5 min to separate plasma.
6. Using a pipette, transfer all available plasma to a new tube for protein digestion. Do not disturb the cell layer interface (*see* **Note 3**).

3.1.2 Protein Digestion

1. Add extracted plasma to an extraction buffer solution. The amount added should be 10 mg of protein per 1 mL of final solution (one part of plasma to five parts buffer).
2. Add proteinase K. Concentration should be between 50 and 100 μg/mL (*see* **Note 4**).
3. Incubate solution in an agitating water bath or oscillating heating block at 37–56 °C for 1 h to overnight.
4. [Optional] Incubate solution at 65 °C for 10 min to inactivate proteinase K.

3.1.3 Purification of DNA

1. Centrifuge solution at 4 °C at 1000 × *g* for 15 min.
2. Pipette the supernatant into a new tube. This tube should have enough spare capacity to contain 4× the current volume.
3. Add 2 volumes of chilled (−20 °C) absolute ethanol.
4. Invert tube several times to mix.
5. [Optional] Use liquid nitrogen to freeze the tube (*see* **Note 5**).
6. Centrifuge solution at 4 °C at 14,000 × *g* for 15 min.
7. Remove and discard supernatant.
8. Allow pellet to air-dry or dry in vacuum dryer.
9. Resuspend pellet in sterile water or buffer as desired. DNA can be kept overnight at 37 °C to ensure complete resuspension.

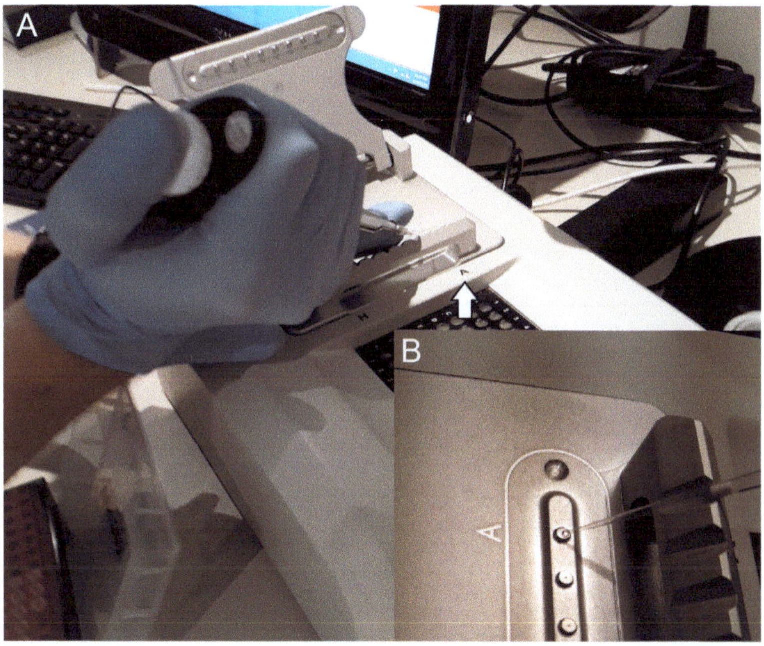

Fig. 2 Loading of sample on a spectrophotometer. Once obtained, DNA should be checked for concentration and purity on a spectrophotometer. After providing a blank sample of whatever solvent the DNA is suspended in, samples to be assayed can be placed within a cuvette for insertion into the spectrophotometer or placed on the sensor location, depending on model. (**a**) Loading a sample into a multi-sensor fiber optic-based spectrophotometer. The white arrow indicates the location of the "A" marked on the instrument on the inset. (**b**) Close-up of the sample being placed on the sensor pedestal. The sample should be pipetted so that the liquid is as close to the center of the sensor pedestal as possible to ensure light to pass through the sample and not air. Use of between 1 and 2 μL is typically enough

10. Quantitate DNA using a spectrophotometer to determine concentration and 260/280 nm absorption ratio. The 260/280 ratio should be as close to 1.8 as possible, and ratios diverging from this value will have less reliable concentration results (Figs. 2 and 3).

3.2 Isolation of DNA from Exosomes

3.2.1 Plasma Separation

1. Collect blood in a vacutainer or equivalent vessel containing EDTA, lithium heparin, or other anticoagulant (*see* **Note 1**).
2. Enough blood should be collected to maximize plasma yield and hence overall DNA produced. You may need to balance this with concerns over the amount of blood removed for other patient collection needs (*see* **Note 2**).
3. At the time of collection, gently invert collection tube 5–10 times to mix blood. Do not shake the blood or subject it to shocks that may cause cell lysis.

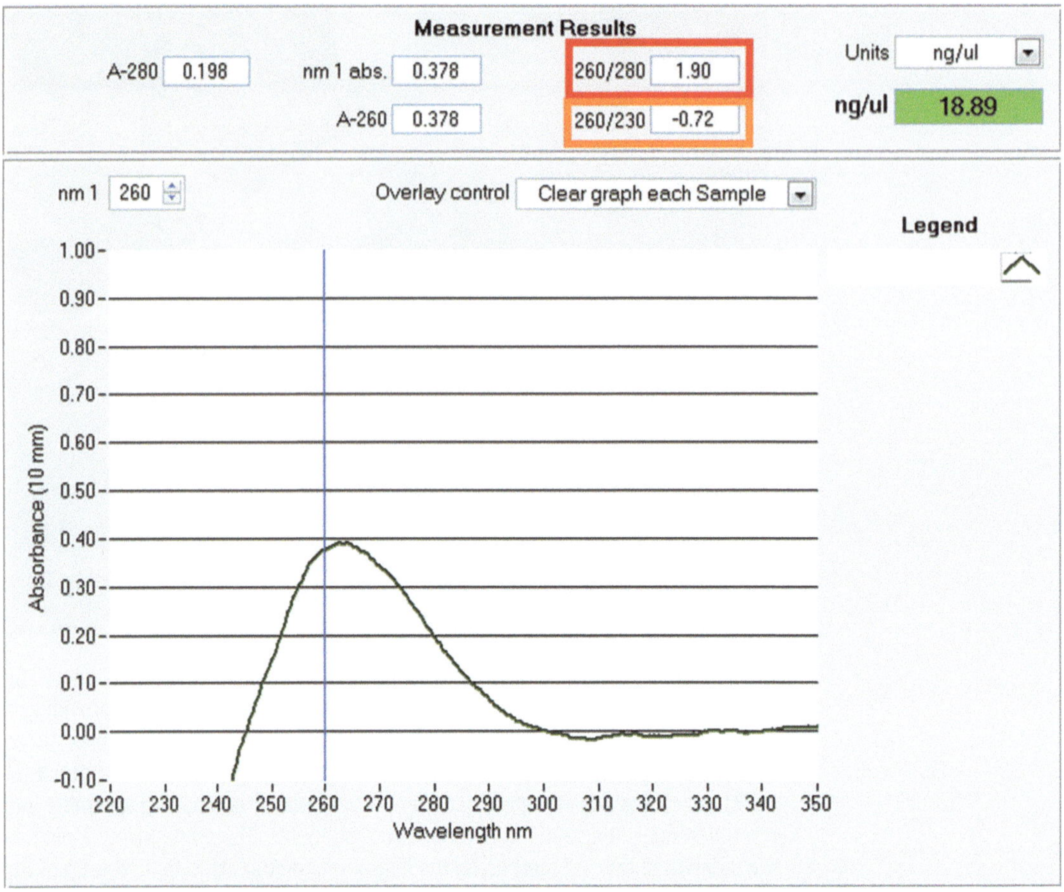

Fig. 3 Example spectrophotometer result. Once complete, the spectrophotometer will provide an estimation of the concentration of DNA used, often directly (green box), but sometimes the user must calculate the value themselves from the raw absorption value (Conc (μg/mL) = Absorption × 50). The spectrophotometer will also provide an $A_{260/280\text{nm}}$ ratio (red box), which should be around 1.8. Significant divergence from this value indicates the presence of contaminants. Similarly, the spectrophotometer may provide an $A_{260/230\text{nm}}$ ratio (orange box), the value of which should be between 2 and 2.2. Significant divergence (as seen here) from this value also indicates the presence of contaminants. If this is the case, additional rounds of DNA purification may be needed

4. Centrifuge blood at 2000 × *g* for 15–20 min, until plasma separates.
5. [Alternative] Centrifuge blood at 250 × *g* for 30 min, followed by centrifugation at 1000 × *g* for 5 min, followed again by centrifugation at 2000 × *g* for 5 min to separate plasma.
6. Using a pipette, transfer all available plasma to a new tube for exosome isolation. Do not disturb the cell layer interface (*see* **Note 3**).

3.2.2 Filtration and Separations of Exosomes

1. Perform centrifugation of plasma at 4 °C at 1000 × *g* for 10 min followed by centrifugation at 4 °C at 10,000 × *g* for 30 min.
2. Remove the supernatant by pipette, and pass through a 0.22 μm filter, using a syringe.
3. Pack a chromatographic separation column with Sepharose 2B beads, and equilibrate it with phosphate-buffered saline (PBS).
4. Add 0.5 mL of the filtrate to the separation column, and passage aliquot through column using 9 mL phosphate-buffered saline.
5. Collect 1 mL aliquots of the separated filtrate.
6. Subject aliquots to spectrophotometry at 280 nm absorbance. Select aliquots with the highest absorbance for further processing. You may wish to perform testing to determine what range of absorbance is most desirable for your application. Other aliquots can be discarded.
7. Subject aliquots to ultracentrifugation at 4 °C at 105,000 × *g* for 2 h.
8. Remove supernatant and discard.
9. Resuspend the exosome pellet in 1 mL phosphate-buffered saline.

3.2.3 Digestion of Proteins and Lysis of Exosomes

1. Add resuspended exosome pellet to the extraction buffer solution. Add approximately 10 mg of protein per 1 mL of final solution (one part of plasma to five parts buffer).
2. Add proteinase K. The concentration should be between 50 and 100 μg/mL (*see* **Note 4**).
3. Incubate the solution in an agitating water bath or oscillating heating block at 37–56 °C overnight.
4. [Optional] Incubate solution at 65 °C for 10 min to inactivate proteinase K.

3.2.4 Purification of DNA

1. Centrifuge solution at 4 °C at 1000 × *g* for 15 min.
2. Pipette the supernatant into a new tube. This tube should have enough spare capacity to contain 4× the current volume.
3. Add 2 volumes of chilled (−20 °C) absolute ethanol.
4. Invert tube several times to mix.
5. [Optional] Use liquid nitrogen to freeze the tube (*see* **Note 5**).
6. Centrifuge solution at 4 °C at 14,000 × *g* for 15 min.
7. Remove and discard supernatant.
8. Allow pellet to air-dry or dry in vacuum dryer.

9. Resuspend pellet in sterile water or buffer as desired. DNA can be kept overnight at 37 °C to ensure complete resuspension.
10. Quantitate DNA using a spectrophotometer to determine concentration and 260/280 nm absorption ratio. The 260/280 ratio should be as close to 1.8 as possible, and ratios diverging from this value will have less reliable concentration results.

4 Notes

1. While preservatives and low-binding tubes may help to improve yields, prompt centrifugation following collection will also provide relatively high levels of cfDNA and/or clean exosomes. Make sure to treat tubes gently to minimize the risk of cell lysis and contamination by cellular DNA.
2. Plasma samples from multiple collection tubes can be pooled for increased DNA yields.
3. To prevent contamination by leukocytes or other DNA-containing cells, it may be useful to leave a small layer of untouched plasma behind at the plasma/cell interface. Pipetting should be performed slowly to avoid disturbing the cell layer, and operators may consider drawing up the first ~75% of available plasma and depositing it in a separate tube before attempting the last ~25%.
4. Use of and incubation time for proteinase K may need to be adjusted depending on the desired downstream application to prevent interference from bound albumin, histones, and similar constituents. More aggressive lysis and protein digestion may be necessary for exosomes due to intrinsic proteins isolated along with exosome-contained DNA.
5. Use of liquid nitrogen freezing and longer centrifugation in the final steps will lead to increased DNA yield but also higher proportions of contaminants. Adjust accordingly.

References

1. Castro C, Peleteiro B, Lunet N (2018) Modifiable factors and esophageal cancer: a systematic review of published meta-analyses. J Gastroenterol 53:37–51
2. Luo H, Li H, Hu Z, Wu H, Liu C, Li Y, Zhang X, Lin P, Hou Q, Ding G, Wang Y, Li S, Wei D, Qiu F, Li Y, Wu S (2016) Noninvasive diagnosis and monitoring of mutations by deep sequencing of circulating tumor DNA in esophageal squamous cell carcinoma. Biochem Biophys Res Commun 471:596–602
3. Li X, Ye M, Zhang W, Tan D, Jaffrezic-Renault N, Yang X, Guo Z (2019) Liquid biopsy of circulating tumor DNA and biosensor applications. Biosens Bioelectron 126:596–607
4. Lianidou E, Pantel K (2019) Liquid biopsies. Genes Chromosomes Cancer 58:219–232
5. Hsieh CC, Hsu HS, Chang SC, Chen YJ (2016) Circulating cell-free DNA levels could predict oncological outcomes of patients undergoing esophagectomy for esophageal

squamous cell carcinoma. Int J Mol Sci 17: E2131

6. Ueda M, Iguchi T, Masuda T, Nakahara Y, Hirata H, Uchi R, Niida A, Momose K, Sakimura S, Chiba K, Eguchi H, Ito S, Sugimachi K, Yamasaki M, Suzuki Y, Miyano S, Doki Y, Mori M, Mimori K (2016) Somatic mutations in plasma cell-free DNA are diagnostic markers for esophageal squamous cell carcinoma recurrence. Oncotarget 7:62280–62291
7. Ruivo CF, Adem B, Silva M, Melo SA (2017) The biology of cancer exosomes: insights and new perspectives. Cancer Res 77:6480–6488
8. Elazezy M, Joosse SA (2018) Techniques of using circulating tumor DNA as a liquid biopsy component in cancer management. Comput Struct Biotechnol J 16:370–378
9. Corcoran RB, Chabner BA (2018) Application of cell-free DNA analysis to cancer treatment. N Engl J Med 379:1754–1765
10. Fettke H, Kwan EM, Azad AA (2019) Cell-free DNA in cancer: current insights. Cell Oncol (Dordr) 42:13–28
11. Alidousty C, Brandes D, Heydt C, Wagener S, Wittersheim M, Schäfer SC, Holz B, Merkelbach-Bruse S, Büttner R, Fassunke J, Schultheis AM (2017) Comparison of blood collection tubes from three different manufacturers for the collection of cell-free DNA for liquid biopsy mutation testing. J Mol Diagn 19:801–804
12. Eisenberger CF, Knoefel WT, Peiper M, Merkert P, Yekebas EF, Scheunemann P, Steffani K, Stoecklein NH, Hosch SB, Izbicki JR (2003) Squamous cell carcinoma of the esophagus can be detected by microsatellite analysis in tumor and serum. Clin Cancer Res 9:4178–4183
13. Ikoma D, Ichikawa D, Ueda Y, Tani N, Tomita H, Sai S, Kikuchi S, Fujiwara H, Otsuji E, Yamagishi H (2007) Circulating tumor cells and aberrant methylation as tumor markers in patients with esophageal cancer. Anticancer Res 27:535–539
14. Ling ZQ, Zhao Q, Zhou SL, Mao WM (2012) MSH2 promoter hypermethylation in circulating tumor DNA is a valuable predictor of disease-free survival for patients with esophageal squamous cell carcinoma. Eur J Surg Oncol 38:326–332
15. Das M, Sharma SK, Sekhon GS, Saikia BJ, Mahanta J, Phukan RK (2014) Promoter methylation of MGMT gene in serum of patients with esophageal squamous cell carcinoma in North East India. Asian Pac J Cancer Prev 15:9955–9960
16. Tomita H, Ichikawa D, Ikoma D, Sai S, Tani N, Ikoma H, Fujiwara H, Kikuchi S, Okamoto K, Ochiai T, Otsuji E (2007) Quantification of circulating plasma DNA fragments as tumor markers in patients with esophageal cancer. Anticancer Res 27:2737–2741
17. Xu Y, Xie Z, Lu H (2018) Detection of epidermal growth factor receptor mutation in the peripheral blood of patients with esophageal carcinoma to guide epidermal growth factor receptor-tyrosine kinase inhibitor treatment. J Cancer Res Ther 14:103–105

Chapter 17

Genome Sequencing in Esophageal Squamous Cell Carcinoma

Suja Pillai, Neven Maksemous, and Alfred K. Lam

Abstract

Technological advances in the form of next-generation sequencing allow sequencing of large numbers of different DNA sequences in a single/parallel reaction compared to conventional sequencing. It is a powerful tool which has enabled comprehensive characterization of esophageal squamous cell carcinoma. Whole-genome sequencing is the most comprehensive but expensive, whereas whole-exome sequencing is cost-effective, but it only works for the known genes. Thus, second-generation sequencing methods can provide a complete picture of the esophageal squamous cell carcinoma genome by detecting and discovering different type of alterations in the cancer which may lead to the development of effective diagnostic and therapeutic approaches for esophageal squamous cell carcinoma.

Key words Next-generation sequencing, Esophageal squamous cell carcinoma

1 Introduction

DNA sequencing is generally referred to the sequencing of nucleotides within a DNA molecule using laboratory methods [1]. Sequencing plays an important role in identifying pathological mutations which are important in understanding the pathogenesis of human diseases as well as planning targeted gene therapies for patients with cancer. First-generation sequencing/Sanger sequencing had limited applications because of technical limitations in its workflow in terms of throughput [2]. Throughput is a function of sequencing reaction time, the number of sequencing reactions that can be run in parallel, and lengths of sequences read by each reaction [2]. Following the successes of human genome project in 2005, a massive parallel sequencing system called the next-generation sequencing (NGS) was developed to reduce the cost and time of genome sequencing [3]. Hence, next-generation sequencing refers to the high-throughput DNA sequencing technologies which are capable of sequencing large numbers of different DNA sequences in a single/parallel reaction [3, 4].

Alfred K. Lam (ed.), *Esophageal Squamous Cell Carcinoma: Methods and Protocols*, Methods in Molecular Biology, vol. 2129, https://doi.org/10.1007/978-1-0716-0377-2_17, © Springer Science+Business Media, LLC, part of Springer Nature 2020

1.1 Influence of Next-Generation Sequencing on ESCC Research

Understanding the tumor biology of esophageal squamous cell carcinoma (ESCC) offers the potential for development of effective diagnostic and therapeutic approaches, thus increasing cure rates and decreasing morbidities associated with this disease.

Simultaneous testing of multiple genes for mutation is affordable and time-efficient compared to conventional Sanger sequencing which is expensive, and single-gene testing is impractical in clinical use [5]. Next-generation sequencing machines first entered the market in 2008–2009 and involve a wet-and-dry laboratory workflow for its application in a research or diagnostic setting [6].

Next-generation sequencing technologies have helped in unveiling the genomic landscape of ESCC by identifying several critical genes and pathways important in the tumorigenesis of ESCC [7]. Depending on the purpose, next-generation sequencing is applied in ESCC research in the form of whole-genome, whole-exome, targeted gene sequencing, RNA sequencing, and ChIP-sequencing [8, 9]. These technologies initiate opportunities to translate the analysis of DNA into tools that can help in the development of effective diagnostic and therapeutic approaches for ESCC [7]. Table 1 summarizes the current NGS studies in ESCC [10,11–13, 14–34].

1.2 Whole-Genome Sequencing (WGS)

Sequencing of the whole human genome or determination of the complete DNA sequence of an organism's genome at a single time is termed as whole-genome sequencing [35]. Capturing approximately six billion nucleotides comprising the human genome, including introns, exons, promoters, and enhancers, whole-genome sequencing is the most comprehensive of the genome sequencing methods [4]. Whole-genome sequencing provides a complete characterization of the cancer genome; also it has the potential to discover driver mutations and chromosomal rearrangements and study complex karyotypes [36].

This method has the ability to discern the full range of genomic alterations including nucleotide substitutions, copy number alterations, and structural rearrangements [11]. Read/sequencing depth in gene sequencing is defined as the number of unique reads in a given nucleotide in the reconstructed sequence [37]. Whole-genome sequencing, because of its high read depth, is considered as the gold standard for gene sequencing as it has the sensitivity to detect driver mutations which are present at frequencies as low as 1% of the tumor cells [37].

Song and colleagues performed the first whole-genome sequencing of seventeen ESCC samples [10]. The study reported several recurrently mutated genes altered in ESCC, thus validating the ability of whole-genome sequencing to detect driver genes in the pathogenesis of ESCC. Another whole-genome sequencing works by Zhang et al. utilized 14 tumors and their matched non-neoplastic tissues which reported focal amplifications of *CBX4* and

Table 1
Next-generation sequencing studies of esophageal squamous cell carcinoma to date

Author/year	Sample number	Platform/ technique	Findings
Agrawal/ 2012 [11]	12	GA IIx/WES	Inactivating mutations of *NOTCH1* were identified in ESCCs
Ma/2012 [14]	3	GA IIx/RNA-seq	PTK6 is significantly downregulated in ESCC
Gao/2014 [13]	113	HiSeq2000/ WES	A mean of 82 non-silent mutations per tumor was identified
Lin/2014 [15]	139	HiSeq2000/ WES, TS	Number of novel gene mutations such as *ESCCFAT1, FAT2, ZNF750,* and *KMT2D* were identified
Lin/2014 [16]	8	Ion Proton™ System/RNA-seq	533 significantly differentially expressed protein-coding and noncoding genes were identified as potential targets for ESCC diagnosis and therapy
Song/2014 [10]	88	HiSeq 2000/ WES, WGS	*ADAM29* and *FAM135B* were identified as two novel genes associated with ESSC
Sun/2014 [17]	1	GA IIx/RNA-seq	Alternative polyadenylation site profiles were generated, 903 genes were identified to have shortened 3′ UTRs, and 917 genes were found to use distal polyA sites
Zhang/2015 [18]	104	HiSeq 2000/ WES, WGS	APOBEC-mediated mutational signature was identified which suggested that APOBEC-catalyzed deamination provides a source of DNA damage in ESCC
Wang/2015 [19]	9	HiSeq 2500/ CGP	ESSC demonstrated enrichment in alterations involving PI3K/AKT/MTOR signaling, and a total of 522 genomic variations were identified
Cheng/2016 [20]	104	HiSeq 2000/ WGS, WES	Identified and validated prevalence of mutations in *NOTCH1*
Kishino/2016 [21]	57	Ion PGM/TS	Non-synonymous somatic mutations and copy number alterations were identified
Nakazato/ 2016 [22]	92	Ion PS/TS	Genetic and epigenetic alterations of the SWI/SNF complex were identified in ESCC
Luo/2016 [23]	55	HiSeq 2000/ WES, TS	Tested the feasibility of plasma-circulating tumor DNA for the noninvasive analysis of tumor mutations in ESCC
Chen/2016 [24]	45	HiSeq 2000/ UDS	Clonal composition of tumor-infiltrating lymphocytes could be analyzed directly from unfractionated ESCC specimens
Pan/2016 [25]	5	HiSeq 2500/ RNA-seq	CASC9 is significantly upregulated in ESCC tissues and may represent a marker of poor prognosis

(continued)

Table 1 (continued)

Author/year	Sample number	Platform/ technique	Findings
Ueda/2016 [26]	64	HiSeq 2000/TS	Next-generation sequencing using a multigene panel is an effective method for detecting somatic mutations in plasma cell-free DNA of ESCC
Hao/2016 [27]	13	HiSeq4000/ WES	Epigenetic and genetic intratumor heterogeneity of ESCC was revealed
Zheng/2016 [28]	35	Ion PGM/TS	Frequent mutations were found in *TP53* and less frequent mutations in *PIK3CA*
Peng/2017 [29]	43	MiSeq/TS	Different methylation levels among ESCC, normal-appearing tissues, and healthy controls were noted
Liu/2017 [30]	227	HiSeq 2500/ WGS, WES, TS	Intraepithelial neoplasia and ESCCs had similar mutations and markers of genomic instability
Forouzanfar/ 2017 [12]	9	GA IIx/WES	Novel and damaging variants of the Notch signaling pathway identified
Yang/2017 [31]	24	HiSeq 2500/TS	Total of 115 genetic alterations and more than one genetic alteration was detected in most patients
Zhang/2017 [18]	15	WES, RNA-seq	Activation of the JAK/STAT pathway is a regulatory mechanism of ADAR1 expression and causes abnormal RNA editing profile in ESCC
Kobayashi/ 2018 [32]	54	Ion Chef™ System/TS	Mutations of *TP53* and *CDKN2A* and *PIK3CA* amplification were common in early esophageal squamous neoplasia, while other mutations accumulated with disease progression
Wang/2018 [33]	7	RNA-seq	mRNA and long noncoding RNA co-expression networks were built, and highly connected networks were identified for the first time in ESCC
Yokota/2018 [34]	126	MiSeq sequencer/TS	*PIK3CA* mutation was identified as a biomarker for favorable prognosis

ESCC esophageal squamous cell carcinoma, *WGS* whole-genome sequencing, *WES* whole-exome sequencing, TS

CBX8 [38]. Following these, whole-genome sequencing of DNA and RNA in 94 ESCC samples identified six mutational signatures, and one of the signatures, E4, was found to be unique in ESCC linked to alcohol intake [39].

Even though whole-genome sequencing is the most comprehensive, it is the most expensive and creates a high amount of redundant data [36]. Nevertheless, in some countries, the costs of the sequencing are now decreasing which could allow the clinical use of it in patients [40].

1.3 Whole-Exome Sequencing

Exome characterizes 1% of the whole-genome region, and approximately 85% of disease-causing mutations are expected to occur within the exome [40]. Whole-exome sequencing (WES) is a technique in which only the coding regions of DNA, which are of interest, are sequenced, though it is possible to target any desired region of the genome [41].

As 1% of the genome is represented by exome, higher sequence coverage could be easily achieved by WES, and it comes with considerably less price than whole-genome sequencing [40]. With this reduced cost, it becomes possible to increase sequencing depth [40].

Agrawal et al. published the first whole-exome sequencing (WES) on 23 esophageal cancers (11 adenocarcinomas and 12 squamous cell carcinomas) reporting significant differences in the spectrum of mutations between the two histological subtypes [11]. The study also confirmed that *TP53* is the most commonly mutated gene in ESCC [11].

In a more recent study, whole-exome sequencing identified novel and damaging variants of the Notch signaling pathway especially *TNRC6B* (Trinucleotide Repeat Containing 6B) mutation as a predisposing factor in familial ESCC pedigrees [12].

Gao et al. performed whole-exome sequencing on 113 matched tumor-nonneoplastic pairs of ESCC and reported mutational profile of ESCC closely resembles those of squamous cell carcinomas of other tissues but differs from that of esophageal adenocarcinoma [13].

Even though whole-exome sequencing eliminates the high redundancy of whole-genome sequencing, however, there are some limitations to this approach, particularly in relation to the study of cancer genomes. Whole-exome sequencing misses regions adjoining the exons such as promoters, enhancers, and transcription factor binding sites, unless the probe set is expanded to cover them [42]. In addition, whole-exome sequencing typically requires large amounts of high-quality DNA at least 3 μg especially from peripheral blood [43]. This requirement of whole-exome sequencing presents practical challenges to studies where such amounts of DNA are unavailable or would exhaust the reserve [43].

Whole-exome sequencing represents an immense reduction in time and resources when compared with whole-genome sequencing, as well as allowing for more effective detection of rare mutations through the improved coverage and hence can be a trustworthy and economical way to identify variations in ESCC cancer genome, and more importantly, the method can help to detect pathogenic mutations in ESCC in the absence of a mutation in susceptibility genes of ESCC. Also, the limitations can be significantly diminished as technologies improve.

1.4 Whole-Transcriptome Sequencing/RNA Sequencing

Transcriptome is defined as complete set of all messenger RNA molecules in a cell or population of cells [44]. Conventional methods of studying transcriptome included microarray methods [44]. The application of next-generation sequencing technology to study the transcriptome at the nucleotide level is known as RNA sequencing [44]. The method involves total conversion of cellular RNA into complementary DNA which is then treated like genomic DNA undergoing WGS/WES sequencing [36]. It is a potent approach for understanding cancer as it helps in detecting intragenic fusions and in-frame fusion in which important events are leading to oncogene activation [36]. Also, gene expression profiles found using RNA-seq are particularly useful for identifying low-level expression for specific transcripts and detecting allele-specific expression bias [44]. Consequently, transcriptome sequencing helps in interpreting the functional elements of the genome, helping in understanding the development of cancer in a better way.

Compared to microarrays, RNA-seq does not require known genes and can include detection of novel transcripts, nonhuman transcripts, and alternative splice forms [44]. Transcriptome sequencing is highly cost-efficient but is limited to the detection of coding fusion transcripts [36]. In a recent study by Xing and colleagues, RNA sequencing was used to identify new serum markers for diagnosis of ESCCs, using six pairs of ESCC and matched nonneoplastic tissues offering new potential markers for the noninvasive diagnosis of ESCC [9].

1.5 Targeted Next-Generation Sequencing

Targeted sequencing is a variation of re-sequencing where only a small subset of the genome is sequenced. In this method of sequencing, known genes/exons are tested by designing custom-made primers to target genes of interest [45]. Even though this approach will not detect structural variants, targeted gene sequencing represents an economic way of identifying somatic mutations in ESCC, making this technology a possibility for clinical use, and provides patient-specific information.

In conclusion, among the four approaches of next-generation sequencing, whole-genome sequencing is the most comprehensive but expensive, whereas whole-exome sequencing is cost-effective, but it only works for the known genes. Thus, second-generation sequencing methods can provide a complete picture of the genome of ESCC by detecting and discovering different type of alterations that would help in diagnostics and will further help in developing personalized medicine in the cancer.

Many instruments could perform next-generation sequencing based on different chemistries. For example, sequencing by synthesis uses specially designed fluorescent-labeled terminator nucleotides, which allow the chain termination process to be reversed. The terminator contains a fluorescent label, which can be detected by a camera generating a temporal series of color images that can be computationally converted into sequence reads [46]. Another technology uses ligation of fluorescently labeled hybridization probes to determine the sequence of a template DNA strand, two bases at a time as a program for sequencing [4]. Alternative method of sequencing is pyrosequencing, which depends on the detection of pyrophosphate released during nucleotide incorporation [46].

In 2010, compact benchtop sequencers were introduced for smaller research and individual laboratories. These sequencers had simplified workflow and short run times compared to big sequencers [47]. Notable among them were Ion Personal Genomic Machine (PGM) released by Ion Torrent and MiSeq launched by Illumina [48].

PGM was the first commercial sequencing machine that did not require fluorescence and camera, resulting in higher speed and throughput, lower cost, and smaller instrument size [47]. However, in genomes with very high A-T content, sequencing by Ion Torrent PGM showed lack of coverage in 30% of the analyzed genome [49]. MiSeq was the only compact next-generation sequencer that integrated amplification, sequencing, and data analysis in a single instrument [47]. In a comparison study, the sequencing accuracy shown by MiSeq was superior to PGM [50]. Among these compact sequencers, Ion Torrent PGM has high throughput. On the other hand, Illumina MiSeq is best with respect to least number of errors [3].

In the following discussion, we would present the workflow of one of the benchtop sequencers based on semiconductor sequencing technology. In this technology, a nucleotide is incorporated into the DNA molecules by the polymerase; a proton is released resulting in the change in pH helping the sequencer to recognize whether a nucleotide is added or not [51]. The platform allows running of both smaller and large gene panels by using different type of chips, and use of cartridge-based consumables enhances consistency, offering flexibility without affecting cost. This approach allows the system to complete sequencing runs in as little as 5 h, a fraction of the time required by traditional first-generation sequencers.

2 Materials

2.1 Library Preparation Reagents and Materials

1. Nucleic acid from various sources—including formalin-fixed paraffin-embedded (FFPE) tissue and cell-free DNA—can be used as the starting material. Please *see* Chapter 8 on Biobanking for preservation of cancer tissue.
2. Custom panels comprise of one or two primer pools for the genes of interest.

3. The Ion AmpliSeq™ Library Kit 2.0 provides reagents for preparing eight libraries. They should be stored at −30 °C to −10 °C. It consists of the following reagents:
   5× Ion AmpliSeq™ HiFi Mix.

   FuPa reagent (used to partially digest primers for ligation).

   Switch Solution (helps to identify changes in PCR during library construction).

   DNA ligase (enzyme to cleave DNA).

   Ion AmpliSeq™ Adapters.

   Platinum™ PCR Super Mix High Fidelity.

   Library Amplification Primer Mix.

   Low TE buffer (Tris-EDTA buffer).

   Barcode Adapters Kit (each kit provides 16 different barcode adapters. These barcode adapters are required to run multiple libraries per sequencing chip).

   96-well thermal cycler.

   Fluorometer (Qubit™).

   Eppendorf™ DNA LoBind™ Microcentrifuge Tubes, 1.5 mL.

   Agencourt™ AMPure™ XP Kit (for purification of DNA libraries).

   DynaMag™-96 Side Magnet or other plate magnet—attract DNA beads that contain:
   The DNA.

   Nuclease-free water.

   70% ethanol.

   Pipettors, 2–200 μL, and low-retention filtered pipette tips.

2.2 Ion Chef™ Reagents and Materials

The Ion Chef™ System is an automated system used to prepare enriched, template-positive ion sphere particles [ISPs] and load them onto the ion chip (Ion 510 Chip, Ion 520 Chip, or Ion 530 Chip). Ion 510 & Ion 520 & Ion 530 Chef Kit supports four Ion Chef runs (two chips/Ion Chef run) and four sequencer initializations (two ion chips/sequencer initialization). It contains:

Tip Cartridge.

Chip adapter.

Enrichment cartridge—used for enrichment of template-positive ion sphere particles.

PCR Plate and Frame Seal—used to cover the PCR plate during template preparation.

Recovery Tube and Recovery Station Disposable Lid Ion S5 Chef Solutions.

Ion 510 & Ion 520 & Ion 530 Chef Reagents (stored at −30 °C to −10 °C).

2.3 Ion S5™ Sequencing Reagents and Materials

Ion GeneStudio S5 Plus System to sequence the loaded chips.

Ion S5 Sequencing Solutions.

Ion S5 Wash Solution 4 × 1.5 L.

Ion S5 Cleaning Solution.

Ion S5 Sequencing Reagents should be stored at (−30 °C to −10 °C).

Ion 530 Chip contains eight chips.

3 Methods

3.1 Overview of Next-Generation Sequencing

Next-generation sequencing involves a wet-and-dry laboratory workflow for its application in a research or diagnostic setting. We describe the workflow of targeted sequencing using a benchtop sequencer. Several different library preparation kits are commercially available. Each one makes use of similar molecular techniques and only vary slightly. The quality of DNA greatly influences the efficacy of library preparation and ultimately sequence output.

3.2 Construction of Library

1. Isolate genomic DNA or RNA.
2. If starting with RNA, reverse-transcribe to make cDNA.
3. For panels with two primer pools, use Table 2 to prepare for each sample a target amplification master mix without primers in a 1.5-mL tube (*see* **Note 1**).

Table 2
Master mix for library preparation

Component	Volume
5× Ion Ampliseq HiFi master mix	2 μL
2× Ion Ampliseq primer Pool	5 μL
G DNA, 10 ng	1 μL
Nuclease-free water	2 μL
Total	10 μL

Table 3
Thermal program for amplification

Stage	Step	Temperature	Time	Cycles
Hold	Activate the enzyme	99 °C	2 min	1
Cycles	Denature Anneal and extend	99 °C 60 °C	15 s 4 min	18
Hold		10 °C	Hold	1

Table 4
Thermal program for digestion of amplicons

Temperature	Time
50 °C	10 min
55 °C	10 min
60 °C	20 min
10 °C	Hold (for up to 1 h)

4. Mix thoroughly by pipetting up and down five times, and then transfer master mixes to two wells of a 96-well PCR plate (Table 2). Always change pipette tips between samples. Pipet viscous solutions slowly, and ensure complete mixing by vortexing or pipetting.
5. The tubes with master mix and DNA should be placed in a thermal cycler and activated according to the thermal program outlined in Table 3 to amplify target genomic regions (*see* **Note 2**).
6. At the completion of amplification, new strip tubes should be obtained for all the samples.
7. Amplification products for each primer pool should be combined into one tube, and the total volume in each tube should be 20 μL.
8. To each combined amplicon pool, 2 μL of FuPa reagent should be added to partially digest primers for ligation. Total reaction volume should be 22 μL.
9. The mixture should be pipetted up and down five times to mix, and the strip tubes should then be placed in a thermal cycler, and temperature should be performed according to the program as indicated in Table 4. We could make this step as STOPPING POINT and store plate at −20 °C for longer periods.

Table 5
Components to be added to the digested amplicons

Component	Volume
Switch solution	4 μL
Ion Ampliseq adapter mix (P1 + barcode)	2 μL
DNA ligase	2 μL
Total volume	15 μL

10. As multiple samples libraries will be loaded for each sequencing chip, each sample must be assigned a unique barcode to enable sample distinction.
11. For each barcode X chosen, a separate mix of Ion P1 Adapter and Ion Xpress™ Barcode X should be made. This consisted of 2 μL Adapter P1, 2 μL Ion Xpress Barcode, and 4 μL nuclease-free water.
12. Diluted adapters could be stored at −20 °C for multiple uses. The designated barcode number should be recorded on the sample tracking sheet.
13. Carefully remove the plate seal, and then add the components in the order listed to each well containing digested amplicons (Table 5). The total volume should be 30 μL including ~22 μL of digested amplicon.
14. Mix by pipetting at least five times before sealing the plate strip tubes should be placed in a thermal cycler (Fig. 1), and temperature program was performed as indicated in Table 6. This could be the STOPPING POINT. Samples can be stored for up to 24 h at 10 °C on the thermal cycler. For longer periods, store at −20 °C.

3.2.1 Library Purification

1. AMPure XP reagent should be brought to room temperature and vortexed thoroughly to disperse the beads before use.
2. The solution should be pipetted slowly, and then 45 μL (1.5× sample volume) of Agencourt AMPure XP Reagent should be added to each library and pipetted up and down five times to thoroughly mix the bead suspension with the DNA.
3. The mixture should then be incubated for 5 min at room temperature.
4. The tube should be placed in a magnetic rack and incubated for 2 min until solution clears.
5. The supernatant must be discarded without disturbing the pellet.

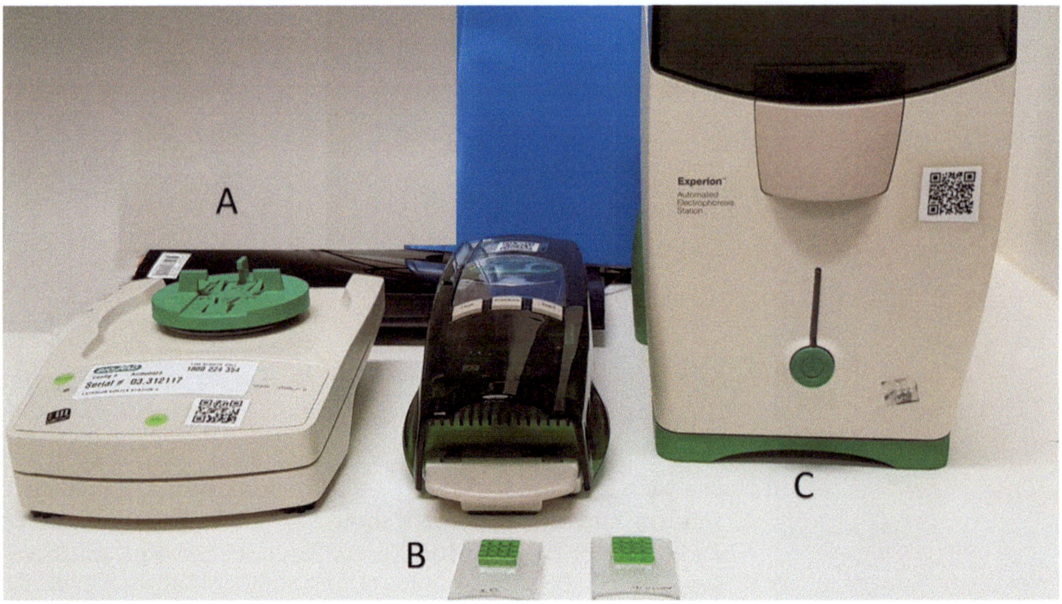

Fig. 1 Automated Electrophoresis System: Platform for analyzing the quantity and quality of DNA through electrophoresis. (**a**) Vortex station—for complete mixing of DNA or RNA samples and for analysis of reagents before electrophoresis. (**b**) Priming station—prepares chips for automated electrophoresis of DNA. (**c**) Electrophoresis station which performs steps of gel-based DNA electrophoresis in one unit

Table 6
Thermal program for adaptor ligation

Temperature	Time
22 °C	30 min
72 °C	10 min
10 °C	Hold

6. 75 μL of freshly prepared 70% ethanol should be added (combine 230 μL of ethanol with 100 μL of nuclease-free water per sample), and the tube should be moved from side to side in the magnet to wash the beads. Then, the supernatant is discarded without disturbing the pellet.
7. **Steps 4–6** should be repeated for a second wash.
8. Ensure that all ethanol droplets are removed from the wells. Keeping the plate in the magnet, air-dry the beads at room temperature for 5 min. Do not overdry (*see* **Note 3**).
9. The constructed libraries can then be stored at −20 for future template preparation.
10. Proceed to library quantification.

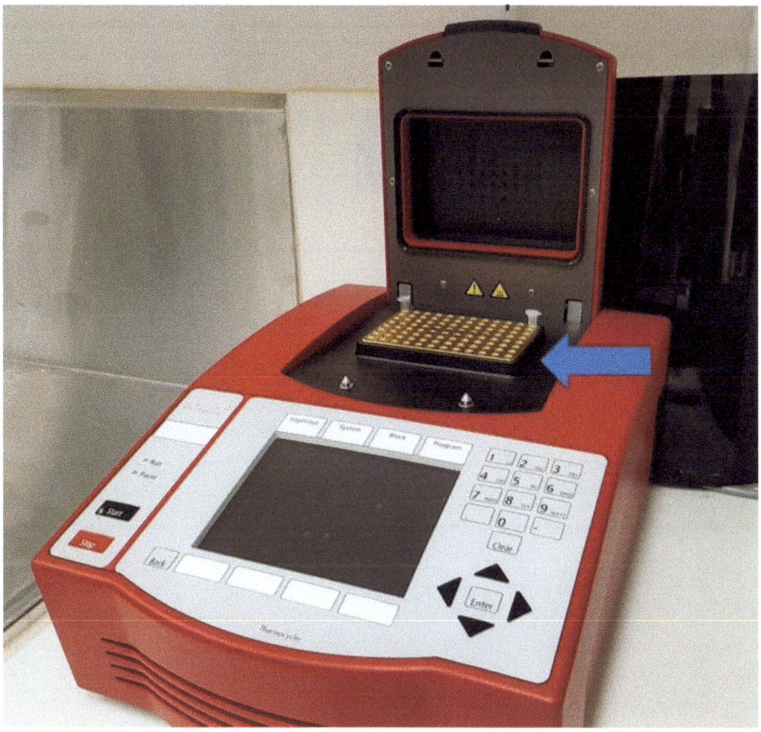

Fig. 2 Thermocycler: This is used for amplification of target genomic DNA regions. The device has thermal block with holes (arrow) where tubes holding the reaction mixture can be inserted. The thermal program for amplification can then be entered by using the touchscreen

3.2.2 Library Quantification

1. Experion 1K DNA kit could be used (Fig. 2). It can also be quantified by qPCR Qubit™ 2.0 or 3.0 Fluorometer or with the Agilent™ 2100 Bioanalyzer™ instrument.
2. Eleven samples can be analyzed on the chip at a time. Samples should be grouped into pools according to previous barcoding and according to experimental design.
3. For each pool, all samples should be diluted to the same concentration (10 ng/μL), and then equal volumes should be added to a single tube, and calculations should be done according to the manual.
4. Based on the calculated library concentration, determine the dilution that results in a concentration of ~100 pM.
5. Dilute library to ~100 pM, combine, and then proceed to template preparation, or libraries can be stored at 4–8 °C for up to 1 month. For longer term, store at −20 °C.

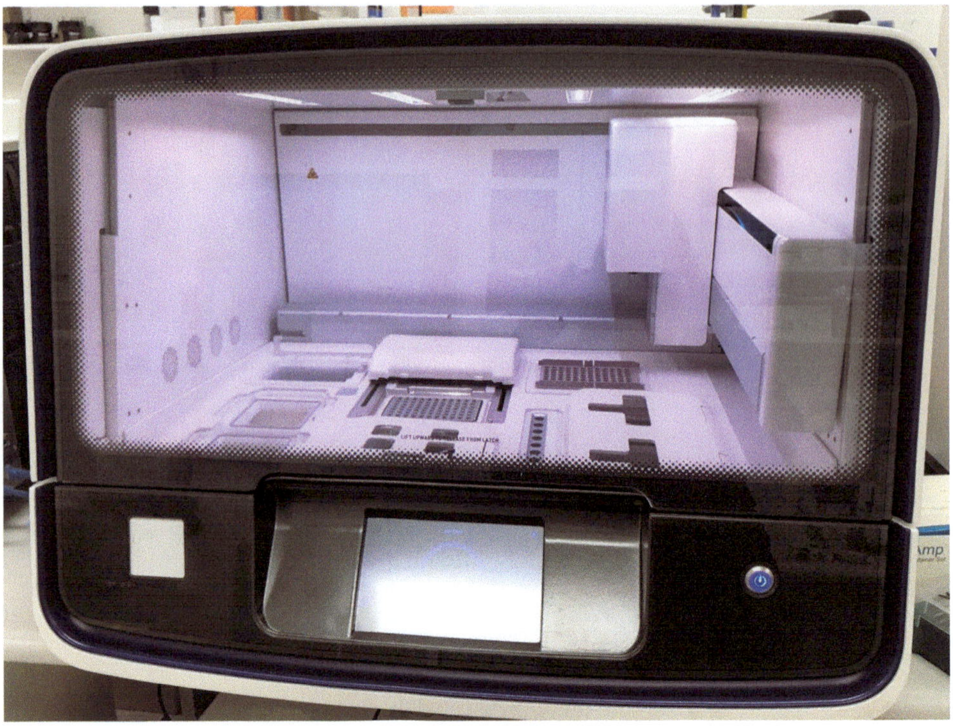

Fig. 3 A Next-generation sequencing equipment (Ion Chef instrument) which provides automated library preparation, template preparation, and chip loading results in significantly higher productivity. *B. Interior* of a next-generation sequencing equipment (Ion Chef instrument) which shows the different stations involved in the preparation of sequencing chips

3.3 Template Preparation and Chip Loading

1. Create a planned run in Torrent Suite™ Software.
2. Fresh dilution of each library or combined library should be prepared before use with the Ion Chef System (Figs. 3a and b) (use the library dilutions within 48 h).
3. Individual or combined stock libraries of 200 bp or 400 bp should be diluted to 50 pM (Table 7).
4. Different template sizes (for example, 200 base and 400 base) shouldn't be mixed in a single templating run.
5. Allow the Ion 510™ & Ion 520™ & Ion 530™ Chef Reagents cartridge to warm to room temperature 45 min prior to use.
6. Ensure that the consumables are free of condensate before loading.
7. Gently tap the reagents and solutions of cartridges on the bench, and centrifuge the tubes containing sodium hydroxide (NaOH; at position C) and diluted libraries at positions A and B of reagents cartridge.
8. Samples (libraries) should be diluted to the same concentration 50 pM and pooled together in a single tube.

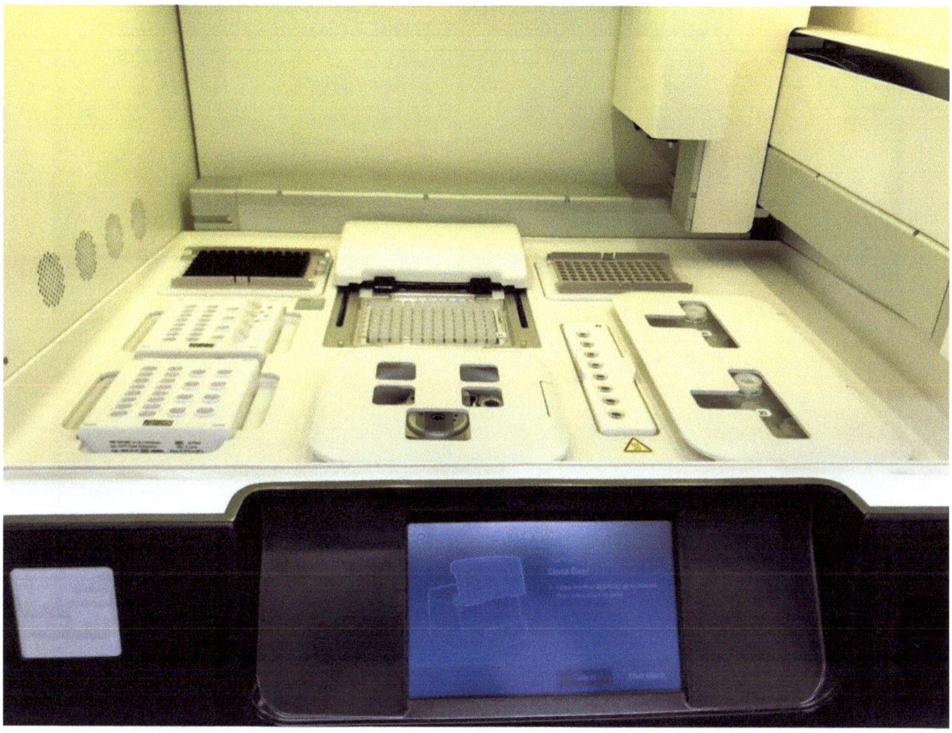

Fig. 3 (continued)

Table 7
Dilution of stock libraries

Library length	Recommended concentration	Molecules per 25 μL input volume	Templating size in planned run setup
<300 bp	25–60 pM	$600–900 \times 10^6$	200
>300 bp	25–60 pM	$600–900 \times 10^6$	400

3.4 Loading the Diluted Libraries to the Ion Chef

25 μL of diluted individual library or combined library should be added to the bottom of the barcoded Sample Tube in positions A and B and then loaded onto the Ion Chef instrument. To set up an Ion Chef run, in the instrument touchscreen, step-by-step option should be selected (Fig. 4).

1. Open the Ion Chef door.
2. A New Tip Cartridge should be loaded in the New Pipette Tip Position.
3. A new PCR plate should be placed into the thermal cycler sample block (Fig. 5).

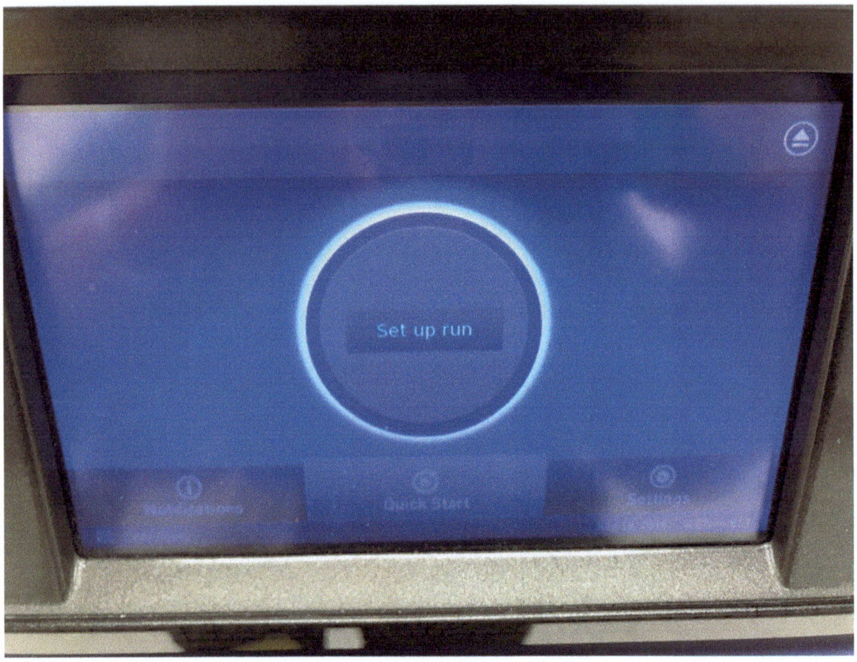

Fig. 4 Touchscreen interface of next-generation sequencing equipment (Ion Chef System). It is a simple interface which provides access to functions like loading the chip, cleaning the instrument, and performing system maintenance and configuration tasks

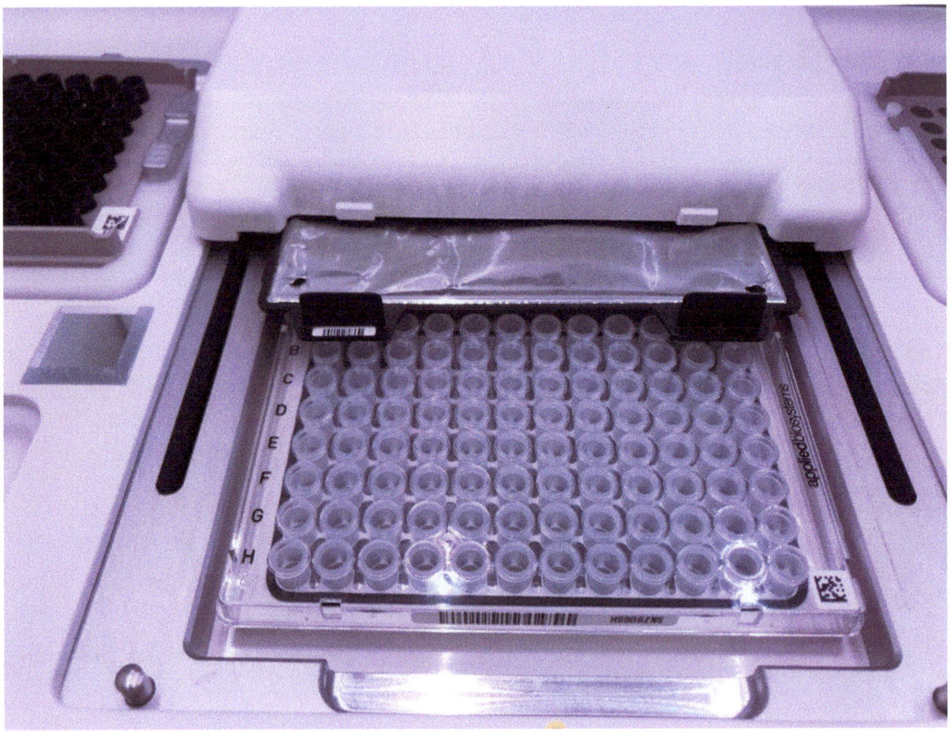

Fig. 5 Thermal cycler sample block of the system. It carry out thermal cycling of the sequencing reactions on a 96-well PCR reaction plate inside the next-generation sequencing equipment (Ion Chef instrument)

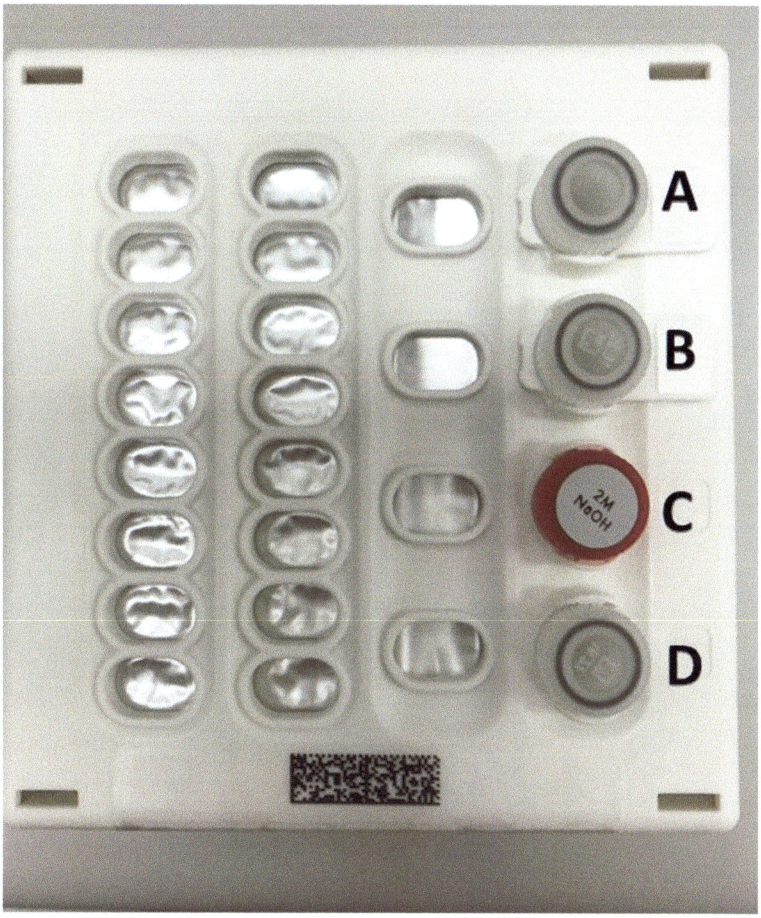

Fig. 6 Reagents cartridge—It is used for the templating of the ion sphere particles. (**a** and **b**) indicates the position of diluted library, (**c**) is for sodium hydroxide (NaOH), and (**d**) indicates the position of empty tube. All tubes must be uncapped for the run

4. The reagents and solutions cartridges should be loaded into the reagents and solution stations. Each cartridge fits only one location on the deck and in one orientation.
5. The two library sample tubes, each containing 25 μL of diluted library, must be inserted into positions A and B on the reagents cartridge. Ensure that all tubes in positions A, B, and C and the empty tube in position D are uncapped (Fig. 6).

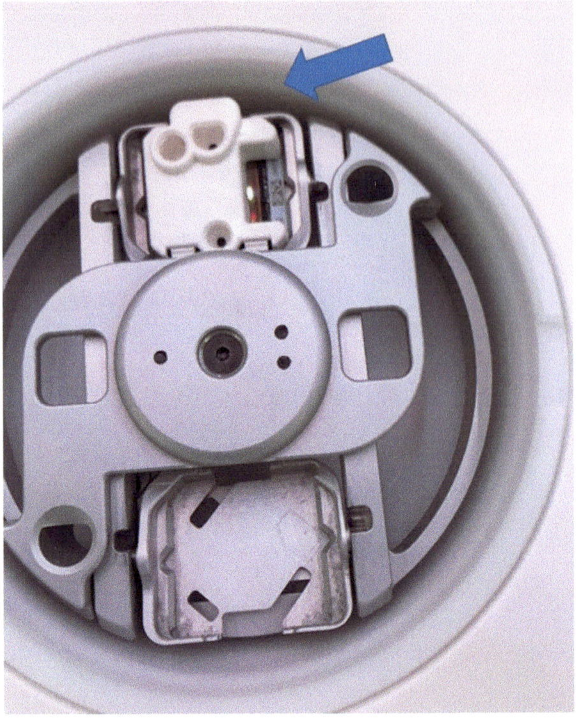

Fig. 7 Chip-loading centrifuge—It is important for the centrifugation of sequencing chips. It is mounted to chip-loading adapters and loaded with template-positive ion sphere particles. The arrow indicates the position of chip in the centrifuge. Single chip can be loaded instead of two provided there is a chip balance of the same series as the instrument

6. Six recovery tubes need to be loaded into each recovery centrifuge (the centrifuge must be load-balanced). Each recovery centrifuge needs to be covered by a recovery station disposable lid with the lid firmly placed.
7. Enrichment cartridge should be properly loaded (with the letters facing right side and upward).
8. Two chips used for templating and sequencing should be loaded into a chip-loading centrifuge bucket (Fig. 7). Then, the two chip adapters must be attached to the assembly (*see* **Note 4**).

3.5 Initialize the Sequencer

3.5.1 Before Initializing the Sequencer

1. The sequencer (Fig. 8) should be initialized at least 50 min before the Ion Chef System finishes chip loading. Ensure that the first chip is immediately sequenced after loading is complete.
2. The sequencer can be initialized up to 24 h before starting a sequencing run.

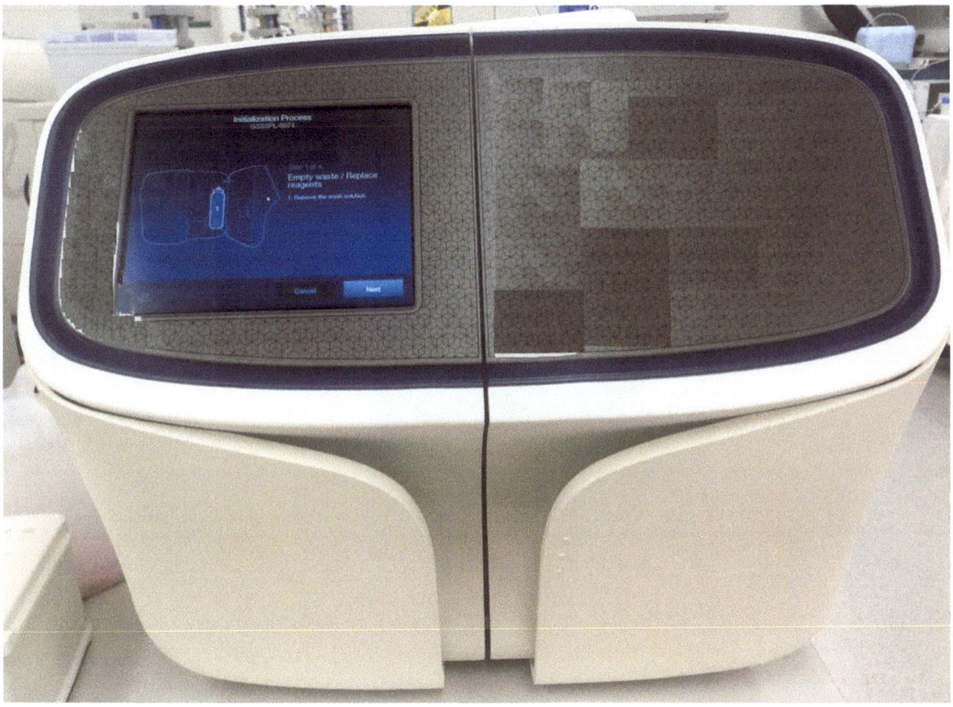

Fig. 8 Benchtop next-generation sequencer which enables a simple targeted sequencing workflow for laboratory. The system is simple to use with cartridge-based reagents enabling the production of high-quality sequencing data

3. When sequencing two runs (two chips) per initialization, the second run must be started within 24-h period.
4. If the first chip cannot be loaded immediately, the chip should be placed into a chip storage container and stored at 4 °C until ready to be sequenced (up to 6–8 h maximum).
5. The new Ion S5 Sequencing Reagents cartridge should be equilibrated to room temperature for at least 45 min before loading into the Ion S5 sequencer.

3.5.2 Initialize the Sequencer

1. Start the instrument.
2. The Ion S5 Wash Solution bottle should be removed and empty the waste reservoir.
3. The empty waste reservoir needs to be reinstalled.
4. The used Ion S5™ Sequencing Reagents cartridge must be replaced with a new cartridge.
5. The new Ion S5 Wash Solution bottle must be thoroughly mixed, and red cap must be removed and installed.
6. For the first step of initialization, the used sequencing chip from any previous run should be properly seated in the chip clamp.

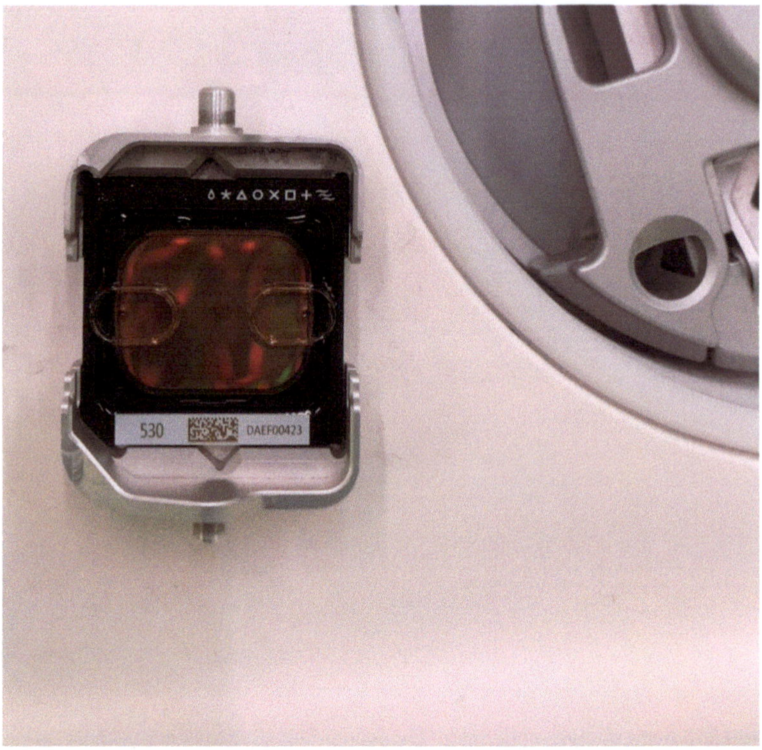

Fig. 9 Chip used for sequencing—It generates millions of sequencing reads on the sequencer using the automated workflow of the next-generation sequencing equipment (Ion Chef System)

7. Close the instrument door.
8. The instrument should confirm that the consumables and chip are properly installed and that the Ion S5 Cleaning Solution contains enough reagent to perform the post-run clean.
9. When initialization is completed (~50 min), then **Home** should be selected from the touchscreen. The S5 instrument is ready for the first sequencing run.

3.5.3 Start Sequencing Run

1. From the instrument touchscreen, select **Run**. The door and chip clamp should be unlocked.
2. The used sequencing chip should be replaced by the chip (Fig. 9) loaded with template-positive ion sphere particles in the chip clamp.
3. Close the instrument door and select **Next** from the touchscreen. Then the corrected planned run should be auto-populated.
4. When sequencing, the first run of two sequencing runs on the same initialization. Deselect post-run clean checkbox, and then select **Review** from the touchscreen. Then, select the **Start run** from the touchscreen to begin the sequencing run (*see* **Note 5**).

3.6 Data Analysis

This part should better be performed by staff with bioinformatics expertise.

1. Sequencing results of the Ion Torrent S5 run were assessed via the Torrent Browser, which is a Web-based user interface on the Torrent Server.
2. The Torrent Browser runs report comprises of the statistics and quality metrics of the run, which include the Ion Sphere Particle (ISP) density, the percentage of polyclonal ISPs (ISPs carrying clones from two or more templates), and low-quality percentage (percentage of ISPs with a low signal).
3. Together, these factors make up the percentage of usable reads, which is the percentage of Library ISPs that are not eliminated by the quality filters for being polyclonal, having low read quality, or the result of primer dimer.
4. These reports were used to evaluate the quality of the Ion Chef run. A good-quality run has at least 30% ISP loading and 30% usable reads.
5. The data from the sequencing runs can be analyzed using the Torrent Suite analysis pipeline, which includes raw sequencing data processing (DAT processing), splitting of the reads according to the barcode for the individual sample output sequence, classification, signal processing, base calling, read filtering, adapter trimming, and alignment quality control.

4 Notes

1. Minimize freeze thaw cycles of panels by aliquoting as needed for your experiments. Panels can be stored at 4 °C for 1 year.
2. If you are using a DNA panel with two primer pools, set up two 10-μL amplification reactions, and then combine them after target amplification to give a volume of 20 μL. Cycle number recommendations in Table 2 are based on 10-ng DNA input. Cycle number can be increased when input material quality or quantity is questionable.
3. Residual ethanol drops could inhibit library amplification. If needed, centrifuge the plate and remove remaining ethanol before air-drying the beads. Under conditions of low relative humidity, the beads could air-dry rapidly. Do not overdry the beads.
4. Loading of the chips can fail if the chip adapter is not attached securely. Ensure that each chip adapter is firmly attached to the centrifuge bucket, and the two buckets are securely seated in the centrifuge rotors. The chips that are loaded in positions 1 and 2 of the instrument are loaded with ion sphere particles

(ISPs) prepared from the DNA libraries. The Ion Chef Library Sample Tube are loaded in Positions A and B, respectively, of the reagents cartridge. For single chip loading, only one diluted library or combined library should be loaded into position A and an empty tube into position B of the reagents cartridge. The instrument door should be closed gently by lifting the door before pulling it down, and ensure that both sides of the door are properly locked after closing it. Select Start from the touchscreen to start Deck Scan. The instrument vision system should scan the barcodes of all consumables and reagents. On the Run options screen, "the default run time could be used." When the run is complete, the Ion Chef instrument should be unloaded and the first chip is sequenced as soon as possible.

5. If the Enable post-run clean checkbox is deselected, then the cleaning is automatically performed after the first run and the second run is not available. When starting the second sequencing run, ensure that the Enable post-run clean checkbox is selected. Then, the post-run cleaning is performed after the second run on a single initialization. The second sequencing run should be started within 24 h of starting the initialization.

References

1. Sanger F, Nicklen S, Coulson AR (1977) DNA sequencing with chain-terminating inhibitors. Proc Natl Acad Sci U S A 74:5463–5467
2. Rizzo JM, Buck MJ (2012) Key principles and clinical applications of "next-generation" DNA sequencing. Cancer Prev Res 5:887–900
3. Pillai S, Gopalan V, Lam AK (2017) Review of sequencing platforms and their applications in phaeochromocytoma and paragangliomas. Crit Rev Oncol Hematol 116:58–67
4. Mardis ER (2013) Next-generation sequencing platforms. Annu Rev Anal Chem 6:287–303
5. Sasaki Y, Tamura M, Koyama R et al (2016) Genomic characterization of esophageal squamous cell carcinoma: insights from next-generation sequencing. World J Gastroenterol 22:2284–2293
6. Lohmann K, Klein C (2014) Next generation sequencing and the future of genetic diagnosis. Neurotherapeutics 11:699–707
7. Golyan FF, Moghaddassian M, Forghanifard MM et al (2019) Whole exome sequencing reveals a novel damaging mutation in human fibroblast activation protein in a family with esophageal squamous cell carcinoma. J Gastrointest Cancer. (In press) https://doi.org/10.1007/s12029-019-00224-x
8. Lin DC, Dinh HQ, Xie JJ et al (2018) Identification of distinct mutational patterns and new driver genes in oesophageal squamous cell carcinomas and adenocarcinomas. Gut 67:1769–1779
9. Xing S, Zheng X, Wei LQ et al (2017) Development and validation of a serum biomarker panel for the detection of esophageal squamous cell carcinoma through RNA transcriptome sequencing. J Cancer 8:2346–2355
10. Song Y, Li L, Ou Y et al (2014) Identification of genomic alterations in oesophageal squamous cell cancer. Nature 509:91–95
11. Agrawal N, Jiao Y, Bettegowda C et al (2012) Comparative genomic analysis of esophageal adenocarcinoma and squamous cell carcinoma. Cancer Discov 2:899–905
12. Forouzanfar N, Baranova A, Milanizadeh S et al (2017) Novel candidate genes may be possible predisposing factors revealed by whole exome sequencing in familial esophageal squamous cell carcinoma. Tumour Biol 39:1010428317699115
13. Gao YB, Chen ZL, Li JG et al (2014) Genetic landscape of esophageal squamous cell carcinoma. Nat Genet 46:1097–1020
14. Ma S, Bao JYJ, Kwan PS et al (2012) Identification of PTK6, via RNA sequencing analysis,

as a suppressor of esophageal squamous cell carcinoma. Gastroenterology 143:675–686
15. Lin DC, Hao JJ, Nagata Y et al (2014) Genomic and molecular characterization of esophageal squamous cell carcinoma. Nat Genet 46:467–473
16. Bainbridge MN, Wang M, Burgess DL et al (2010) Whole exome capture in solution with 3 Gbp of data. Genome Biol 11:R62
17. Sun M, Ju H, Zhou Z (2014) Pilot genome-wide study of tandem 3' UTRs in esophageal cancer using high-throughput sequencing. Mol Med Rep 9:1597–1605
18. Zhang J, Chen Z, Tang Z et al (2017) RNA editing is induced by type I interferon in esophageal squamous cell carcinoma. Tumour Biol 39:1010428317708546
19. Wang K, Johnson A, Ali SM et al (2015) Comprehensive genomic profiling of advanced esophageal squamous cell carcinomas and esophageal adenocarcinomas reveals similarities and differences. Oncologist 20:1132–1139
20. Cheng C, Cui H, Zhang L et al (2016) Genomic analyses reveal FAM84B and the NOTCH pathway are associated with the progression of esophageal squamous cell carcinoma. Gigascience 5:1
21. Kishino T, Niwa T, Yamashita S et al (2016) Integrated analysis of DNA methylation and mutations in esophageal squamous cell carcinoma. Mol Carcinog 55:2077–2088
22. Nakazato H, Takeshima H, Kishino T et al (2016) Early-stage induction of SWI/SNF mutations during esophageal squamous cell carcinogenesis. PLoS One 11:e0147372
23. Luo H, Li H, Hu Z et al (2016) Noninvasive diagnosis and monitoring of mutations by deep sequencing of circulating tumor DNA in esophageal squamous cell carcinoma. Biochem Biophys Res Commun 471:596–602
24. Welander J, Andreasson A, Juhlin CC et al (2014) Rare germline mutations identified by targeted next-generation sequencing of susceptibility genes in pheochromocytoma and paraganglioma. J Clin Endocrinol Metab 99:1352–1360
25. Pan Z, Mao W, Bao Y et al (2016) The long noncoding RNA CASC9 regulates migration and invasion in esophageal cancer. Cancer Med 5:2442–2447
26. Ueda M, Iguchi T, Masuda T et al (2016) Somatic mutations in plasma cell-free DNA are diagnostic markers for esophageal squamous cell carcinoma recurrence. Oncotarget 7:62280–62291
27. Hao JJ, Lin DC, Dinh HQ et al (2016) Spatial intratumoral heterogeneity and temporal clonal evolution in esophageal squamous cell carcinoma. Nat Genet 48:1500–1507
28. Zheng H, Wang Y, Tang C et al (2016) TP53, PIK3CA, FBXW7 and KRAS mutations in esophageal cancer identified by targeted sequencing. Cancer Genomics Proteomics 13:231–238
29. Quail MA, Smith M, Coupland P et al (2012) A tale of three next generation sequencing platforms: comparison of ion torrent, Pacific biosciences, and Illumina MiSeq sequencers. BMC Genomics 13:341
30. Liu X, Zhang M, Ying S et al (2017) Genetic alterations in esophageal tissues from squamous dysplasia to carcinoma. Gastroenterology 153:166–177
31. Yang JW, Choi YL (2017) Genomic profiling of esophageal squamous cell carcinoma (ESCC)-basis for precision medicine. Pathol Res Pract 213:836–841
32. Kobayashi S, Yamaguchi T, Maekawa S et al (2018) Target sequencing of cancer-related genes in early esophageal squamous neoplasia resected by endoscopic resection in Japanese patients. Oncotarget 9:36793–36803
33. Lin ZW, Gu J, Liu RH et al (2014) Genome-wide screening and co-expression network analysis identify recurrence-specific biomarkers of esophageal squamous cell carcinoma. Tumour Biol 35:10959–10968
34. Yokota T, Serizawa M, Hosokawa A et al (2018) PIK3CA mutation is a favorable prognostic factor in esophageal cancer: molecular profile by next-generation sequencing using surgically resected formalin-fixed, paraffin-embedded tissue. BMC Cancer 18:826
35. van El CG, Cornel MC, Borry P et al (2013) Whole-genome sequencing in health care: recommendations of the European Society of Human Genetics. Eur J Hum Genet 21:1–5
36. Meyerson M, Gabriel S, Getz G (2010) Advances in understanding cancer genomes through second-generation sequencing. Nat Rev Genet 11:685–696
37. Sims D, Sudbery I, Ilott NE et al (2014) Sequencing depth and coverage: key considerations in genomic analyses. Nat Rev Genet 15:121–132
38. Zhang L, Zhou Y, Cheng C et al (2015) Genomic analyses reveal mutational signatures and frequently altered genes in esophageal squamous cell carcinoma. Am J Hum Genet 96:597–611
39. Chang J, Tan W, Ling Z et al (2017) Genomic analysis of oesophageal squamous-cell carcinoma identifies alcohol drinking-related

mutation signature and genomic alterations. Nat Commun 8:15290

40. Chen Z, Zhang C, Pan Y et al (2016) T cell receptorβ-chain repertoire analysis reveals intratumour heterogeneity of tumour-infiltrating lymphocytes in oesophageal squamous cell carcinoma. J Pathol 239:450–458
41. Rabbani B, Tekin M, Mahdieh N (2014) The promise of whole-exome sequencing in medical genetics. J Hum Genet 59:5–15
42. Parla JS, Iossifov I, Grabill I et al (2011) A comparative analysis of exome capture. Genome Biol 12:97
43. Zhu Q, Hu Q, Shepherd L et al (2015) The impact of DNA input amount and DNA source on the performance of whole-exome sequencing in cancer epidemiology. Cancer Epidemiol Biomark Prev 24:1207–1213
44. Wang Z, Gerstein M, Snyder M (2009) RNA-Seq: a revolutionary tool for transcriptomics. Nat Rev Genet 10:57–63
45. Peng X, Xue H, Lü L et al (2017) Accumulated promoter methylation as a potential biomarker for esophageal cancer. Oncotarget 8:679–691
46. Margulies M, Egholm M, Altman WE et al (2005) Genome sequencing in microfabricated high-density picolitre reactors. Nature 43:376–380
47. Pareek CS, Smoczynski R, Tretyn A (2011) Sequencing technologies and genome sequencing. J Appl Genet 52:413–435
48. Li X, Buckton AJ, Wilkinson SL et al (2013) Towards clinical molecular diagnosis of inherited cardiac conditions: a comparison of bench-top genome DNA sequencers. PLoS One 8: e67744
49. Ballester LY, Luthra R, Kanagal-Shamanna R et al (2016) Advances in clinical next-generation sequencing: target enrichment and sequencing technologies. Expert Rev Mol Diagn 16:357–372
50. Wang W, Wei C, Li P et al (2018) Integrative analysis of mRNA and lncRNA profiles identified pathogenetic lncRNAs in esophageal squamous cell carcinoma. Gene 661:169–175
51. Moorthie S, Mattocks CJ, Wright CF (2011) Review of massively parallel DNA sequencing technologies. HUGO J 5:1–12

Chapter 18

Roles of MicroRNAs in Esophageal Squamous Cell Carcinoma Pathogenesis

Farhadul Islam, Vinod Gopalan, and Alfred K. Lam

Abstract

MicroRNAs (miRNAs) are 20–22 nucleotides long single-stranded noncoding RNAs. They regulate gene expression posttranscriptionally by base pairing with the complementary sequences in the 3′-untranslated region of their targeted mRNA. Aberrant expression of miRNAs leads to alterations in the expression of oncogenes and tumor suppressors, thereby affecting cellular growth, proliferation, apoptosis, motility, and invasion capacity of gastrointestinal cells, including cells of esophageal squamous cell carcinoma (ESCC). Thus, alterations in miRNAs expression associated with the pathogenesis and progression of ESCC. In addition, expression profiles of miRNAs correlated with various clinicopathological factors, including pathological stages, histological differentiation, invasion, metastasis of cancer, as well as survival rates and therapy response of patients with ESCC. Consequently, expression profiles of miRNAs could be useful as diagnostic, prognostic, and prediction biomarkers in ESCC. Herein, we describe the quantitative reverse transcriptase polymerase chain reaction (qRT-PCR) and microarray methods for detection and quantitate miRNAs in ESCC. In addition, we summarize the roles of miRNAs in ESCC pathogenesis, progression, and prognosis.

Key words MicroRNAs, Cancer pathogenesis, Prognosis, qRT-PCR, Microarray

1 Introduction

MicroRNAs (miRNAs) are 20–22 nucleotides long small single-stranded RNA molecules, transcribed by RNA polymerase II from miRNA genes [1, 2]. Firstly, they form a several hundred to thousand nucleotides long miRNA called primary-miRNA (pri-miRNA) [3]. Then, the pri-miRNA precursor is processed by Drosha (RNA polymerase III) into 60–70 nucleotide double-stranded precursor miRNA (pre-miRNA). Subsequently, the pre-miRNA interacts with Dicer (an endonuclease or helicase with RNase activity) and becomes mature, single-stranded, 20–22 nucleotide miRNA (miRNA) [3, 4]. This mature miRNA interacts with RNA-induced silencing complex (RISC) containing Dicer and many associated proteins, including Argonaute (Ago) protein

Alfred K. Lam (ed.), *Esophageal Squamous Cell Carcinoma: Methods and Protocols*, Methods in Molecular Biology, vol. 2129,
https://doi.org/10.1007/978-1-0716-0377-2_18,

family, which in turn directs the complex for miRNA's target mRNA [5]. These Ago proteins contain two conserved domains: a PAZ domain that can bind single-strand 3′ of mature miRNAs and a PIWI domain that interacts with 5′ end of the guide strand [6]. Thus, they bind to the mature miRNA through RISC complex and orient it for interaction with target mRNA. miRNAs-mediated gene silencing occurs either by directly cleaving target mRNAs or by preventing mRNAs for being translated [6]. Base pairing between miRNA and mRNA directs the ways of gene silencing, i.e., complete complementarity between miRNA and target mRNA sequence leads Ago2-mediated direct cleavage and degradation of target mRNA, whereas incomplete complementarity leads silencing of target gene by preventing translation [7].

The function of miRNAs is gene regulation by being the complementary of one or more mRNAs; thus, their expression is critical for cellular process such as cell proliferation, apoptosis, and differentiation during mammalian development [8]. Therefore, alterations or aberrant expression of miRNAs is associated with various diseases and pathophysiological conditions, including neurological disorders, cardiovascular diseases, infections, inflammatory diseases, and cancers [9, 10].

In esophageal squamous cell carcinoma (ESCC), miRNAs have many roles in the pathogenesis by regulating the expression of oncogenes and tumor suppressors, affecting the proliferation, apoptosis, migration, and invasion capacities of cells in ESCC [11, 12]. Accordingly, overexpression or upregulation and repression or downregulation of certain miRNAs have been associated with the occurrence, staging, prognosis, and recurrence of ESCC [13–15]. In addition, miRNAs are released into the blood and are highly stable, which could be used as a noninvasive test for screening cancers. Thus, various miRNAs could have the potential to be used as biomarkers for ESCC.

miRNAs are very short and exist in different forms; thereby, accurate detection and quantification of miRNA could be challenging. However, various cutting-edge techniques, e.g., Northern blot analysis, quantitative RT-PCR, and microarray hybridization, have been developed to detect as well as quantitate the miRNA expression in biological and clinical samples. The purpose of this chapter is to overview the roles of miRNA in ESCC's pathogenesis, progression, and prognosis and describe the methods such as miRNAs microarray and qRT-PCR for detection and quantification of miRNAs in ESCC.

1.1 Aberrant miRNAs Expression and Pathogenesis of ESCC

Since miRNAs regulate genes expression associated with cellular growth, proliferation, apoptosis, and differentiation of gastrointestinal cells, thus deregulations of miRNAs contributed to the development and progression of ESCC. Downregulation of tumor-suppressive miRNAs, normally targeting the expression of

Table 1
miRNAs associated with the pathogenesis of esophageal squamous cell carcinoma

miRNA	Targets	Role in ESCC	References
miRNA-92a	CHD1/E-cadherin	Migration and invasion	[27]
miRNA-296	Cyclin D1, p27	Cell proliferation	[28]
miRNA-498	FOXO1, KLF6	Cell proliferation, migration, and invasion	[14]
miRNA-205	ZEB2	Migration and invasion	[28, 29]
miRNA-143/145	FSCN1	Metastasis	[26]
miRNA-518b	RAP1b	Cell proliferation and invasion	[30]
miRNA-1288	FOXO1	Cell proliferation, migration, and invasion	[15]
miRNA-133a/b	FSCN1, MMP14	Cell proliferation and invasion	[31]
miRNA-98/214	EZH2	Migration and invasion	[32]
miRNA-21	PDCD4, PTEN, FASL, TIMP3, RECK	Cell proliferation, migration, invasion, and apoptosis	[21–24]
miRNA-25	CHD1	Migration and invasion	[33]
miRNA-150	ZEB1	Epithelial-mesenchymal transition (EMT)	[34]
miRNA-99a/100	mTOR	Apoptosis and cell proliferation	[35]
miRNA-375	PDK1, IGFIR, CHAP31, LDHB	Migration, tumorigenesis, and metastasis	[36, 37]
miRNA-139	NR5A2, Cyclin E1, MMP9	Invasion, tumor growth, and proliferation	[38]
miRNA-195	CDC42	Invasion and metastasis	[39]
miRNA-126	ADAM9	Cell proliferation and migration	[40]
miRNA-19a	TNF-α	Apoptosis and tumor growth	[41]
miRNA-208	SOX6, p21	Cell cycle kinetics and cell proliferation	[42]
miRNA-655	ZEB1, TGFBR2	Apoptosis, tumor growth, and EMT	[43]
miRNA-1294	c-MYC	Cell proliferation, migration, and invasion	[44]
miRNA-9	c-MYC, CHD1, CD44	Migration and metastasis	[45]
miRNA-22	RAD51	Therapy resistance	[46]
miRNA-200b	Kindlin-2	Migration and invasion	[47]

oncogenes, causes elevated expression of several oncogenes. On the other hand, amplification or overexpression of onco-miRNAs, which target several kinds of tumor suppressor genes, thereby stimulating cancer hallmarks, e.g., sustained proliferation, evasion of growth suppressors, avoidance of immune destruction, replicative immortality, tumor-promoting inflammation, activation of invasion and metastasis, induced angiogenesis, along with genome instability and mutation, resulting in resistance to cell death and deregulation of cellular proliferation in ESCC [14–20].

Fu et al. reported that 12 miRNAs are differentially expressed in ESCC when compared to that of adjacent nonneoplastic mucosae [20]. Among them, miR-1, miR29c, miR-100, miR-133a, miR-133b, miR-143, miR-145, and miR-195 were downregulated, whereas miR-7, miR-21, miR-223, and miR-1246 were upregulated. These alterations associated with invasion, metastasis, and differentiation of ESCC [20].

Table 1 summarizes the representative miRNAs expression profiles associated with ESCC pathogenesis with their target genes. For instance, overexpression of miRNA-1288 correlated with advanced pathological stages and increased cell proliferation, colony formation, enhanced cell migration, and increased cell invasion properties in ESCC cells [15]. In addition, overexpression of miRNA-498 correlated with reduction of cell proliferation, barrier penetration, and colony formation when compared to control and wild-type ESCC cells [14]. The miR expression was significantly reduced in the ESCC when compared to the nonneoplastic esophageal tissues [14]. Furthermore, reduced expression of miRNA-143/145 correlated with lymph node metastasis of patients with ESCC [21].

Therefore, miRNAs dysregulation in ESCC strongly associated with ESCC development; thereby, they could be used as diagnostic markers for ESCC at the early stages of the disease.

1.2 miRNAs in Prognosis of Patients with ESCC

Profiling of miRNAs has the potential to be used as a tool to predict the progression and treatment response in ESCC. Table 2 summarizes the miRNAs associated with the prognosis of patients with ESCC. For instance, overexpression of miRNA-21 associated with advanced clinical stages, lymph node metastasis, and poor survival of patients with ESCC [22, 23]. The miRNA regulates proliferation, survival, apoptosis, and invasion of ESCC cells by regulating the expression of several genes, including tropomyosin 1, phosphatase and tensin homolog, mapsin and programmed cell death 4, Fas ligand, tissue inhibitor of metalloproteinase 3, and reversion-inducing-cysteine-rich protein with kazal motifs [24, 25]. In addition, advanced stages ESCC having lower *miR-498* expression had poorer survival rates when compared to that of high miR-498 expression [14].

Table 2
miRNAs associated with the prognosis of patients with esophageal squamous cell carcinoma

miRNA	Method (s)	Size of sample	Expression type	Prognosis	Reference(s)
miRNA-33a/b	qRT-PCR	100	Underexpression	Poor prognosis	[21]
miRNA-92a	qRT-PCR	107	Overexpression	Poor prognosis	[27]
miRNA-296	WB, qRT-PCR	25	Overexpression	Poor prognosis	[28]
miRNA-518b	qRT-PCR	30	Underexpression	Good prognosis	[30]
miRNA-21	qRT-PCR	178	Overexpression	Poor prognosis	[21–24]
miRNA-25	qRT-PCR	62	Overexpression	Poor prognosis	[33]
miRNA-150	qRT-PCR	108	Underexpression	Poor prognosis	[34]
miRNA-99a	qRT-PCR	101	Underexpression	Poor prognosis	[35]
miRNA-375	qRT-PCR	300	Underexpression	Poor prognosis	[36, 37]
miRNA-139	qRT-PCR	106	Overexpression	Poor prognosis	[38]
miRNA-655	qRT-PCR	22	Overexpression	Good prognosis	[43]
miRNA-22	qRT-PCR	100	Underexpression	Poor prognosis	[46]
miRNA-19a	RT-PCR	105	Overexpression	Poor prognosis	[41]
miRNA-9	qRT-PCR	67	Overexpression	Poor prognosis	[45]
miRNA-133b	qRT-PCR	100	Underexpression	Poor prognosis	[31]
miRNA-195	qRT-PCR	98	Underexpression	Poor prognosis	[39]
miRNA-200b	qRT-PCR	88	Underexpression	Poor prognosis	[47]
miRNA-1294	RT-PCR	79	Underexpression	Poor prognosis	[44]
miRNA-508	qRT-PCR	207	Overexpression	Poor prognosis	[48]
miRNA-126	MISH	185	Underexpression	Good prognosis	[40]
miRNA-181b	qRT-PCR	178	Overexpression	Poor prognosis	[49]
miRNA-146b	qRT-PCR	178	Overexpression	Poor prognosis	[49]
miRNA-942	qRT-PCR	158	Overexpression	Poor prognosis	[50]
miRNA-100	qRT-PCR	120	Underexpression	Good prognosis	[51]
miRNA-223	qRT-PCR	109	Overexpression	Poor prognosis	[52]
miRNA-17a	qRT-PCR	105	Overexpression	Poor prognosis	[53]
miRNA-142	qRT-PCR	91	Overexpression	Poor prognosis	[54]
miRNA-302b	qRT-PCR	50	Underexpression	Good prognosis	[55]

qRT-PCR quantitative reverse transcriptase polymerase chain reaction, *MISH* miRNA in situ hybridization, *WB* Western blots miRNA-133a and miRNA-133b were frequently downregulated in ESCC and were associated with poor differentiation of the cancer. The overall survival of ESCC patients with miR-133a-low/miR-133b-low expression has the worse prognosis. They also associated with advanced stages and chemotherapy response, thereby acting as an independent predictive factor for therapy in patients with ESCC [26].

Overall, altered expression level of miRNAs provides information for the evaluation of detection, stages, progression, and treatment response of patients with ESCC, which suggests that miRNAs might serve as biomarkers for early detection of the disease as well as prognostic and predictive markers of the disease.

2 Materials

2.1 Isolation of Total RNA

1. Total RNA extraction kit.
2. Chloroform.
3. 1.5 μL tube.
4. RNase-free water.
5. 100% ethanol.
6. Centrifuges.
7. Ice.
8. Vortex.
9. Sterile-filtered water.

2.2 Microarray

2.2.1 Post-processing

1. Metal slide racks rehydration trays.
2. Centrifuge with slide rack adaptors.
3. Succinic anhydride.
4. 1-methyl-2-pyrrolidinone.
5. 1 M sodium borate solution, pH 8.0 (adjust pH with NaOH).
6. Diamond-tipped glass-etching pen.
7. Stratalinker for ultraviolet cross-linking.
8. 2x saline sodium citrate (SSC): 0.30 M sodium chloride (NaCl), 0.030 M trisodium citrate.

2.2.2 Labelling of RNA

1. miRNA array labelling kit.
2. Dimethyl sulfoxide (DMSO).

2.2.3 Hybridization

1. Labelled RNA.
2. Hybridization chamber.
3. Water bath at 42 °C.

4. Heat block at 100 °C.
5. Hybridization buffer: 100 mM 2-(*N*-morpholino) ethanesulfonic acid, 1 M sodium chloride (NaCl), 20 mM ethylenediaminetetraacetic acid (EDTA), 0.01% Tween 20. Do not autoclave. Store at 2–8 °C.
6. miRNA Bioarray Essentials Kit.
7. 22 × 25 mm lifter slips.

2.2.4 Washing and Scanning

1. Metal slide rack.
2. Four glass slide boxes with covers.
3. Centrifuge rotor adaptors for metal slide racks.
4. Microarray scanner.
5. Wash buffer: 1× SSC, 0.2% SDS (sodium dodecyl sulfate).

2.3 qRT-PCR

1. RNase-free, sterile filtered water.
2. miRNA isolation kit.
3. 20× miRNA assay mix.
4. 10× reverse transcription buffer: 0.75 M potassium chloride (KCl), 0.1 M magnesium chloride ($MgCl_2$), 0.5 M Tris–HCl. Adjust pH to 8.6 at 25 °C.
5. dNTP mix w/dTTP (100 mM total).
6. RNase inhibitor (20 U/μL).
7. Reverse transcriptase.
8. miRNA reverse transcription primer.
9. Universal PCR Master Mix.
10. Real-time thermal cycler.
11. Standard thermal cycler.
12. Centrifuge with plateholders.
13. Microcentrifuge.
14. Vortex.
15. Polypropylene tube.
16. Reagent tubes with caps.
17. 96-well optical reaction plates.
18. Optical adhesive covers.
19. Primers for target miRNAs.
20. Internal control primer.

3 Methods

3.1 Extraction of Total RNA Including miRNAs from Tissue, Blood, or Cells

1. Select and collect the tissue samples from patients/healthy controls, from storage (*see* **Note 1**) or cells from culture. In the case of frozen tissue, allow it to thaw enough so that tissues can be removed from the RNA later. Deparaffinize the samples for paraffin-embedded formalin-fixed tissues by 56 °C heating with gentle shaking. For cultured cells, collect the cells by trypsinization.
2. Add 700 μL lysis buffer (triazole) onto the specimen or cells and homogenize the samples using vortex.
3. After complete homogenization of the samples, incubate them on benchtop at room temperature for 5 min.
4. Add 140 μL chloroform to the homogenate and cap securely. Vortex the tubes vigorously for mixing the component for 30 s.
5. Keep the tubes on benchtop for 2–3 min, and then centrifuge the samples for 15 min at 12,000 × *g* at 4 °C (*see* **Note 2**).
6. Take the aqueous phase into a new 1.5 μL tubes.
7. Add 1.5 volumes (usually 525 μL) of 100% ethanol, and mix thoroughly by pipetting up and down several times.
8. Put 700 μL of the samples to the isolating column, close the lid, centrifuge at 8000 × *g* for 30 s at room temperature, and repeat this step with remaining samples.
9. After that, add 700 μL wash buffer to the column, and centrifuge at 8000 × *g* for 30 s at room temperature (repeat the washing twice).
10. Finally, transfer the column into new 1.5 μL collection tubes, and elute with 30–50 μL RNase-free water by centrifuging 1 min at 8000 × *g* at room temperature.

3.2 miRNAs Microarray: A microarray Used for miRNAs Expression has 5 Steps

1. Isolation of small RNAs from sample (*see* Subheading 3.1).
2. Post-processing.
3. Labelling of RNA.
4. Hybridization.
5. Washing and scanning (*see* **Note 3**).

3.3 Post-processing

1. Take 100 mL 0.5× SSC into hydration tray. Set the warmer to 37 °C and warm on slide warmer.
2. Preheat a heating block at max (>100 °C) for 5 min.
3. Hold the diamond pen perpendicular to the slide, and mark the boundaries of the array on back side of the slide. Since after processing the arrays will not be visible, their boundaries need to be marked.

4. Set slide array side down on the hydration tray, and observe spots until full hydration is achieved (this will look like a light layer of condensation covering the array). Do not rehydrate more than 1 min.
5. Dry the slides by flipping one at a time onto the heating block with the array face up. Do this in one smooth motion and with one hand, pinching the array at one end and flipping it over as you move it to the hot plate. Bright light at the right angle indicates the slide is drying. Dry the array within 1–2 s.
6. Remove the slide and place into a metal slide rack.
7. Put UV cross-link the arrays at 60 mJ (if you are using a Stratalinker, push the energy button, lighting up the indicator for ujoulesx100, enter 600, and then press start).
8. Measure 335 mL of 1-methyl-2-pyrrolidinone into a clean, dry 500 mL beaker. Dissolve 5.5 g of succinic anhydride in the 1-methyl-2-pyrrolidinone using a stir bar. Note that the stock bottle of solid succinic anhydride should be stored under desiccation and vacuumed.
9. Mix 15 mL of 1 M sodium borate pH 8.0 with dissolved succinic anhydride.
10. Quickly pour the buffered blocking solution into a clean, dry glass slide dish. Plunge the slides rapidly into blocking solution and vigorously shake.
11. Keep the tops of the slides under the level of solution, and after 30 s of plunge mixing, put a lid on the glass box, and shake gently on a rotator for 15 min.
12. Transfer slide rack to a glass jar filled with distilled water.
13. Plunge the slides up and down a few times in the water.
14. Transfer the rack to a glass dish of 95% ethanol and plunge several times to rinse.
15. Make sure the ethanol is crystal clear.
16. Spin slide rack in a benchtop centrifuge for 1 min at 200 × *g*.
17. Repeat spinning and washing with ethanol if the slides are not clean and dry.

3.4 Labelling

1. Thaw the components of labelling kit on ice followed by vortexing, and then spin them down (*see* **Note 4**) using table microcentrifuge machine for 30 s.
2. Mix the microRNA array labelling kit components (e.g., Cy5 or Cy3 according to the kit manual), and spike in miRNA (3 μL of total RNA) in an RNase-free microcentrifuge tube (*see* **Note 5**).

3. After adding the miRNA, pipette up and down several times to ensure all elements have been mixed thoroughly.
4. Incubate the mixtures at 37 °C for 30 min and then at 95 °C for 5 min.
5. Immediately cool the samples on ice, and briefly spin the sample and place back on ice (*see* **Note 6**).
6. Add 3 μL labelling buffer, 1 μL labelling enzyme, and 2 μL dimethyl sulfoxide (DMSO) (or alternative according to the kit manual).
7. Mix them again by pipetting up and down several times, and ensure that all reagents have been mixed thoroughly.
8. Incubate at 16 °C for 120 min and then at 65 °C for 15 min, and leave the reaction at 4 °C (*see* **Note 7**).
9. Perform hybridization on the array within 1–2 h.

3.5 Hybridization

1. Preheat 3× hybridization buffer at 65 °C for 5 min and vortex to resuspend.
2. Add 5–10,100 μL drops of 2× SSC in the bottom of the hybridization chamber to prevent the arrays from drying out.
3. Put the slides in the hybridization chamber by keeping array side up.
4. Add the lifter slip over the arrays (this is where the diamond pen marking comes in handy) (*see* **Note 8**).
5. Define the volume of eluted RNA (should be around 20 μL), and add half of this volume in hybridization buffer (i.e., for a 20 μL sample, add 10 μL) (*see* **Note 9**).
6. Denature the samples by heating at 95 °C in heat block for 2 min.
7. Cool them down, spin the samples for 30 s, and immediately apply sample.
8. Finally, close the hybridization chamber and carefully transfer them to a 42 °C water bath for 12–16 h.

3.6 Washing and Scanning

1. Prepare four slide boxes with washing solutions (*see* **Note 10**).
2. Remove the hybridization chamber from the water bath.
3. Remove slides one at a time from the chamber, tip off lifter slip in first low-strength washing buffer, and then place the slides metal rack sitting in the second low-strength buffer.
4. Wash the slides in the low-strength buffer for 1 min.
5. Then wash in high-strength buffer for 1 min.
6. Spin slide rack in a benchtop centrifuge for 3 min at 400 × *g*.
7. Put the slides in a plastic slide box and scan immediately.

3.7 Quantitative Real-Time Polymerase Chain Reaction (qRT-PCR)

1. Take the samples from storage, and thaw them on ice.
2. Label the tubes or 96-well plate ideally, allowing for comparison with a reference miRNA, controls, and replicates (*see* **Note 11**).

3.7.1 Performing the Reverse Transcription Reaction

3. Allow enough time to thaw the required components for preparing cDNA on ice (*see* **Note 12**).
4. Make the reverse transcription master mix by mixing 0.075 μL 100 mM dNTPs, 0.5 μL reverse transcriptase, 0.75 μL 10× buffer, 0.095 μL RNase inhibitor, 2.08 μL water, and 1.5 μL of miRNA reverse transcription primer for both miRNAs in polypropylene tubes (*see* **Note 13**).
5. Make a total of four master mixes with a negative and a positive reverse transcriptase batch for each miRNA (multiply the volume by the number of wells for each corresponding well).
6. Mix and centrifuge briefly the master mixes (*see* **Note 14**).
7. Add 5.0 μL of reaction mix/master mixes into each corresponding well.
8. Add 2.5 μL of either experimental or reference miRNAs into each 96-well reverse transcription reaction plate.
9. Close the plate, mix, and centrifuge briefly.
10. Put the plate on ice for 5 min.
11. Place the plate on ice until you are ready to perform the reverse transcription reaction.
12. Finally, run reverse transcription reaction on a 96-well PCR platform, with sequential incubations at 16 °C for 30 min, 42 °C for 30 min, and 85 °C for 5 min.
13. Allow the plate to cool down, and centrifuge for a brief time to bring down the sample bottom.

3.7.2 Performing the Polymerase Chain Reaction (PCR)

1. Label your PCR strips or tubes 96-well plate for polymerase chain reaction.
2. Add 10 μL 2× Universal PCR Master Mix to 7.67 μL nuclease-free water for a total of 17.67 μL on ice into a polypropylene tube labelled PCR reaction (*see* **Note 15**).
3. Mix and centrifuge with benchtop machine for 15 s.
4. Add 1.0 μL (or alternative according to the kit manual) of 20× microRNA assay mix into the corresponding PCR reaction tube.
5. Add this into corresponding wells.
6. Add 1.33 μL of the reverse transcription product from the 96-well reverse transcription plate into the 96-well PCR plate, and seal with optical adhesive cover.

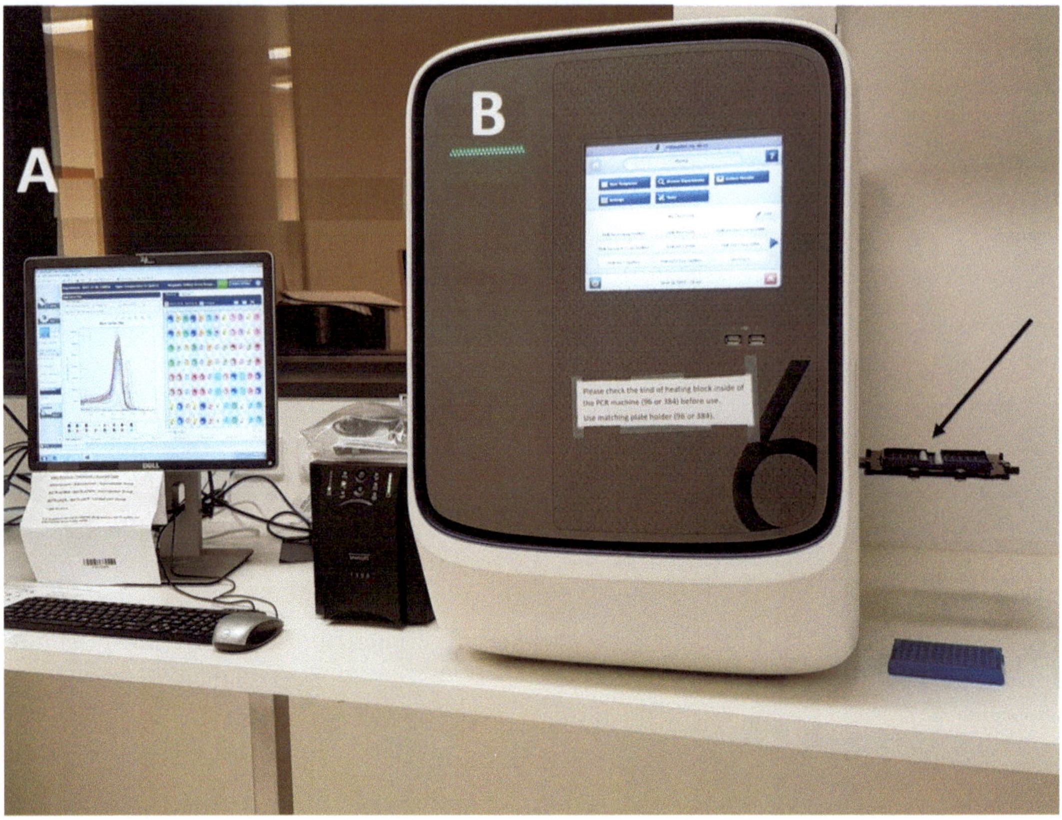

Fig. 1 A setup of quantitative real-time PCR system. (**a**) On-screen melt curve plot in the user interface of PCR system. (**b**) The machine for PCR reactions. Note: The tray contain the tubes/plate of reaction mixture which would be inserted into the machine for analysis (arrow)

7. Mix and centrifuge with benchtop machine for 15 s.
8. Place the PCR plate/tubes, and run real-time PCR (Fig. 1) at standard conditions: 1 cycle of 10 min at 95 °C for enzyme activation and 40 cycles of PCR (15 s at 95 °C, followed by 60 s at 60 °C) (*see* **Note 16**).
9. After completion of PCR, do the analysis and transfer the results to Excel or an alternative spreadsheet and analysis software (Fig. 2).

4 Notes

1. In case of tissues, measure the tissue weight. Do not take more than 50 mg of tissues, and do not thaw tissues before adding lysis reagents.
2. After centrifugation, the sample separates into three layers: an upper aqueous phase containing RNA including small

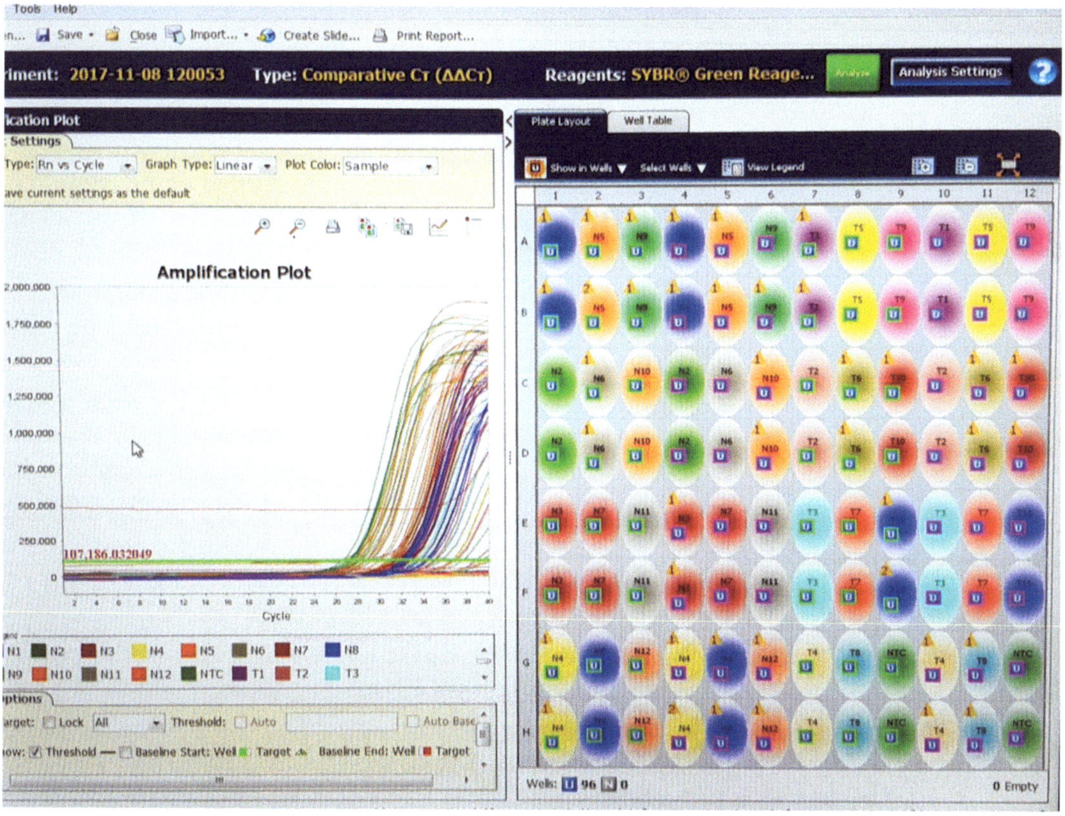

Fig. 2 A higher magnification on screen showing the amplification plots of the samples after analysis. The different colors represent different samples that were put in different wells of the system

miRNAs, a white interphase, and a lower red organic phase. The volume of the aqueous phase should be approximately 350 μL.

3. Need to apply RNA directly to the array, always use gloves when handling the arrays, and arrays should be stored desiccated at room temperature.
4. Instead of thawing the enzymes in this step, you should flick the enzyme tubes three to four times, and subsequently spin them down using a table microcentrifuge machine. Do not vortex enzymes.
5. 3 μL of total RNA should contain approximately between 0.25 and 1.5 μg, and if not sure of the concentration, quantitate RNA sample using a quantitation kit.
6. You can leave on ice for a minimum of 2 min and a maximum of 15 min.
7. Make sure the sample is protected from light to not interfere with the dye.

8. A flat metal spatula can be helpful to align one side of the lifter slip so that we can gently drop the other side down. Use the spatula to align the lifter slip over the array, and be careful not to scratch the array surface.
9. The amount of RNA to use for hybridization will vary depending on the concentration of the miRNAs that you're trying to visualize. Hybridizing with the small RNAs isolated from 20 μg of total RNA might be a good starting point.
10. The first two washes should be with low-strength buffer (0.1× SSC, 0.2% SDS), and the second two washes should be with high strength buffer (1× SSC, 0.2% SDS).
11. Recommended controls for this reaction should include a well where water replaces RNA in the reverse transcription reaction and wells with no reverse transcriptase as negative control. In addition, adjust controls according to the experiment design and aims.
12. Prior to opening the reverse transcription primer tubes, thaw them on ice and mix and centrifuge them.
13. In the negative reverse transcriptase batch, replace the reverse transcriptase volume with RNase-free water.
14. Reverse transcription master mix should be kept on ice while preparing the microRNA samples.
15. Adjust these volumes for the appropriate number of reverse transcription reactions, and prepare separate batches for experimental miRNA and reference miRNA.
16. Use the amplification plots of the reference miRNA reaction to ensure that the assay is performing correctly.

References

1. Ambros V (2004) The functions of animal microRNAs. Nature 431:350–355
2. Bartel DP (2004) MicroRNAs: genomics, biogenesis, mechanism, and function. Cell 116:281–297
3. Lee Y, Kim M, Han J, Yeom KH, Lee S, Baek SH, Kim VN (2004) MicroRNA genes are transcribed by RNA polymerase II. EMBO J 23:4051–4060
4. Bernstein E, Caudy AA, Hammond SM, Hannon GJ (2001) Role for a bidentate ribonuclease in the initiation step of RNA interference. Nature 409:363–366
5. Rana TM (2007) Illuminating the silence: understanding the structure and function of small RNAs. Nat Rev Mol Cell Biol 8:23–36
6. Pratt AJ, MacRae IJ (2009) The RNA-induced silencing complex: a versatile gene-silencing machine. J Biol Chem 284:17897–17901
7. Lim LP, Lau NC, Garrett-Engele P, Grimson A, Schelter JM, Castle J, Bartel DP, Linsley PS, Johnson JM (2005) Microarray analysis shows that some microRNAs downregulate large numbers of target mRNAs. Nature 433:769–773
8. He L, Hannon GJ (2004) MicroRNAs: small RNAs with a big role in gene regulation. Nat Rev Genet 5:522–531
9. Alvarez-Garcia I, Miska EA (2005) MicroRNA functions in animal development and human disease. Development 132:4653–4662
10. Xiao C, Rajewsky K (2009) MicroRNA control in the immune system: basic principles. Cell 136:26–36

11. Song JH, Meltzer SJ (2012) MicroRNAs in pathogenesis, diagnosis, and treatment of gastroesophageal cancers. Gastroenterology 143:35–47.e2
12. Guo Y, Chen Z, Zhang L, Zhou F, Shi S, Feng X, Li B, Meng X, Ma X, Luo M, Shao K, Li N, Qiu B, Mitchelson K, Cheng J, He J (2008) Distinctive microRNA profiles relating to patient survival in esophageal squamous cell carcinoma. Cancer Res 68:26–33
13. Lu J, Getz G, Miska EA, Alvarez-Saavedra E, Lamb J, Peck D, Sweet-Cordero A, Ebert BL, Mak RH, Ferrando AA, Downing JR, Jacks T, Horvitz HR, Golub TR (2005) MicroRNA expression profiles classify human cancers. Nature 435:834–838
14. Islam F, Gopalan V, Law S, Tang JC, Chan KW, Lam AK (2017) MiR-498 in esophageal squamous cell carcinoma: clinicopathological impacts and functional interactions. Hum Pathol 62:141–151
15. Gopalan V, Islam F, Pillai S, Tang JC, Tong DK, Law S, Chan KW, Lam AK (2016) Overexpression of microRNA-1288 in oesophageal squamous cell carcinoma. Exp Cell Res 348:146–154
16. Harada K, Baba Y, Ishimoto T, Shigaki H, Kosumi K, Yoshida N, Watanabe M, Baba H (2016) The role of microRNA in esophageal squamous cell carcinoma. J Gastroenterol 51:520–530
17. Mei LL, Qiu YT, Zhang B, Shi ZZ (2017) MicroRNAs in esophageal squamous cell carcinoma: potential biomarkers and therapeutic targets. Cancer Biomark 19:1–9
18. Matsushima K, Isomoto H, Kohno S, Nakao K (2010) MicroRNAs and esophageal squamous cell carcinoma. Digestion 82:138–144
19. Chu Y, Zhu H, Lv L, Zhou Y, Huo J (2013) MiRNA s in oesophageal squamous cancer. Neth J Med 71:69–75
20. Fu HL, Wu DP, Wang XF, Wang JG, Jiao F, Song LL, Xie H, Wen XY, Shan HS, Du YX, Zhao YP (2013) Altered miRNA expression is associated with differentiation, invasion, and metastasis of esophageal squamous cell carcinoma (ESCC) in patients from Huaian, China. Cell Biochem Biophys 67:657–668
21. Liu R, Liao J, Yang M, Sheng J, Yang H, Wang Y, Pan E, Guo W, Pu Y, Kim SJ, Yin L (2012) The cluster of miR-143 and miR-145 affects the risk for esophageal squamous cell carcinoma through co-regulating fascin homolog 1. PLoS One 7:e33987
22. Hezova R, Kovarikova A, Srovnal J, Zemanova M, Harustiak T, Ehrmann J, Hajduch M, Svoboda M, Sachlova M, Slaby O (2015) Diagnostic and prognostic potential of miR-21, miR-29c, miR-148 and miR-203 in adenocarcinoma and squamous cell carcinoma of esophagus. Diagn Pathol 10:42
23. Akagi I, Miyashita M, Ishibashi O, Mishima T, Kikuchi K, Makino H, Nomura T, Hagiwara N, Uchida E, Takizawa T (2011) Relationship between altered expression levels of MIR21, MIR143, MIR145, and MIR205 and clinicopathologic features of esophageal squamous cell carcinoma. Dis Esophagus 24:523–530
24. Li P, Mao WM, Zheng ZG, Dong ZM, Ling ZQ (2013) Down-regulation of PTEN expression modulated by dysregulated miR-21 contributes to the progression of esophageal cancer. Dig Dis Sci 58:3483–3493
25. Wang N, Zhang CQ, He JH, Duan XF, Wang YY, Ji X, Zang WQ, Li M, Ma YY, Wang T, Zhao GQ (2013) MiR-21 down-regulation suppresses cell growth, invasion and induces cell apoptosis by targeting FASL, TIMP3, and RECK genes in esophageal carcinoma. Dig Dis Sci 58:1863–1870
26. Chen G, Peng J, Zhu W, Tao G, Song Y, Zhou X, Wang W (2014) Combined downregulation of microRNA-133a and microRNA-133b predicts chemosensitivity of patients with esophageal squamous cell carcinoma undergoing paclitaxel-based chemotherapy. Med Oncol 31:263
27. Chen ZL, Zhao XH, Wang JW, Li BZ, Wang Z, Sun J, Tan FW, Ding DP, Xu XH, Zhou F, Tan XG, Hang J, Shi SS, Feng XL, He J (2011) microRNA-92a promotes lymph node metastasis of human esophageal squamous cell carcinoma via E-cadherin. J Biol Chem 286:10725–10734
28. Hong L, Han Y, Zhang H, Li M, Gong T, Sun L, Wu K, Zhao Q, Fan D (2010) The prognostic and chemotherapeutic value of miR-296 in esophageal squamous cell carcinoma. Ann Surg 251:1056–1063
29. Matsushima K, Isomoto H, Yamaguchi N, Inoue N, Machida H, Nakayama T, Hayashi T, Kunizaki M, Hidaka S, Nagayasu T, Nakashima M, Ujifuku K, Mitsutake N, Ohtsuru A, Yamashita S, Korpal M, Kang Y, Gregory PA, Goodall GJ, Kohno S, Nakao K (2011) MiRNA-205 modulates cellular invasion and migration via regulating zinc finger E-box binding homeobox 2 expression in esophageal squamous cell carcinoma cells. J Transl Med 9:30
30. Zhang M, Zhou S, Zhang L, Zhang J, Cai H, Zhu J, Huang C, Wang J (2012) miR-518b is down-regulated, and involved in cell proliferation and invasion by targeting Rap1b in

esophageal squamous cell carcinoma. FEBS Lett 586:3508–3521
31. Akanuma N, Hoshino I, Akutsu Y, Murakami K, Isozaki Y, Maruyama T, Yusup G, Qin W, Toyozumi T, Takahashi M, Suito H, Hu X, Sekino N, Matsubara H (2014) MicroRNA-133a regulates the mRNAs of two invadopodia-related proteins, FSCN1 and MMP14, in esophageal cancer. Br J Cancer 110:189–198
32. Huang SD, Yuan Y, Zhuang CW, Li BL, Gong DJ, Wang SG, Zeng ZY, Cheng HZ (2012) MicroRNA-98 and microRNA-214 post-transcriptionally regulate enhancer of zeste homolog 2 and inhibit migration and invasion in human esophageal squamous cell carcinoma. Mol Cancer 11:51
33. Xu X, Chen Z, Zhao X, Wang J, Ding D, Wang Z, Tan F, Tan X, Zhou F, Sun J, Sun N, Gao Y, Shao K, Li N, Qiu B, He J (2012) MicroRNA-25 promotes cell migration and invasion in esophageal squamous cell carcinoma. Biochem Biophys Res Commun 421:640–645
34. Yokobori T, Suzuki S, Tanaka N, Inose T, Sohda M, Sano A, Sakai M, Nakajima M, Miyazaki T, Kato H, Kuwano H (2013) MiR-150 is associated with poor prognosis in esophageal squamous cell carcinoma via targeting the EMT inducer ZEB1. Cancer Sci 104:48–54
35. Sun J, Chen Z, Tan X, Zhou F, Tan F, Gao Y, Sun N, Xu X, Shao K, He J (2013) MicroRNA-99a/100 promotes apoptosis by targeting mTOR in human esophageal squamous cell carcinoma. Med Oncol 30:411
36. Isozaki Y, Hoshino I, Nohata N, Kinoshita T, Akutsu Y, Hanari N, Mori M, Yoneyama Y, Akanuma N, Takeshita N, Maruyama T, Seki N, Nishino N, Yoshida M, Matsubara H (2012) Identification of novel molecular targets regulated by tumor suppressive miR-375 induced by histone acetylation in esophageal squamous cell carcinoma. Int J Oncol 41:985–994
37. Kong KL, Kwong DL, Chan TH, Law SY, Chen L, Li Y, Qin YR, Guan XY (2012) MicroRNA-375 inhibits tumour growth and metastasis in oesophageal squamous cell carcinoma through repressing insulin-like growth factor 1 receptor. Gut 61:33–42
38. Liu R, Yang M, Meng Y, Liao J, Sheng J, Pu Y, Yin L, Kim SJ (2013) Tumor-suppressive function of miR-139-5p in esophageal squamous cell carcinoma. PLoS One 8:e77068
39. Sun N, Ye L, Chang T, Li X, Li X (2014) microRNA-195-Cdc42 axis acts as a prognostic factor of esophageal squamous cell carcinoma. Int J Clin Exp Pathol 7:6871–6879
40. Liu R, Gu J, Jiang P, Zheng Y, Liu X, Jiang X, Huang E, Xiong S, Xu F, Liu G, Ge D, Chu Y (2015) DNMT1-microRNA126 epigenetic circuit contributes to esophageal squamous cell carcinoma growth via ADAM9-EGFR-AKT signaling. Clin Cancer Res 21:854–863
41. Liu M, Wang Z, Yang S, Zhang W, He S, Hu C, Zhu H, Quan L, Bai J, Xu N (2011) TNF-α is a novel target of miR-19a. Int J Oncol 38:1013–1022
42. Li H, Zheng D, Zhang B, Liu L, Ou J, Chen W, Xiong S, Gu Y, Yang J (2014) Mir-208 promotes cell proliferation by repressing SOX6 expression in human esophageal squamous cell carcinoma. J Transl Med 12:196
43. Harazono Y, Muramatsu T, Endo H, Uzawa N, Kawano T, Harada K, Inazawa J, Kozaki K (2013) miR-655 Is an EMT-suppressive microRNA targeting ZEB1 and TGFBR2. PLoS One 8:e62757
44. Liu K, Li L, Rusidanmu A, Wang Y, Lv X (2015) Down-regulation of MiR-1294 is related to dismal prognosis of patients with esophageal squamous cell carcinoma through elevating C-MYC expression. Cell Physiol Biochem 36:100–110
45. Song Y, Li J, Zhu Y, Dai Y, Zeng T, Liu L, Li J, Wang H, Qin Y, Zeng M, Guan XY, Li Y (2014) MicroRNA-9 promotes tumor metastasis via repressing E-cadherin in esophageal squamous cell carcinoma. Oncotarget 5:11669–11680
46. Wang XC, Zhang ZB, Wang YY, Wu HY, Li DG, Meng AM, Fan FY (2013) Increased miRNA-22 expression sensitizes esophageal squamous cell carcinoma to irradiation. J Radiat Res 54:401–408
47. Zhang HF, Zhang K, Liao LD, Li LY, Du ZP, Wu BL, Wu JY, Xu XE, Zeng FM, Chen B, Cao HH, Zhu MX, Dai LH, Long L, Wu ZY, Lai R, Xu LY, Li EM (2014) miR-200b suppresses invasiveness and modulates the cytoskeletal and adhesive machinery in esophageal squamous cell carcinoma cells via targeting Kindlin-2. Carcinogenesis 35:292–301
48. Lin C, Liu A, Zhu J, Zhang X, Wu G, Ren P, Wu J, Li M, Li J, Song L (2014) miR-508 sustains phosphoinositide signalling and promotes aggressive phenotype of oesophageal squamous cell carcinoma. Nat Commun 5:4620
49. Zhao Y, Schetter AJ, Yang GB, Nguyen G, Mathé EA, Li P, Cai H, Yu L, Liu F, Hang D, Yang H, Wang XW, Ke Y, Harris CC (2013) microRNA and inflammatory gene expression

as prognostic marker for overall survival in esophageal squamous cell carcinoma. Int J Cancer 132:2901–2909

50. Ge C, Wu S, Wang W, Liu Z, Zhang J, Wang Z, Li R, Zhang Z, Li Z, Dong S, Wang Y, Xue Y, Yang J, Tan Q, Wang Z, Song X (2015) miR-942 promotes cancer stem cell-like traits in esophageal squamous cell carcinoma through activation of Wnt/β-catenin signalling pathway. Oncotarget 6:10964–10977
51. Zhou S, Yang B, Zhao Y, Xu S, Zhang H, Li Z (2014) Prognostic value of microRNA-100 in esophageal squamous cell carcinoma. J Surg Res 192:515–520
52. Kurashige J, Watanabe M, Iwatsuki M, Kinoshita K, Saito S, Hiyoshi Y, Kamohara H, Baba Y, Mimori K, Baba H (2012) Overexpression of microRNA-223 regulates the ubiquitin ligase FBXW7 in oesophageal squamous cell carcinoma. Br J Cancer 106:182–188
53. Xu XL, Jiang YH, Feng JG, Su D, Chen PC, Mao WM (2014) MicroRNA-17, microRNA-18a, and microRNA-19a are prognostic indicators in esophageal squamous cell carcinoma. Ann Thorac Surg 97:1037–1045
54. Lin RJ, Xiao DW, Liao LD, Chen T, Xie ZF, Huang WZ, Wang WS, Jiang TF, Wu BL, Li EM, Xu LY (2012) MiR-142-3p as a potential prognostic biomarker for esophageal squamous cell carcinoma. J Surg Oncol 105:175–182
55. Zhang M, Yang Q, Zhang L, Zhou S, Ye W, Yao Q, Li Z, Huang C, Wen Q, Wang J (2014) miR-302b is a potential molecular marker of esophageal squamous cell carcinoma and functions as a tumor suppressor by targeting ErbB4. J Exp Clin Cancer Res 33:10

Chapter 19

Mass Spectrometry for Biomarkers Discovery in Esophageal Squamous Cell Carcinoma

Farhadul Islam, Vinod Gopalan, and Alfred K. Lam

Abstract

Mass spectrometry-based proteomics analysis could categorize proteins and study their interactions in large scale in human cancers. By this method, many proteins are upregulated or downregulated in esophageal squamous cell carcinoma (ESCC) when compared to nonneoplastic esophageal mucosae. The method can also be used to identify novel, effective biomarkers for early diagnosis or predict prognosis of patients with ESCC. These changes are associated with different clinical and pathological parameters. Different biological matrices such as pathological tissue, body fluids, and cancer cell lines-based proteomics have widely been used. Herein, we described cell line-based label-free shotgun proteomics (in-solution tryptic digestion) to identify the protein biomarkers differently expressed in ESCC.

Key words Label-free proteomics, Shotgun proteomics, ESCC, Cancer, Biomarkers

1 Introduction

Proteomics are the approach of cataloguing, analyzing of proteins in large scale to determine when a protein is expressed, how much is made, and with what other proteins it can interact. It is the systematic analysis of protein profiles of cells or tissues, which are complements of genomics analysis [1]. In addition, proteomics analysis may provide insight into posttranslational modifications affecting cellular function not identified by genomics analysis. Identifying global protein expression as well as changes in specific proteins expression in cancer-related processes is important as these proteins could be biomarkers in early cancer diagnosis [2]. Thus, proteomics analysis of biological matrices has been studied in different cancers, including from the pancreas, nasopharynx, thyroid, lung, oral cavity, large intestine, breast, and melanomas for biomarker (s) identifications [3–11].

Mass spectrometry (MS)-based proteomics technologies are powerful tools used for large-scale protein identification and quantitation for biomarker discovery and development [12]. Among

Alfred K. Lam (ed.), *Esophageal Squamous Cell Carcinoma: Methods and Protocols*, Methods in Molecular Biology, vol. 2129, https://doi.org/10.1007/978-1-0716-0377-2_19, © Springer Science+Business Media, LLC, part of Springer Nature 2020

various biological matrices, cell culture-based models are suitable approach to identify biomarkers at initial stage because the body fluids such as plasma or serum are highly complex at the protein level and pose various limitations [13]. The proteins secreted from cancers comprise only a minuscule component of the proteome. Many other proteins in these body fluids masked the cancer-related proteins [13]. In addition, the target protein(s) of the body fluids may derive not just from cancer cells but also from any distant tissue or organ [14]. In tissues, presence of fibroblasts, inflammatory cells, and other nonmalignant cells pose difficulties in analyzing the specific contribution by cancer cells [15]. Therefore, identifying candidate biomarkers from enriched conditioned medium of cancer cells in culture represents a simple and reliable approach toward screening for the cancer protein biomarker.

A number of mass spectrometric-based approaches including MALDI-TOF/TOF (matrix-assisted laser desorption/ionization-time-of-flight), MALDI-TOF-MS (matrix-assisted laser desorption/ionization-time-of-flight mass spectrometry), SELDI-TOF-MS (surface-enhanced laser desorption/ionization-time-of-flight mass spectrometry), SILAC-TOF (stable isotope labelling with amino acids in cell culture-time-of-flight), and label-free shotgun proteomics are being for biomarker discovery [13, 16–23]. Among these, label-free shotgun proteomics is highly effective for the identification of peptides, subsequently obtaining the global protein profile of the tested sample. This label-free shotgun proteomics is suitable for applications in complex biological systems and generates faster, cleaner, and simpler results [24, 25].

Table 1 shows the summary of studies carried out in esophageal squamous cell carcinoma (ESCC) using proteomics techniques. Proteome analysis using mass spectrometry unveiled that many proteins are upregulated or downregulated in ESCC in comparison to that of nonneoplastic esophageal mucosae. This aberrant expression of proteins in ESCC deregulates the key events involved in cells' growth and development, thereby leading to the initiation of carcinogenesis and disease progression. These changes also correlated with disease stage, progression, therapeutic response, and cancer recurrence.

In the present chapter, we describe the label-free shotgun proteomics combined with MS to compare the protein expression profiles in cultured ESCC cells. Fig. 1 illustrates the experimental workflow for label-free shotgun proteomics analysis in ESCC. In the first step, we culture ESCC and nonneoplastic esophageal cells. Subsequently, we collect the cell lysate. Then, we analyze the lysates using liquid chromatography coupled with tandem mass spectrometry (LC-MS/MS) followed by in-solution tryptic digestion. Finally, the resulting peptide mass data searches against the National Center for Biotechnology Information (NCBI) *Homo*

Table 1
Mass spectrometry-based proteomics used in ESCC for biomarker discovery

Biological matrices	Key findings	Techniques	References
Patient's sera	Loss of clusterin in ESCC	2-DE and MALDI-TOF-MS	[26]
ESCC and adjacent nonneoplastic epithelia	28 proteins aberrantly expressed in ESCC compared to nonneoplastic epithelia	Ion trap mass coupled with HPLC	[21]
ESCC and adjacent nonneoplastic epithelia	15 proteins were upregulated and 5 proteins were downregulated significantly in ESCC	MADLI-TOF-MS	[27]
ESCC and adjacent nonneoplastic epithelia	18 proteins differentially expressed in ESCC	2-DE and MALDI-TOF-MS	[17]
ESCC and adjacent nonneoplastic epithelia	17 proteins were upregulated and 5 proteins were downregulated significantly in ESCC	2-DE and MALDI-TOF-MS	[16]
Patient's and healthy control's sera	31 proteins differently expressed in ESCC in comparison to healthy individuals	SELDI-TOF-MS and CM10 protein chip	[28]
Cell lines and sera from ESCC and healthy controls	Identified autoantibody against *Hsp70* in patients with ESCC	2-DE and MALDI-TOF-MS TOF-MS	[19]
Cell lines	33 proteins were differentially expressed in ESCC cell lines	MALDI-TOF-MS	[22]
Patient's and age- and gender-matched control's sera	Identified autoantibody against *CDC25B* in ESCC sera	2-DE and MALDI-TOF	[29]
ESCC tissues	22 proteins were differentially expressed in ESCC and TGM3 expression correlated with survival	2D-DIGE and LTQ-MS	[20]
Patient's and age- and gender-matched control's sera	Six protein peaks were identified as diagnostic pattern with a sensitivity of 97.12% and a specificity of 83.87%	SELDI-TOF-MS and CM10 protein chip	[23]
Patient's and healthy control's sera	Glycosylation of 16 proteins were significantly different in ESCC	Lectin-based antibody-microarray	[30]
ESCC and adjacent normal epithelia	12 proteins were upregulated and 17 proteins were downregulated in ESCC	2-DE and MALDI-TOF-MS	[31]
Secretome of ESCC and non-ESCC	120 proteins were upregulated in fluids secreted by ESCC cells	2DE and SILAC-TOF-MS	[13]

(continued)

Table 1
(continued)

Biological matrices	Key findings	Techniques	References
ESCC and adjacent nonneoplastic epithelia	257 proteins were differentially expressed in ESCC	iTRAQ labeling and LC-MS/MS	[32]
ESCC and adjacent nonneoplastic epithelia	4 proteins were differentially expressed in ESCC	2-DE and MALDI-TOF/TOF-MS	[33]
Plasma from patients with ESCC	16 proteins were upregulated and 15 proteins were down regulated in ESCC	2DE-DIGE and MALDI-TOF/TOF-MS	[34]

2-DE two-dimensional gel electrophoresis, *MALDI-TOF-MS* matrix-assisted laser desorption/ionization-time-of-flight mass spectrometry, *HPLC* high-performance liquid chromatography, *SELDI-TOF-MS* surface-enhanced laser desorption/ionization time-of-flight mass spectrometry, *2D-DIGE* two-dimensional differential gel electrophoresis, *LTQ-MS* linear trap quadrupole-mass spectrometry, *SILAC* stable isotope labeling with amino acids in cell culture, *iTRAQ* isobaric tags for relative and absolute quantitation

sapiens database using appropriate software to identify differential expression of proteins in ESCC and nonneoplastic esophageal cells.

2 Materials

All the chemicals and reagents are of analytical grade. Prepare solutions using ultrapure water, and store all the reagents and solution at room temperature unless otherwise indicated. Strictly follow the guidelines and regulations of waste disposal during disposing waste materials, and use the appropriate personal protective equipment during experiments to escape the laboratory hazards.

2.1 Cell Culture

1. Human ESCC and nonneoplastic esophageal epithelial cell lines.
2. Cell culture medium: Dulbecco's Modified Eagle's Medium (DMEM), 2 mM glutamine. Add about 900 mL water to a glass beaker. With gentle stir, add 13.5 g DMEM powder media with glutamine to the water. Stir the mixture until completely. Weigh 3.7 g of sodium bicarbonate and add to the media. Stir for complete dissolving, and adjust the pH with 1 N HCl (hydrogen chloride) and NaOH (sodium hydroxide). Finally, add water up to mark 1 L, and sterilize the media using 0.22-μm membrane filter to aseptically transfer media into sterile container and store at 4 °C.
3. 10% fetal bovine serum (FBS) in media and store at 4 °C.

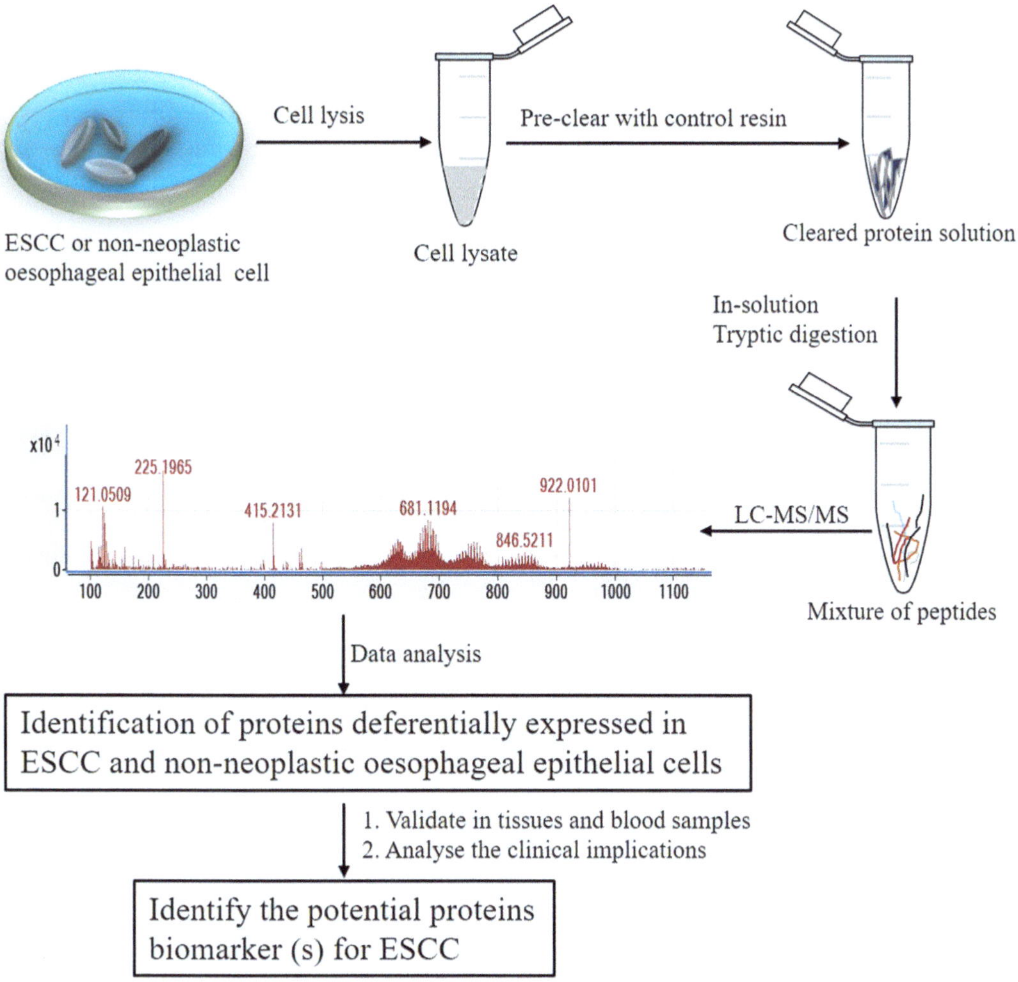

Fig. 1 Experimental workflow of the current study. Schematic illustration of the experiments followed to identify the potential biomarker(s) in ESCC. Both ESCC and nonneoplastic esophageal epithelial cells were cultured, and whole cell lysates were collected. Peptide fingerprints of ESCC and nonneoplastic epithelial cells were generated by in-solution tryptic digestion of the samples followed by preclear. Finally, differentially expressed proteins in ESCC and nonneoplastic epithelial cells were identified by mass spectrometry

4. 1% penicillin and streptomycin antibiotic in media and store at 4 °C.
5. Cell washing buffer: Phosphate buffer saline (PBS) at pH 7.4. Measures 8.0 g NaCl, 0.2 g KCl, 1.42 g Na_2HPO_4, and 0.24 g KH_2PO_4, and add in a glass beaker. Dissolves all the salts in 800 mL water, and adjust the pH with 1 N HCl. Adjust the volume to 1 L with distilled water. Then, sterilize and store at 4 °C.
6. 0.25% trypsin-ethylenediaminetetraacetic acid (EDTA), pH 7.2–8 cell dissociation solution. Preserve at −20 °C.

7. 25 cm^2 and 75 cm^2 polystyrene cell culture flasks.
8. 12-well polystyrene cell culture plates.
9. 15 mL and 50 mL falcon conical centrifuge tubes.
10. Hemocytometer, microscope, and centrifuge machines.
11. 80% ethanol in water (v/v).

2.2 Cell Lysis

1. Cell lysis buffer: 150 mM sodium chloride, 1.0% NP-40 or Triton X-100, 0.5% sodium deoxycholate, 0.1% SDS (sodium dodecyl sulfate), 50 mM Tris, pH 8.0.
2. Protease inhibitors: 1 mM phenylmethylsulfonyl fluoride (PMSF), 5 mM ethylenediaminetetraacetic acid (EDTA), 1 mM ethylene glycol tetraacetic acid (EGTA), and 5–10 mM sodium fluoride.
3. Bicinchoninic acid assay (BCA) protein assay kit.

2.3 Protein Digestion and Mass Spectrometry

1. 0.5 mL tubes.
2. In-solution tryptic digestion kit.
3. 50 mM ammonium bicarbonate.
4. 10 mM dithiothreitol (DTT).
5. 15 mM iodoacetamide (IAA).
6. C18 Ziptips.
7. 60% acetonitrile (ACN).
8. 0.1% trifluoroacetic acid (TFA).
9. 0.1% formic acid.
10. Amber vials with cap.
11. Incubator.
12. Mass acquisition system.

2.4 Data Analysis

1. Data analysis software compatible to the data acquisition system.
2. Internet access to the National Center for Biotechnology Information (NCBI) *Homo sapiens* database.
3. Hi-speedy computer.

3 Methods

3.1 Cell Culture

1. Take the cryovial containing ESCC and nonneoplastic esophageal epithelial cells from liquid nitrogen facility, and transfer them into a 37 °C water bath.
2. Quickly thaw the cells by gently swirling the vial in water bath at 37 °C (*see* **Note 1**).

3. Transfer the vial into a biosafety cabinet, and wipe out site of the vial with 80% ethanol.
4. Add pre-warmed complete growth media (2 mL) in a 15 mL centrifuge tube, and add the thaw cells dropwise into the tube.
5. Centrifuge the cell suspension at approximately 400 × *g* for 3–5 min.
6. Check the cell pellet after centrifugation, and aseptically decant the supernatant without disrupting the cells pellet.
7. Add 2 mL PBS and resuspend the cells pellet with slow pipetting.
8. Centrifuge the suspension at 400 × *g* for 3–5 min and discard the supernatant.
9. Resuspend the cell pellets in complete growth media (containing FBS), transfer them into an appropriate cell culture flask containing recommended growth media, and incubate in the CO_2 incubator at appropriate conditions (*see* **Note 2**).

3.2 Cell Lysis

1. Grow the EAC cells up to 70–80% confluency, and harvest the cells after trypsinization.
2. Take the flask(s) inside biosafety cabinet, discard the media, and rinse with 2 × PBS.
3. Vacuum off the PBS, add 0.25% trypsin-EDTA to the flask, and incubate for 5–10 min or until disassociation of cells (*see* **Note 3**).
4. After completing the detachment of cells from the flask, add growth media to neutralize EDTA.
5. Rinse the flask and pipette off cells to ensure maximum collection of cells.
6. Centrifuge for 3–5 min at 400 × *g*, discard the media, and wash the cells with ice-cold PBS.
7. Extract proteins using cell lysis RIPA buffer from ESCC and nonneoplastic epithelial cells. For this, first add 2–5% protease inhibitors to ice-cold cell lysis buffer, and then add the mixture to cells (1 mL per 10^7 cells/100 mm dish/150 cm^2 flask) for lysis.
8. Keep the cells on ice for 30 min and vortex in every 5 min.
9. Centrifuge the tube for 20 min at 13,000 × *g* at 4 °C. After centrifugation, aspirate the supernatant in a new tube on ice. For storage, keep the protein at −80 °C.
10. Measure the protein concentrations using bicinchoninic acid assay (BCA) protein assay kit.

3.3 Protein Digestion and Mass Spectrometry

1. Dispense 5 μg of protein into 500 μL tubes in duplicate.
2. Add 50 mM ammonium bicarbonate and 10 mM dithiothreitol (DTT) to each tube, and incubate at 95 °C for 5 min to reduce the proteins.
3. Add 15 mM of iodoacetamide (IAA) to the samples, and incubate for 20 min in the dark at room temperature for alkylation.
4. Add 5 ng/μL of trypsin in each tubes, incubate at 37 °C for 3 h, then add more trypsin (increasing the total concentration to 10 ng/μL), and incubate the samples at 30 °C overnight (*see* **Note 4**).
5. Desalt and concentrate the samples using C18 Ziptips.
6. Pool the samples and elute in 60% acetonitrile (ACN) and 0.1% trifluoroacetic acid (TFA).
7. Dry down the samples to remove all solvent.
8. Finally, resuspend the samples in 100 μL of 0.1% formic acid, and transfer to amber vials for LC-MS/MS analysis.
9. Perform the data acquisition, and analyze using mass spectrometry analysis facility.

3.4 Data Analysis

1. Analyze using appropriate tools, and search the resulting peptide mass data against the National Center for Biotechnology Information (NCBI) *Homo sapiens* database (*see* **Note 5**).
2. Define the false discovery rate (FDR) analysis function, and only proteins matched within the 1% FDR bracket should be considered for further analysis (*see* **Note 6**).
3. Exclude the nonspecific proteins using the Protein Alignment Template (*see* **Note** 7).

4 Notes

1. Thawing procedures are stressful for the frozen cells, and using the good techniques and fast thawing at 37 °C ensure high proportion of the cells survive the procedures. Dilute the frozen cells with pre-warmed complete media, and mix with slow pipette up and down.
2. Flask size depends on the number of frozen cells present in the cryovial, and culture conditions vary based on cell type and media used. Generally, cells seeded at 10,000 cells/cm^2, in 5% CO_2, at 37 °C are used for routine culture and passages.
3. Add 2 mL and 5 mL 0.25% trypsin-EDTA in 25 cm^2 and 75 cm^2 flask, respectively. Monitor the cells in every 2 min until they are starting to disassociate. Tap gently the flask to get maximum disassociation and recovery of the cells. Do not

put cells in trypsin for a long time, which may cause reduced viability of the cells.

4. Incomplete digestions of protein may occur if there is insufficient enzyme used and/or insufficient enzyme activity. Enzyme activity can decrease due to long time or inappropriate storage. Increased incubation time and/or use of new stock of trypsin can overcome incomplete digestion of samples.
5. Perform all the experiments in triplicates with at least two biological replicates. The samples from each experimental trial should be run on different days to obtain more reliable peptide mass data.
6. To identify potential biomarkers, proteins identified exclusively in the target ESCC samples should be sought.
7. The identified protein lists from each sample need to be matched against each other in all possible combinations in order to identify proteins expressed exclusively in the target ESCC cells, not in nonneoplastic esophageal epithelial cells or control, indicating they are true potential biomarkers for ESCC. Only proteins that could be identified in at least two of the three independent runs should be short-listed for further analysis.

References

1. Anderson NL, Anderson NG (1998) Proteome and proteomics: new technologies, new concepts, and new words. Electrophoresis 19:1853–1861
2. Tyers M, Mann M (2003) From genomics to proteomics. Nature 422:193–197
3. Gronborg M, Kristiansen TZ, Iwahori A, Chang R, Reddy R, Sato N et al (2006) Biomarker discovery from pancreatic cancer secretome using a differential proteomic approach. Mol Cell Proteomics 5:157–171
4. Wu HY, Chang YH, Chang YC, Liao PC (2009) Proteomics analysis of nasopharyngeal carcinoma cell secretome using a hollow fiber culture system and mass spectrometry. J Proteome Res 8:380–389
5. Iannetti A, Pacifico F, Acquaviva R, Lavorgna A, Crescenzi E, Vascotto C et al (2008) The neutrophil gelatinase-associated lipocalin (NGAL), a NF-kappa-B-regulated gene, is a survival factor for thyroid neoplastic cells. Proc Natl Acad Sci U S A 105:14058–14063
6. Zhong L, Roybal J, Chaerkady R, Zhang W, Choi K, Alvarez CA et al (2008) Identification of secreted proteins that mediate cell-cell interactions in an in vitro model of the lung cancer microenvironment. Cancer Res 68:7237–7245
7. Weng LP, Wu CC, Hsu BL, Chi LM, Liang Y, Tseng CP et al (2008) Secretome-based identification of mac-2 binding protein as a potential oral cancer marker involved in cell growth and motility. J Proteome Res 7:3765–3775
8. Kobayashi R, Deavers M, Patenia R, Rice-Stitt-T, Halbe J, Gallardo S et al (2009) 14-3-3 zeta protein secreted by tumor associated monocytes/macrophages from ascites of epithelial ovarian cancer patients. Cancer Immunol Immunother 58:247–258
9. Wu CC, Chen HC, Chen SJ, Liu HP, Hsieh YY, Yu CJ et al (2008) Identification of collapsin response mediator protein-2 as a potential marker of colorectal carcinoma by comparative analysis of cancer cell secretomes. Proteomics 8:316–332
10. Dombkowski AA, Cukovic D, Novak RF (2006) Secretome analysis of microarray data reveals extracellular events associated with proliferative potential in a cell line model of breast disease. Cancer Lett 241:49–58
11. Paulitschke V, Kunstfeld R, Mohr T, Slany A, Micksche M, Drach J et al (2009) Entering a new era of rational biomarker discovery for early detection of melanoma metastases: secretome analysis of associated stroma cells. J Proteome Res 8:2501–2510
12. Cravatt BF, Simon GM, Yates JR III (2007) The biological impact of mass-spectrometry-based proteomics. Nature 450:991–1000

13. Kashyap MK, Harsha HC, Renuse S, Pawar H, Sahasrabuddhe NA, Kim MS et al (2010) SILAC-based quantitative proteomic approach to identify potential biomarkers from the esophageal squamous cell carcinoma secretome. Cancer Biol Ther 10:796–810
14. Xue H, Lu B, Lai M (2008) The cancer secretome: a reservoir of biomarkers. J Transl Med 6:52
15. Zhang W, Matrisian LM, Holmbeck K, Vick CC, Rosenthal EL (2006) Fibroblast-derived MT1-MMP promotes tumor progression in vitro and in vivo. BMC Cancer 6:52
16. Du XL, Hu H, Lin DC, Xia SH, Shen XM, Zhang Y et al (2007) Proteomic profiling of proteins dysregulated in Chinese esophageal squamous cell carcinoma. J Mol Med 85:863–875
17. Fu L, Qin YR, Xie D, Chow HY, Ngai SM, Kwong DL et al (2007) Identification of alpha-actinin 4 and 67 kDa laminin receptor as stage-specific markers in esophageal cancer via proteomic approaches. Cancer 110:2672–2681
18. Fujita Y, Nakanishi T, Hiramatsu M, Mabuchi H, Miyamoto Y, Miyamoto A et al (2006) Proteomics-based approach identifying autoantibody against peroxiredoxin VI as a novel serum marker in esophageal squamous cell carcinoma. Clin Cancer Res 12:6415–6420
19. Fujita Y, Nakanishi T, Miyamoto Y, Hiramatsu M, Mabuchi H, Miyamoto A et al (2008) Proteomics-based identification of autoantibody against heat shock protein 70 as a diagnostic marker in esophageal squamous cell carcinoma. Cancer Lett 263:280–290
20. Uemura N, Nakanishi Y, Kato H, Saito S, Nagino M, Hirohashi S et al (2009) Transglutaminase 3 as a prognostic biomarker in esophageal cancer revealed by proteomics. Int J Cancer 124:2106–2115
21. Zhou G, Li H, Gong Y, Zhao Y, Cheng J, Lee P, Zhao Y (2005) Proteomic analysis of global alteration of protein expression in squamous cell carcinoma of the esophagus. Proteomics 5:3814–3821
22. Breton J, Gage MC, Hay AW, Keen JN, Wild CP, Donnellan C et al (2008) Proteomic screening of a cell line model of esophageal carcinogenesis identifies cathepsin D and aldo-keto reductase 1C2 and 1B10 dysregulation in Barrett's esophagus and esophageal adenocarcinoma. J Proteome Res 7:1953–1962
23. Xu SY, Liu Z, Ma WJ, Sheyhidin I, Zheng ST, Lu XM (2009) New potential biomarkers in the diagnosis of esophageal squamous cell carcinoma. Biomarkers 14:340–346
24. Bauer KM, Lambert PA, Hummon AB (2012) Comparative label-free LC-MS/MS analysis of colorectal adenocarcinoma and metastatic cells treated with 5-fluorouracil. Proteomics 12:1928–1937
25. Islam F, Chaousis S, Wahab R, Gopalan V, Lam AK (2018) Protein interactions of FAM134B with EB1 and APC/beta-catenin in vitro in colon carcinoma. Mol Carcinog 57:1480–1491
26. Zhang LY, Ying WT, Mao YS, He HZ, Liu Y, Wang HX et al (2003) Loss of clusterin both in serum and tissue correlates with the tumorigenesis of esophageal squamous cell carcinoma via proteomics approaches. World J Gastroenterol 9:650–654
27. Qi Y, Chiu JF, Wang L, Kwong DL, He QY (2005) Comparative proteomic analysis of esophageal squamous cell carcinoma. Proteomics 5:2960–2971
28. Wang SJ, Zhang LW, Yu WF, Yu JK, Zheng S, Li YS et al (2007) Establishment of a diagnostic model of serum protein fingerprint pattern for esophageal cancer screening in high incidence area and its clinical value. Zhonghua Zhong Liu Za Zhi 29:441–443
29. Liu WL, Zhang G, Wang JY, Cao JY, Guo XZ, Xu LH et al (2008) Proteomics-based identification of autoantibody against CDC25B as a novel serum marker in esophageal squamous cell carcinoma. Biochem Biophys Res Commun 375:440–445
30. Shao CCS, Chen L, Cobos E, Wang J, Haab BB, Gao W (2009) Antibody microarray analysis of serum glycans in esophageal squamous cell carcinoma cases and controls. Proteomics Clin Appl 3:923–931
31. Chen JY, Xu L, Fang WM, Han JY, Wang K, Zhu KS (2017) Identification of PA28β as a potential novel biomarker in human esophageal squamous cell carcinoma. Tumour Biol 39:1010428317719780
32. Pawar H, Kashyap MK, Sahasrabuddhe NA, Renuse S, Harsha HC, Kumar P et al (2011) Quantitative tissue proteomics of esophageal squamous cell carcinoma for novel biomarker discovery. Cancer Biol Ther 12:510–522
33. Yazdian-Robati R, Ahmadi H, Riahi MM, Lari P, Aledavood SA, Rashedinia M et al (2017) Comparative proteome analysis of human esophageal cancer and adjacent normal tissues. Iran J Basic Med Sci 20:265–271
34. Zhao J, Fan YX, Yang Y, Liu DL, Wu K, Wen FB et al (2015) Identification of potential plasma biomarkers for esophageal squamous cell carcinoma by a proteomic method. Int J Clin Exp Pathol 8:1535–1544

Chapter 20

Immunoblotting in Detection of Tumor-Associated Antigens in Esophageal Squamous Cell Carcinoma

Farhadul Islam, Vinod Gopalan, and Alfred K. Lam

Abstract

Tumor-associated antigens (TAAs) can be used as cancer markers and as signposts of therapeutic targets since their inimitable expression in cancer or significant overexpression in esophageal squamous cell carcinoma (ESCC) correlates with the initiation and progression of the diseases. Immunoblotting, also known as Western blotting or protein blotting, is a core technique in cell and molecular biology to detect proteins and glycoproteins. The technique allows detection of TAAs from complex protein samples such as in serum, aspirate, or solid tumor homogenate. In the process, proteins are separated according to the molecular weight. They were visualized within a gel matrix and then transferred to a supporting membrane. Finally, they are probed for binding with corresponding antibodies and identified the target proteins. Herein, we describe the Western blots analysis to detect protein or glycoprotein in samples from patients with esophageal squamous cell carcinoma (ESCC) or cells derived from ESCC.

Key words Tumor-associated antigen, Immunoblots, Western blots, Protein blots, ESCC

1 Introduction

Proteins involve in the occurrence, initiation, transformation, and progression of cancer are known as tumor-associated antigens (TAAs). These proteins are either unique in cancer cells (they do not exist in normal tissues or cells) or can exist with significant overexpressed in cancer cells [1]. A large number of TAAs have been identified using proteomics or serological analysis of recombinant cDNA expression libraries in different cancers [1]. However, large percentages of these identified TAAs have no direct association with cancer [2, 3]. Therefore, it is critical to identify and validate the candidate TAAs as diagnostic and/or prognostic marker or therapeutic target. Interestingly, TAAs evoke an immune response and generated autoantibodies against them [2]. The immune response evoked by TAA (s) can be detected by immunoassays such as Western blotting or enzyme-linked immunoassay in samples from cancer patients and control, thereby identifying

Alfred K. Lam (ed.), *Esophageal Squamous Cell Carcinoma: Methods and Protocols*, Methods in Molecular Biology, vol. 2129, https://doi.org/10.1007/978-1-0716-0377-2_20,

candidate TAAs [4]. In addition, the TAAs present in complex biological or clinical samples such as serum, aspirate, or solid tumor homogenate, cell lysate can be detected with these immunoassays.

TAAs and anti-TAAs autoantibodies are closely associated with the prognosis and recurrence of cancer [5, 6]. Thus, they can be used as biomarker for cancer diagnosis or monitoring diseases progress and predicting prognosis of various cancer, including esophageal squamous cell carcinoma (ESCC) [2–6]. In ESCC, demonstration of proteins by ESCC is important in studying the pathogenesis as well as assessing the prognosis and therapeutic effects in patients with ESCC.

Western blots could be used to study the expression of oncoproteins and tumor suppressor proteins. For instance, it is used to study the expressions of proteins (vascular endothelial growth factor receptor 1 and 2 [VEGFR-1 and VEGF-2]) in ESCC [7] as well as expression of family with Sequence Similarity 134, Member B (FAM134B) protein in ESCC [8]. In ESCC, various proteins involving the AKT (protein kinase B) signaling pathway are important in the pathogenesis of ESCC. Yu and colleagues noted that DnaJ (Hsp40) homolog, subfamily B, member 6 (DNAJB6a) and the proteins in the AKT signaling pathway, as studied by Western blots, suggest DNAJB6 as potential marker for progression [9]. In addition, expression of nidogen-2 (NID2) protein by Western blots was used to study the suppressor effect of cancer metastases in ESCC [10]. NID2 suppresses the EGFR/Akt and integrin/FAK/PLCγ metastasis-related pathways in ESCC. Furthermore, Li and colleagues have demonstrated epithelial to mesenchymal transition (EMT) through E-cadherin and N-cadherin expressions and phosphorylated AKT proteins in ESCC [11].

microRNAs are important in the pathogenesis of ESCC. For instance, Gopalan and colleagues have studied the regulation of forkhead box O1 (FOXO1) tumor suppression protein in ESCC by miR-1288 [12]. In addition, miR-498 overexpression increased p21 protein, FOXO1, and Kruppel-like factor 6 (KLF6) in ESCC [13]. On therapeutic aspect, in the study of immunotherapy, Western blots are used to study the expression of programmed death-ligand 1 (PD-L1) protein induced by chemotherapy in ESCC [14].

In this chapter, we use FAM134B protein as example to show how Western blotting could use to detect protein in serum and cell ones from patients with ESCC. Fig. 3 illustrated the outline of the method (Fig. 3a) and FAM134B expression pattern in ESCC cell lines.

2 Materials

2.1 Western Blotting

The aim of this method is to detect TAAs in serum from patients with ESCC and ESCC cell line(s). The materials required for this method include:

1. Cell lysis buffer: 150 mM sodium chloride, 1.0% Nonidet-P40 (NP-40) or Triton X-100, 0.5% sodium deoxycholate, 0.1% SDS (sodium dodecyl sulfate), 50 mM Tris, pH 8.0.
2. Protease inhibitors: 1 mM phenylmethylsulfonyl fluoride (PMSF), 5 mM ethylenediaminetetraacetic acid (EDTA), 1 mM ethylene glycol tetraacetic acid (EGTA), and 5–10 mM sodium fluoride.
3. Cell scraper.
4. 1.5 mL tubes.
5. Ice.
6. Phosphate-buffered saline (PBS).
7. ESCC cell line and nonneoplastic esophageal epithelial cell line (as control).
8. MilliQ water.
9. Serum cleanup kit.
10. Bicinchoninic acid (BCA) protein assay kit.
11. 4–15% 2D polyacrylamide gel electrophoresis (PAGE) gel.
12. Gel electrophoresis system.
13. Loading buffer: 100 mM Tris–HCl (pH 6.8), 4% (w/v) SDS, 0.2% (w/v) bromophenol blue, 200 mM and 200 mM β-mercaptoethanol.
14. Protein solutions: Protein extracted from serum of patients with ESCC, normal individuals, and ESCC cell lines (*see* **Note 1**).
15. Coomassie brilliant blue dye.
16. Loading tips.
17. Protein standard ladder.
18. Polyvinylidene fluoride (PVDF) membrane.
19. Blotting buffer: 10 mM Tris–HCl (pH 8.0) and 1 mM EDTA (pH 8.0). Add milliQ water up to 1 L.
20. 10× TBS: 24.2 g Tris and 87.6 g NaCl. Make up to IL with milliQ water. Adjust pH to 7.6 by adding hydrochloric acid.
21. Wash buffer: Tris-buffered saline and Tween 20 (TBST) buffer. 125 mL 10× TBS in 1168 mL milliQ water and add 7.5 mL 20% Tween 20.

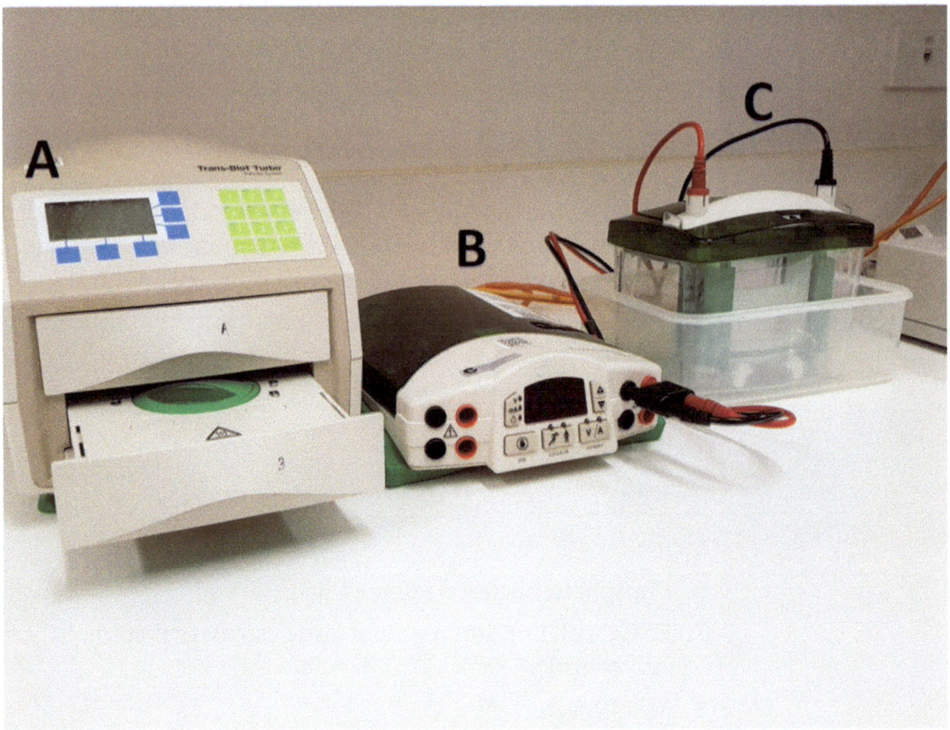

Fig. 1 An example of the setup for Western blotting. (**a**) Gel transfer system (transfer the separated protein samples from gel to membrane). (**b**) Power supply. (**c**) Gel electrophoresis tank (separate the mixture of protein according to the size and charge)

22. Blocking buffer: 5% (w/v) milk powder solution. 5 g milk powder and make it 100 mL with TBST.
23. Primary antibody (e.g., mouse anti-FAM134B antibody).
24. Secondary antibody: horseradish peroxidase conjugate (e.g., anti-mouse secondary antibody).
25. Loading control antibody (e.g., β-actin, GAPDH, lamin B1, etc.).
26. Western blotting signal detection reagents (e.g., enhanced chemiluminescence Western blotting substrate).
27. Power supply and gel transfer system (Fig. 1).
28. Image development and detection system (Fig. 2).
29. Image J software or other software as appropriate.

3 Methods

All the chemicals and reagents are of analytical grade, and prepare solutions using ultrapure water. First, this method required culture of ESCC and nonneoplastic esophageal epithelial cells (control) as

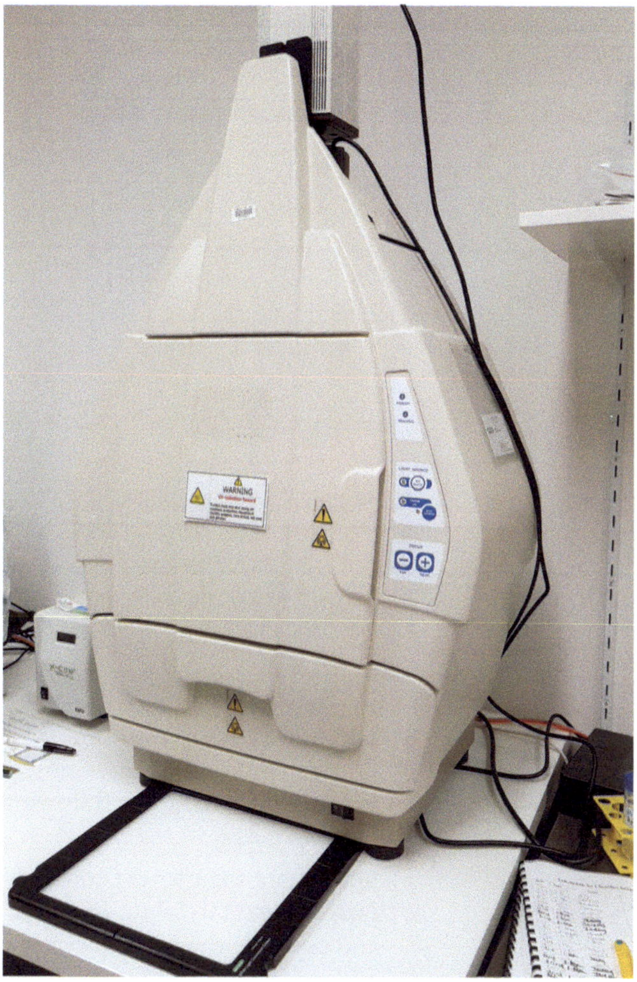

Fig. 2 Image development and detection system. The signal(s) or band of the samples of interest needs to be detected using the system followed by the appropriate enzyme substrate solution (e.g., ECL) on the blot

well as separation of serum from patients with ESCC and healthy donors (controls). Then, extract total proteins from cancer and control samples. The steps involved in this method are as below:

1. Grow the ESCC cells and nonneoplastic esophageal epithelial cells in appropriate medium up to 80% confluence.
2. Discard the media and wash the cells twice with ice-cold PBS.
3. Collect the cells in 1.5 mL tubes by scrapping using cell scraper on ice, and lyse using cell lysis buffer. For this, keep the cells on ice for 30 min and vortex for 15 s in every 5 min. Then collect the whole cell proteins followed by centrifugation at 14,000 × *g* for 15 min. Finally, add 1% protease inhibitors to the protein solution and keep on ice.

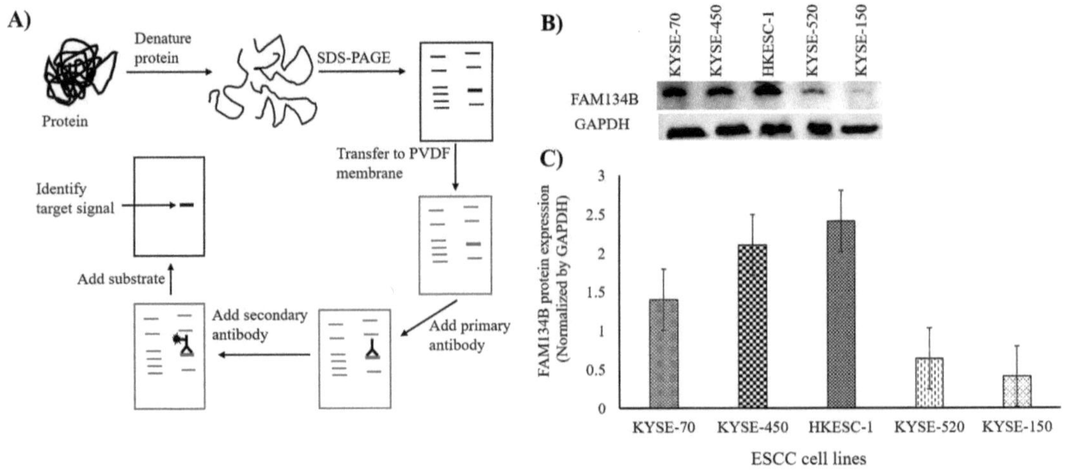

Fig. 3 Detection of protein using Western blotting. (**a**) Schematic of Western blot for detection of protein. (**b**) Protein bands of TAAs FAM134B in different ESCC cell lines (HKESC-1, KYSE-70, KYSE-150, KYSE-450, and KYSE-520). Differential expression of FAM134B was noted in different cell lines, which is implied by the protein bands intensities. GAPDH was used as loading or internal housekeeping control in this experiment. (**c**) Bar graph represented the protein band intensities of FAM134B in ESCC cells followed by GAPDH normalization

4. For serum samples from patients with ESCC and healthy donors, preclear the serum by removing IgG and albumin with serum cleanup kit following the manufacturer's guidelines (*see* **Note 2**).
5. Quantitate the protein concentrations by BCA kit or as appropriate. Take 10–50 μg of whole cell proteins in 1.5 mL tubes, and equalize the protein concentration of different samples by adding blotting buffer (*see* **Note 3**).
6. Mix the protein samples with loading buffer (*see* **Note 4**).
7. Boil the protein to denature them at 95–100 °C for 5 min, and cool them at room temperature for 5–10 min.
8. Load the proteins (10–50 μL), and ladder (2–5 μL), and separate the total proteins using 4–16% polyacrylamide gel at 100 V and 300 A in blotting buffer. Stop running the gel when proteins reach to the bottom line.
9. Transfer the proteins onto the polyvinylidene difluoride (PVDF) membrane using gel transfer system (e.g., Transblot, iBlot, iBlot 2, etc.) (*see* **Note 5**).
10. Check the protein transferred to the membrane by staining the blot with Coomassie brilliant blue dye for 10 min, and then destain completely by washing with distilled water.
11. Block the PVDF membrane using blocking buffer for 90 min at room temperature with gentle shaking (*see* **Note 6**).

12. Wash the blot with wash buffer for 5 min three times. Then add primary antibody (e.g., mouse anti-FAM134B antibody) diluted (1:100 to 1:1000) in wash buffer, and incubate for 2 h at room temperature or overnight at 4 °C with gentle shaking (*see* **Note 7**).
13. After the incubation, collect the primary antibody solution, and wash the membrane for 10 min trice with PBST with agitation.
14. Add secondary antibody diluted (1:500 to 1:5000) in wash buffer, and incubate at room temperature for 30–90 min at dark.
15. Then wash the membrane with gentle agitation as follows: 5 min three times in wash buffer, 5 min three times in PBST, and 5 min two times in PBS.
16. Finally, add appropriate enzyme substrate solution (e.g., ECL), and incubate as recommended (usually 2–5 min at dark) by the manufacturer to visualize protein bands/signals under the detection system.
17. Detect the protein bands/signals according to molecular size, and measure the band intensity by densitometry scanning using appropriate software (e.g., Image J 1.45 s, National Institute of Health, USA) (*see* **Note 8**).
18. Develop the blot again with loading control antibody (β-actin, GAPDH, lamin B1, etc.) diluted (1:200 to 1000) in wash buffer, and normalize the signals of protein of interest (Fig. 3).

4 Notes

1. Measure the protein concentration with BCA kit or by other methods as appropriate. At least 30 μg protein was from each group. Avoid too diluted protein solution to overflow the gel's well. Concentrate the proteins by freeze-drying or by the methods as appropriate if the concentration is very low. In case serum protein concentrations may be very high, need to dilute it to get good signal.
2. Strong background will appear if serum proteins improperly precleared. Difficulties will happen in detecting the signal of interest.
3. If the protein amount varies among the tested samples, the signal of the intended protein (s) will mislead. In addition, signal from loading control will be different. Therefore, normalization of the signal will be difficult.

4. When loading buffer content of hazardous chemicals such as bromophenol blue and β-mercaptoethanol, the fume hood should be used during preparation and applications.
5. For low-molecular-weight protein of interest, run the PAGE at lower voltage, e.g., 60 V for 20 min, and then increase the voltage to 100 for better separation.
6. Blocking conditions such as time, concentration of blocking buffer, room temperature, or 4 °C may need to be optimized. Following the instruction for troubleshooting of the antibody manufacturers could help to get good signal. Insufficient blocking can generate strong background, whereas excessive blocking minimizes the signal of interest.
7. The amount or concentration of antibody varies on source and clonality of the antibody. Generally, 1–10 μg/mL is acceptable, but need to check datasheets for precise recommendations of the supplier. Incubate time may need to be optimized to get good signal.
8. High-protein expression is correlated with a strong/thick band, and lower expression of proteins is represented as a thin/weak band.

References

1. Harao M, Mittendorf EA, Radvanyi LG (2015) Peptide-based vaccination and induction of CD8+ T-cell responses against tumor antigens in breast cancer. BioDrugs 29:15–30
2. Gao HJ, Yue ZG, Zheng M, Zheng ZX (2012) Identification and expression of a tumor-associated antigen in esophageal squamous cell carcinoma. Zhongguo Yi Xue Ke Xue Yuan Xue Bao 34:244–248
3. Lee SY, Jeoung D (2007) The reverse proteomics for identification of tumor antigens. J Microbiol Biotechnol 17:879–890
4. Fernandez MF, Tang N, Alansari H, Karvonen RL, Tomkiel JE (2005) Improved approach to identify cancer-associated autoantigens. Autoimmun Rev 4:230–235
5. Liu CC, Yang H, Zhang R, Zhao JJ, Hao DJ (2017) Tumour-associated antigens and their anti-cancer applications. Eur J Cancer Care 26: e12446
6. Zhang JY, Looi KS, Tan EM (2009) Identification of tumor-associated antigens as diagnostic and predictive biomarkers in cancer. Methods Mol Biol 520:1–10
7. Xu WW, Li B, Lam AK, Tsao SW, Law SY, Chan KW, Yuan QJ, Cheung AL (2015) Targeting VEGFR1- and VEGFR2-expressing non-tumor cells is essential for esophageal cancer therapy. Oncotarget 6:1790–1805
8. Islam F, Gopalan V, Law S, Tang JC, Lam AK (2019) FAM134B promotes esophageal squamous cell carcinoma in vitro and its correlations with clinicopathologic features. Hum Pathol 87:1–10
9. Yu VZ, Wong VC, Dai W, Ko JM, Lam AK, Chan KW, Samant RS, Lung HL, Shuen WH, Law S, Chan YP, Lee NP, Tong DK, Law TT, Lee VH, Lung ML (2015) Nuclear localization of DNAJB6 is associated with survival of patients with esophageal cancer and reduces akt signaling and proliferation of cancer cells. Gastroenterology 149:1825–1836.e5
10. Chai AW, Cheung AK, Dai W, Ko JM, Ip JC, Chan KW, Kwong DL, Ng WT, Lee AW, Ngan RK, Yau CC, Tung SY, Lee VH, Lam AK, Pillai S, Law S, Lung ML (2016) Metastasis-suppressing NID2, an epigenetically-silenced gene, in the pathogenesis of nasopharyngeal carcinoma and esophageal squamous cell carcinoma. Oncotarget 7:78859–78871
11. Li B, Xu WW, Lam AKY, Wang Y, Hu HF, Guan XY, Qin YR, Saremi N, Tsao SW, He QY, Cheung ALM (2017) Significance of PI3K/AKT signaling pathway in metastasis of esophageal squamous cell carcinoma and its

potential as a target for anti-metastasis therapy. Oncotarget 8:38755–38766

12. Gopalan V, Islam F, Pillai S, Tang JC, Tong DK, Law S, Chan KW, Lam AK (2016) Overexpression of microRNA-1288 in oesophageal squamous cell carcinoma. Exp Cell Res 348:146–154
13. Islam F, Gopalan V, Law S, Tang JC, Chan KW, Lam AK (2017) MiR-498 in esophageal squamous cell carcinoma: clinicopathological impacts and functional interactions. Hum Pathol 62:141–151
14. Ng HY, Li J, Tao L, Lam AK, Chan KW, Ko JMY, Yu VZ, Wong M, Li B, Lung ML (2018) Chemotherapeutic treatments increase PD-L1 expression in esophageal squamous cell carcinoma through EGFR/ERK activation. Transl Oncol 11:1323–1333

Chapter 21

Immunohistochemistry for Protein Detection in Esophageal Squamous Cell Carcinoma

Kais Kasem and Alfred K. Lam

Abstract

Immunohistochemistry is the identification of a cell protein by a specific antibody targeting that protein. It is the most common ancillary test to study the pathology of cancer. Immunohistochemical protein markers are used to differentiate poorly differentiated squamous cell carcinoma from poorly differentiated adenocarcinoma or neuroendocrine carcinomas. They could be used to identify and type the carcinoma in metastatic locations. Importantly, immunodetection of markers also helps in prediction of response to therapies as well as assessing the different biomarkers related to the pathogenesis and clinical behavior of esophageal squamous cell carcinoma. Successful application of the immunochemistry depends on understanding the mechanisms and principles as well as the limitations of the procedure. Automation of the procedure by different models of automatic stainers is widely used in diagnostic laboratories. The use of autostainers streamlines the workflows and certainly reduces the labor, time, and cost of using immunohistochemistry in clinical and research settings.

Key words Immunohistochemical, Immunohistochemistry, Esophagus, Squamous cell carcinoma, Autostainer

1 Introduction

1.1 Concept of Use of Immunohistochemistry

The basic mechanism of immunohistochemistry is to detect the target protein (antigen) in a tissue by an antibody. The success of the detection depends on applying the basic principles to enhance the specificity and sensitivity of the process. Immunohistochemistry is widely used in studying protein expression in cancer, including esophageal squamous cell carcinoma in pathological diagnostic works and in research.

Compared with other methods such as Western blots or mass spectrometric analysis of proteins (Chapters 19 and 20), immunohistochemistry allows the identification of the cellular and subcellular location of the proteins. This is a more objective method to

Kais Kasem and Alfred K. Lam contributed equally to this work.

Alfred K. Lam (ed.), *Esophageal Squamous Cell Carcinoma: Methods and Protocols*, Methods in Molecular Biology, vol. 2129,
https://doi.org/10.1007/978-1-0716-0377-2_21,

localize the tumor-related proteins as the proteins could be seen in the tumor cells in contrast to the adjacent nonneoplastic tissue or tumor stroma. The non-cancer cells could give more reliable results in other quantitative method, such as Western blots. The later method gives a thick band in gel (*see* Chapter 20) but not able to subcellular location of the protein. The most important advantage is immunohistochemistry works well on formalin-fixed paraffin-embedded tissue. Formalin-fixed paraffin-embedded tissue is the most common method to process the cancer tissue for clinical pathological management of patients with cancer.

The uses of immunohistochemical techniques vary significantly in methods, scope, and purpose depending on the specific use in clinical diagnostic or research applications. The variability between different manufacturers and commercial products is also considerable. Antibodies of clinical diagnostic use are under audit and have high sensitivity and specificity when compared with those used solely for research purposes.

Compared to decades before, the use of immunohistochemistry is a routine in diagnostic laboratories. With the maturing and improvement of techniques, immunohistochemistry is one of the most reliable tests in the diagnostic settings. In the recent decade, nearly all the clinical diagnostic laboratories adopt autostainer for immunohistochemistry. The automation provides streamline and standardized approach to do the staining as well as less labor-intensive than the manual approach. It is decided for diagnostic laboratories that handle a high volume of different immunohistochemical analyses daily. In research on large number of cases, automation is also recommended. This reduce the chance of manual errors such as missing of application of solutions or antibodies in some slides. In addition, the experimental conditions are more uniform by doing large number of slides in one run in autostainer rather than doing several runs of the experiments with small number of slides by manual approach.

1.2 Application of Immunohistochemistry in Esophageal Squamous Cell Carcinoma

It is often difficult to differentiate a poorly differentiated squamous cell carcinoma from other carcinomas in endoscopic biopsies (*see* Chapter 5) because of the limitation in size or representativeness of the samples. This situation also occurs in surgical specimen after neoadjuvant therapy as the residual carcinoma could be small and underwent morphological changes related to the preoperative chemoradiation (*see* Chapter 2). In addition, esophageal squamous cell carcinoma has extensive lymphatic permeation, often involves the lymph nodes, and could be seen in approximately 64% of patients with the tumor at the time of surgery [1]. Immunostains are sometimes needed to identify the presence of tiny metastases (positive to cytokeratin such as AE1/3) as well as the type of carcinoma (squamous cell carcinoma versus adenocarcinoma).

In the scenario of squamous cell carcinoma versus adenocarcinoma, a panel of antibodies could be employed. Squamous cell carcinoma is often positive for p40 and cytokeratin 5/6 (Fig. 1), whereas adenocarcinoma is positive for cytokeratin 7 on immunohistochemistry [2]. In rare circumstances, neuroendocrine carcinomas (large cell and small cell carcinoma) occur in the esophagus, and they can mimic poorly differentiated esophageal squamous cell carcinoma [3]. In contrast to squamous cell carcinoma, neuroendocrine carcinomas are positive for neuroendocrine markers such as chromogranin, synaptophysin, and CD56. Overall, immunodetection of these markers is important in confirming the diagnosis of poorly squamous cell carcinoma. It is important to use a panel of markers as sometimes a carcinoma may contain low level of antigens. A marker, chromogranin is specific for neuroendocrine tumor but of relatively low sensitivity.

Immunotherapy emerges to play important roles in treatment of increasing number of cancers especially in metastasizing carcinoma. Although it is not widely adopted as mainstream therapy for esophageal squamous cell carcinoma, clinical trials are ongoing for this cancer (*see* Chapter 24). It is important to test the presence of the relevant proteins by immunohistochemistry. In addition, a pathologist trained in the interpretation of the stain should score the positivity of PD-L1 protein in cancer cells as the positivity is related to the sensitivity of the therapy. It is worth noting the expression of PD-L1 in esophageal squamous cell carcinoma is affected by chemoradiation [4]. Nevertheless, the staining of PD-L1 protein is not optimal for interpretation as compared to other immunostains [5]. Recently, microsatellite instability high tumors are noted to be associated with better response to immunotherapy [6]. The microsatellites instabilities markers are easier to have high quality in routine diagnostic laboratories. The use of this markers needs to be validated.

In research on esophageal squamous cell carcinoma, thousands of studies were based on immunohistochemical detection of proteins. Tissue microarray technique and whole slide scanning allow a greater number of cases to be studied (*see* Chapters 9 and 10). Immunohistochemical studies are often used to confirm the involvement of genomic changes detected in ESCC at protein levels. Many of the studies use the protein expression detected by immunohistochemical method to study the correlations with clinical and pathological features and more importantly to predict cancer recurrence, survival, as well as response to drugs. Examples found in esophageal squamous cell carcinoma include the testing of different oncoproteins and their interactions (such as FAM134B, NID2, DNAJB6, CAPN10, Fas, p21, p53) [7–14], proliferative marker (Ki-67) [15, 16], and receptors (e.g., VEGFR1 and VEGFR2) [17].

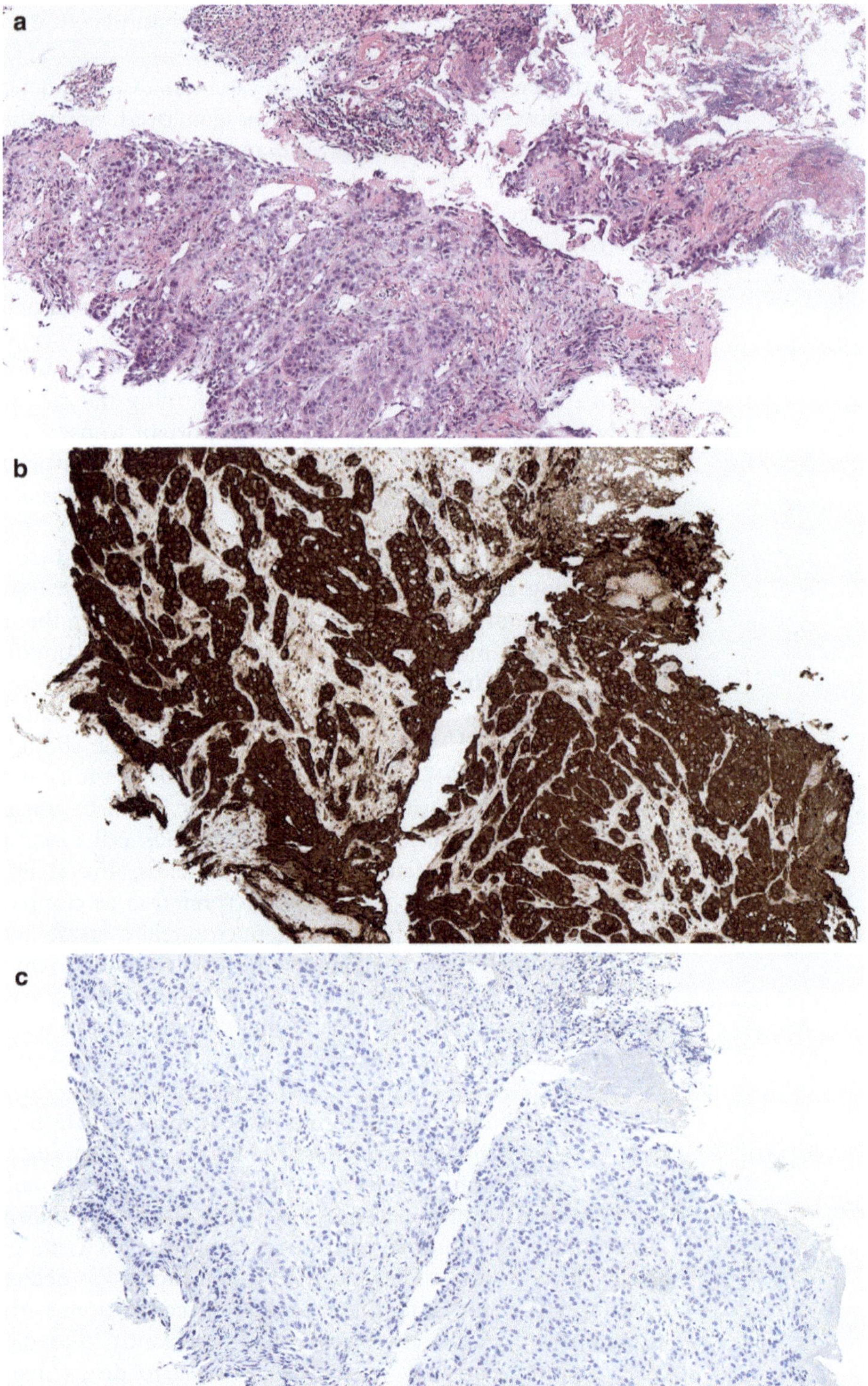

Fig. 1 Expression of markers in endoscopic biopsy of esophageal squamous cell carcinoma. (**a**) Squamous cell carcinoma (hematoxylin and eosin ×6). (**b**) Squamous cell carcinoma with positive staining (brown color) to CK5/6 (hematoxylin and eosin ×6). (**c**) Squamous cell carcinoma with negative staining (blue color) to CK7 (hematoxylin and eosin ×6)

1.3 Principles of Immunohistochemistry for Formalin-Fixed Paraffin-Embedded Tissue

The most commonly applied principles in immunohistochemistry for formalin-fixed paraffin-embedded tissue samples are as follows [18–20]:

1.3.1 Tissue Fixation

Samples first need to be fixed to preserve cellular integrity. This is usually achieved by putting the tissue into a paraformaldehyde or neutral buffered formalin overnight. This is followed by washing of the tissue in 1× phosphate-buffered saline (PBS).

1.3.2 Paraffin Embedding

Because paraffin is immiscible with water, tissue must be dehydrated before adding paraffin wax. This is achieved by immersion in increasing concentrations of alcohol. The gradual change in hydrophobicity minimizes cell damage. The tissue is then incubated with xylene to clear any remaining ethanol. Paraffin is typically heated for embedding and is subsequently allowed to harden.

1.3.3 Sectioning

The tissue is then cut with a sharp blade into ultrathin (up to 5 μm thickness) slices by a microtome. Sections are then dried onto coated microscope glass slides.

1.3.4 Dewaxing

As most staining solutions are aqueous, paraffin-embedded tissue first needs to be dewaxed to replace the wax with water. The slides are agitated in a dish containing dewaxing agent (xylene) and then moved through dishes containing decreasing concentration of ethanol. The slides are then rinsed in water to remove any remaining alcohol.

1.3.5 Antigen Retrieval

The purpose of antigen retrieval is to unmask antigens that have been obscured during the fixation process by forming hydrogen bonding in the antigens. The need for and conditions of antigen retrieval depend on multiple variables, including the target antigen, the antibody used, the type of tissue, and the method and duration of fixation. It is crucial to find the most suitable antigen retrieval method for the specific target. Two methods of antigen retrieval are available: heat-mediated (also known as heat-induced epitope retrieval or HIER) and enzymatic (protease-induced epitope retrieval or PIER). HIER, being the most common, is carried out by placing the slides in a pressure cooker containing an antigen retrieval buffer. The time and temperature vary depending on the specific target. The slides must be washed after the antigen retrieval process.

1.3.6 Blocking

The tissue sections then need to be blocked to minimize nonspecific interaction of the antibody and block endogenous enzymes that can result in false positives. This is usually done by applying blocking solutions, such as bovine serum albumin or peroxidase, directly to the tissue. The slides are then washed again at the end of this step.

1.3.7 Incubating with Antibody

The critical feature of a primary antibody is specificity for the epitope. To achieve a robust and specific signal, a high-quality antibody that exhibits minimal cross-reactivity should be employed. Primary antibody concentration, diluent, incubation time, and temperature all impact the quality of staining. These variables need to be optimized for each antibody and tissue types to achieve specific staining and low background. This step involves incubating the sections in antibodies, which can be directly conjugated primaries or more commonly sequential incubations in both primary and secondary antibodies (fluorescent or enzyme-linked) to increase the sensitivity of the reaction by amplification of signals. If an enzyme-linked secondary is used, a further incubation in substrate will be required. The antibody then needs to be washed off.

1.3.8 Detection

This step involves developing with chromogen, such as 3,3-diaminobenzidine (DAB) for 10 min at room temperature, following by rinsing the tissue in water. DAB causes a visible brown precipitate to form at the site of antigen-antibody binding in the subcellular sites. The slides are then counterstained, commonly with hematoxylin. The aim is to achieve a good balance between DAB reaction product (brown) and hematoxylin (blue). The tissue is then rinsed in water for the last time.

1.3.9 Mounting and Covering

The tissue is dehydrated by moving the slides through dishes containing increasing concentration of ethanol. The last step involves washing in xylene, followed by adding a mounting solution to the slide and gently lowering a coverslip over the tissue. The slides are ready to be examined and interpreted microscopically.

In this chapter, a description of immunohistochemical technique in clinical diagnostic practice using automated stainer and commercially available kits will be discussed. Most laboratories use automated stainer platform and commercially available kits, the majority of which utilize the basic principles of polymer-based immunohistochemistry (polymer with attached enzymes and secondary antibody).

2 Materials

2.1 Specimens

1. Fixation

   10% buffered formalin is most often used for fixation of tissue samples of squamous cell carcinoma (*see* **Note 1**). This is followed by embedding in paraffin.

2. Sectioning

   A microtome, tissue blocks, ice, water bath, coated adhesion slides, and slide rack are all used to produce the sections for staining.

   Chill paraffin-embedded tissue blocks on ice before sectioning, which allows thinner sections to be obtained. A water bath should be filled with water and heated to 40–45 °C. After placing the blade in the holder of the microtome, ensure it is secure and set the clearance angle (*see* **Note 2**). Coated glass slides and slide rack should be ready for the sections [21].

3. Control Tissue

   A section of the appropriate positive control tissues is placed on each test slide for staining. Multiple tissue control blocks are constructed. The appropriate control/s should be selected based on the antibody used (Fig. 2). The presence of controls is essential for accurate interpretation (*see* **Note 3**). An example of a multi-tissue control block contains several tissue

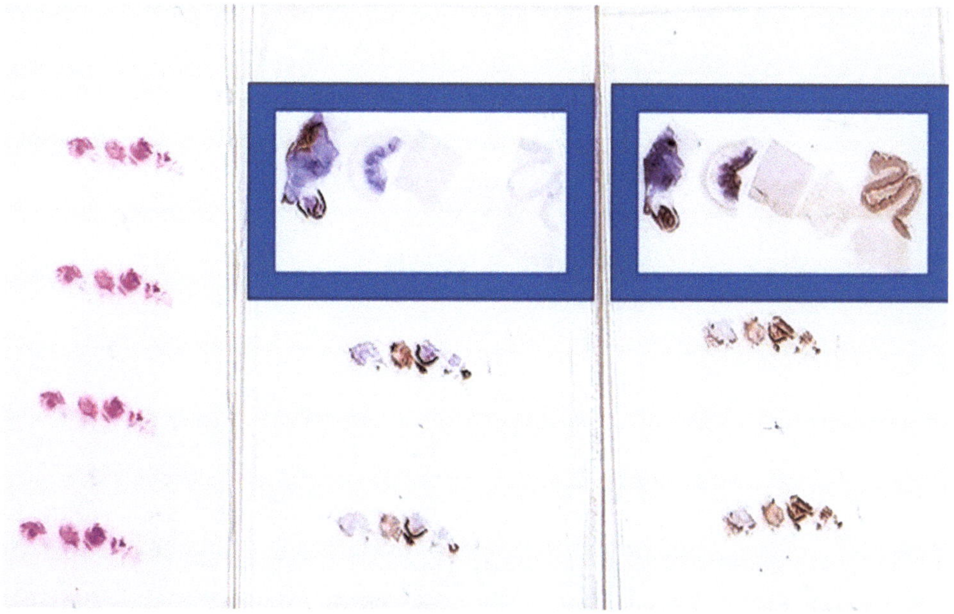

Fig. 2 The slide on the left side is a hematoxylin and eosin-stained slide of esophageal squamous cell carcinoma. The slides on the center and right are sections from the same tissue stained with different immunostains. Note the control tissues (blue boxes) and tested tissues (lower)

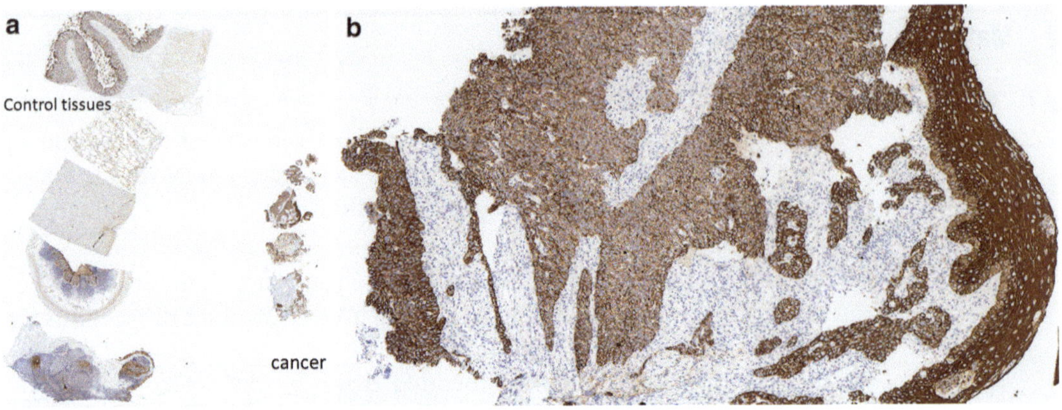

Fig. 3 Control tissues and esophageal squamous cell carcinoma. (**a**) Control tissues (from different organs) and esophageal squamous cell carcinoma (AE1/3 stain). (**b**) Higher magnification of the squamous cell carcinoma in (**a**) showing the positive staining (brown color)

samples, such as appendix, tonsil, liver, pancreas, and skin tissue (Fig. 3) [22]. These control tissues were obtained from selection of tissues sent for pathological examination that have underwent same fixation procedures as the tested tissues.

2.2 Reagents

1. Buffers

   The following commercially available buffers are used, both usually need to be diluted before use:

   (a) Wash buffer (stored in the refrigerator).

   (b) Target Retrieval Solution.

2. Solutions

   The following commercially available solutions are used:

   DAB (3,3-diaminobenzidine) Chromogen Kit (*see* **Note 4**).

   DAB substrate buffer and DAB chromogen (gently mixed and stored at 2–8 °C).

   Alkaline phosphatase kit.

   Distilled water.

   Ethanol.

   Xylene.

   Hematoxylin.

3. Antibodies

   Most of the antibodies used are prediluted, for those that do require dilution. In practice, a reference table is provided for ease of use (*see* **Note 5**).

2.3 Equipment

1. A typical automated stainer including racks, bulk solution bottles, and computer with accompanying software.
2. Pretreatment system (*see* **Note 6**).

3. Slide printer.
4. Wash station trough.
5. 20–200 μL pipette and tips.
6. Automatic coverslipper (optional).

3 Method

Firstly, treat slides with antigen retrieval steps to unmask antigenic sites. The masking is caused by cross-linking of disulfide bonds due to formalin fixation [23]. A peroxidase step is then employed to minimize any endogenous peroxidase activity. The primary antibody is applied and after appropriate incubation, a polymer with attached enzymes and secondary anti-mouse or anti-rabbit antibodies. Finally, the color reagents mostly give brown color, DAB (3,3-diaminobenzidine), or red color, AEC (3-amino-9-ethylcarbazole). The peroxidase enzyme will react with the DAB in the presence of hydrogen peroxide, reducing it to give a stable brown color, at the antigenic sites [24].

3.1 Preparing Tissue Sections

1. The tissue sections should be cut at 3–4 μm and mounted on coated adhesion slides (*see* **Note 7**).
2. A section of the correct control tissue should be also present on the test slide.
3. The sections should be allowed to heat in the hotbox for a minimum of 50 min.

3.2 Entering Case Identification Information

1. The identifications should be pre-entered in automatic stainer. After logging onto the computer and selecting the programming grid panel, slide information such as patient surname, case identification number, and slide number should be entered. The number of slides needed for each case should also be specified.
2. After all cases have been entered, the specific antibodies required for each case should be selected.
3. The entered information then is saved on the hard disk, and slide labels are printed.
4. Once the labels are generated, they should be applied to the appropriate slides.
5. The labeled slides should then be clipped into the slide racks, keeping the slides in numerical order.

3.3 Heat-Induced Epitope Retrieval

This step is carried out using a pretreatment system module (Fig. 4). This instrument is a programmable water bath that is used to perform antigen retrieval using a pretreatment solution (*see* **Note 8**). The programmed steps include preheating, dewaxing,

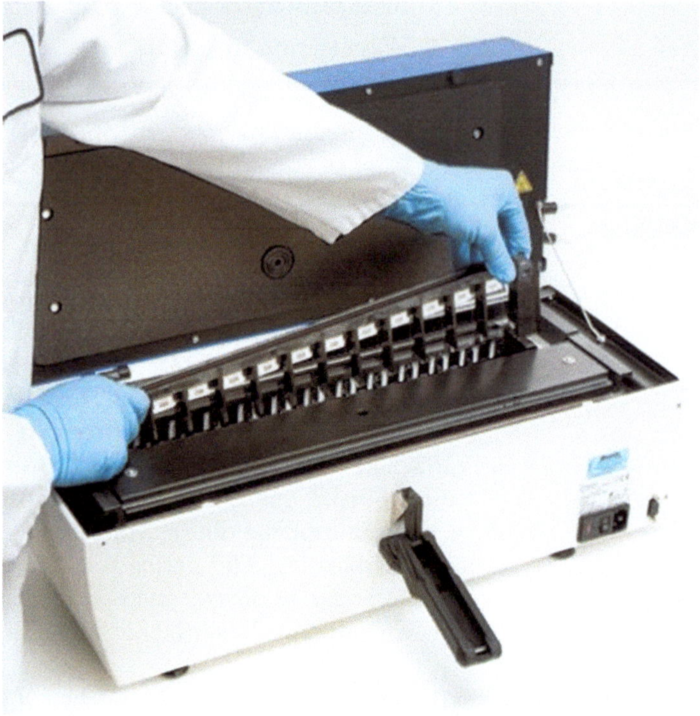

Fig. 4 An example of pretreatment system for antigen retrieval

antigen retrieval temperatures, and cooling down. Antigen retrieval steps are carried out at 95 °C for 15 min. These parameters can be modified through the equipment main menu.

After the cooling down phase is complete, the pretreatment module will alarm. At this point, the lid of the wash station trough containing wash buffer and the lid of the pretreatment module should be removed without delay. The rack of slides in the pretreatment module should be rapidly removed and quickly plunged into the wash buffer. The slides should stay in the buffer for at least 10 min and may stay there overnight if that suites the workflow requirements.

3.4 Setting up the Antibodies

After the slides have been placed in the pretreatment module, the antibody tubes should be placed in the racks of the automatic stainer by following the map generated after setting up of the slides has been completed (Figs. 5 and 6). All the volumes of the antibodies need to be correct, and DAB chromogen needs to be added to the DAB substrate (*see* **Note 9**).

3.5 Starting a Run

The slide racks should be removed from the wash buffer and placed in the automatic stainer, ensuring placing them in the right location based on the generated grid (Fig. 7). In the software provided,

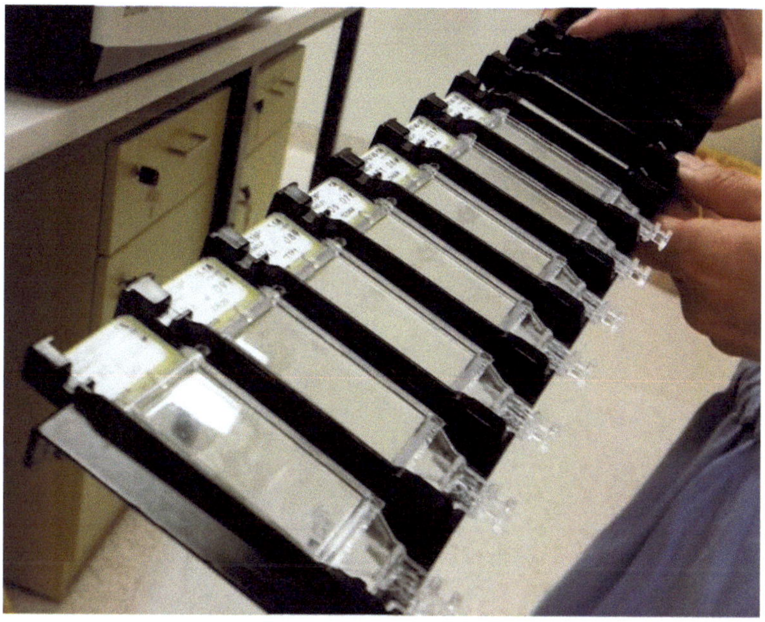

Fig. 5 Slides arranged in a rack ready to be inserted into an automated stainer

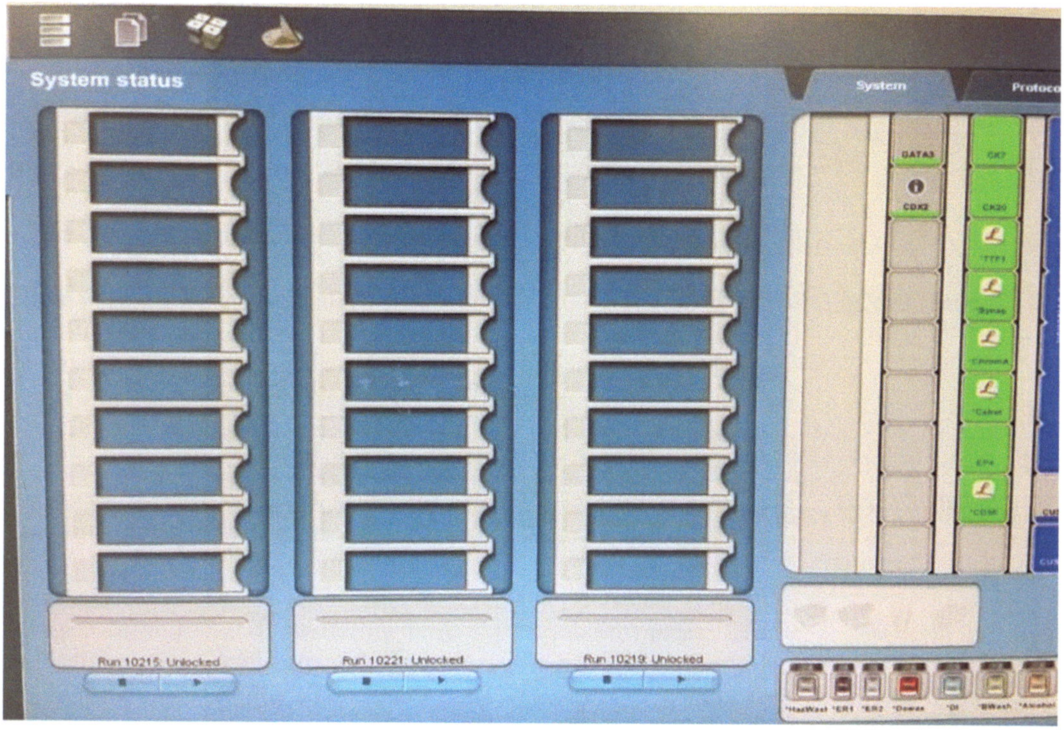

Fig. 6 Automated stainer software interface, allowing selection of antibodies and arrangement of slides in the racks

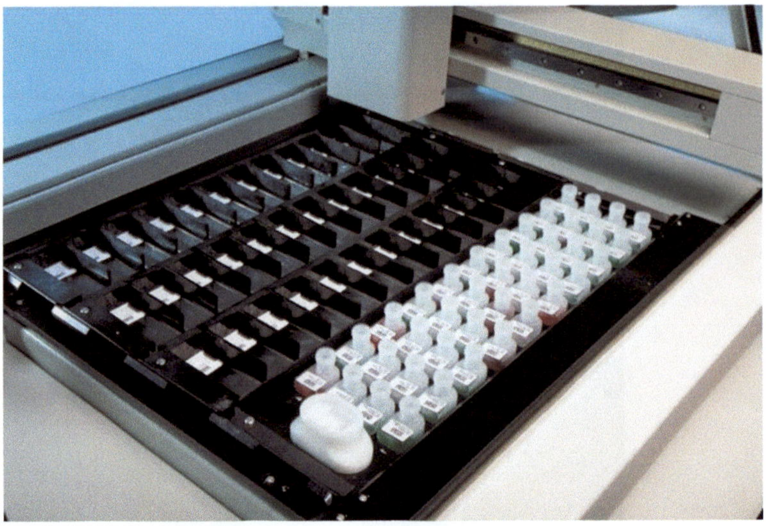

Fig. 7 An example of an automated stainer with reagents, multiple antibodies (left lower), and three roles of slides in their allocated slots (right upper) is demonstrated here. The white bottle in lower part next to the reagents and antibodies is buffer

follow the prompts to start the run and scanning the slides. The pump needs to be primed with deionized water if it is the first run of the day (*see* **Note 10**).

3.6 Completing a Run

On completion of a program, the stainer will alarm. Once the run is complete, wash buffer should be applied on them. The slides are then should be removed from the rack and then washed in running tap water for 3 min.

3.7 Counterstaining

The program for counterstaining with hematoxylin stain should then be performed on the slide stainer. The combination of DAB with hematoxylin is used to stain nuclei. After immunochemical staining, mounting media are used to adhere a coverslip to a tissue section (*see* **Note 11**).

3.8 Staining Results

Typical staining results for this method are a positive reaction when the tissue is stained brown with DAB or red with AEC, while the nuclei with a negative reaction are stained blue.

3.9 DAB Disposal

DAB should be appropriately disposed of. The common disposal method is for DAB to be diluted 100x and flushed down the sink with constant running water. A list of all the hazardous substances, their risk assessment, and the control measures are provided in Table 1.

Table 1
Hazardous substances and risk assessment

Agent/ procedure	Associated hazard	Control measures
Xylene	Moderately flammable liquid which is a mild eye and mucous membrane irritant. It is a primary skin irritant and a central nervous system depressant. It will defat skin and may cause dermatitis. Overexposure has led to death from respiratory failure	Avoid contact with skin and eyes. Use in fume hood as appropriate to volume handled
Absolute ethanol	Flammable liquid and should never be handled close to heat or naked flame. The vapor is heavier than air and can travel for a considerable distance along the ground to a source of ignition and flashback. Ethanol is regarded as one of the safest industrial solvents because although it possesses narcotic properties, vapor concentrations enough to produce narcosis are rarely, if ever, reached in a medical laboratory. Ethanol is rapidly oxidized in the body to carbon dioxide and water and does not produce permanent damage to the central nervous system	*Flammable*. Avoid contact with skin. Keep away from ignition sources
Hematoxylin	The toxic properties of this compound have not been thoroughly investigated. Possibly toxic via oral inhalation or absorption	Wear gloves, mask, eyewear, and gown when handling dry powder
3,3-Diamino benzidine (DAB)	Harmful by inhalation, in contact with skin, and if swallowed. Irritating to eyes, respiratory system, and skin	*Possible Carcinogen*. Wear gloves, gown, and eye protection. Do not breathe in dust. Use in a fume hood

4 Notes

1. Fixation in formalin immobilizes antigens while retaining cellular and subcellular structure. Buffered formalin is excellent at preserving cell structure but may somewhat reduce the antigenicity of some cell components as the cross-linking can obstruct antibody binding. The ideal fixation time depends on the size of the tissue block and the type of tissue, but generally fixation between 18 and 24 h is suitable for most applications. Underfixation can result in edge staining, with strong signal on the edges of the section and no signal in the middle portion of tissue. Overfixation, on the other hand, can mask the epitope, in which case additional antigen retrieval techniques may be

required to help overcome this masking. If the tissue, however, has been fixed for a prolonged period (i.e., over a weekend), there may be no signal detected even after antigen retrieval [25].

2. Setting the clearance angle properly prevents contact between the knife facet and the face of the block, which is set following the manufacturer's instructions. Insert the paraffin block, and orientate it so that the blade will cut straight across the block. Then carefully approach the block with the blade, and cut a few thin sections to ensure the positioning is correct. Adjust the block orientation if necessary. Trim the block to expose the tissue surface to a level where a representative section can be cut, which is normally done at a thickness of 10–30 μm. The sections should be cut at a thickness of about 3–4 μm. Using tweezers, pick up the ribbons of sections, float them on the surface of the water in the hot water bath, and ensure they are flattened out. Pick the sections out of the water bath using microscope slides, and store upright in a slide rack ready for immunohistochemical analysis.
3. An immunohistochemical assay that lacks controls cannot be validly interpreted. The absence of a positive and negative controls that work as expected can lead to erroneous scientific conclusions and clinical misdiagnoses.
4. Chromogenic detection methods often use a conjugated enzyme to visualize epitope-antibody interactions. When using this method of detection, the endogenous activity of the same enzyme must be blocked. Protocols that include alkaline phosphatase often require reagents to prevent nonspecific signals. Alkaline phosphatase, usually isolated from calf intestine, is an enzyme that catalyzes the hydrolysis of phosphate groups from a substrate molecule, resulting in a colored product or the release of light as one product of the reaction.
5. Primary antibody concentration, incubation time, diluent, and temperature all impact the quality of staining. All these variables need to be optimized for each antibody and sample to achieve specific staining and low background signal. Optimization is commonly done by maintaining a constant incubation time and temperature while varying the antibody concentration in order to determine when an optimal signal is achieved with low background noise.
6. Pretreatment systems allow the entire pretreatment process of deparaffinization, rehydration, and epitope retrieval to be combined into a well-documented, 3-in-1 specimen preparation procedure. Preheat mode holds the buffer solution at a user-selectable temperature. To perform epitope retrieval, the desired parameters for time and temperature need to be set, and the run can then begin.

7. Coated adhesion slides are preferred. There are electrostatically charged adhesion slides with excellent adhesive properties and are highly reliable in instrument-based applications.
8. The pretreatment solution can be used for a certain number of slides, after which the solution needs to be discarded and a fresh pretreatment solution be used.
9. Some antibodies must be purchased as a concentrate due to either supplier restrictions or cost. These then need to be diluted into a specific concentration for optimal. Each antibody will need a "workup" to identify the optimal concentration for staining before it is placed into routine use.
10. It is important to check all buffer and deionized water volumes are adequate and the waste drums have enough free volume before starting a run.
11. It is important to ensure the dehydrating alcohols are clean and free of any eosin from previous runs.

References

1. Lam KY, Ma LT, Wong J (1996) Measurement of extent of spread of oesophageal squamous carcinoma by serial sectioning. J Clin Pathol 49:124–129
2. Lam AK, Kumarasinghe MP (2019) Adenocarcinoma of the oesophagus and oesophagogastric junction NOS. In: Odze RD, Lam AK, Ochiai A, Washington MK (eds) WHO classification of tumours, 5th edn, pp 38–43, Chapter 2
3. Lam KY, Law S, Tung PH, Wong J (2000) Esophageal small cell carcinomas: clinicopathologic parameters, p53 overexpression, proliferation marker, and their impact on pathogenesis. Arch Pathol Lab Med 124:228–233
4. Ng HY, Li J, Tao L, Lam AK, Chan KW, Ko JM, Yu VZ, Wong M, Li B, Lung ML (2018) Chemotherapeutic treatments increase PD-L1 expression in esophageal squamous cell carcinoma through EGFR/ERK activation. Transl Oncol 11:1323–1333
5. Patel SP, Kurzrock R (2015) PD-L1 expression as a predictive biomarker in cancer immunotherapy. Mol Cancer Ther 14:847–856
6. Nebot-Bral L, Coutzac C, Kannouche PL, Chaput N (2019) Why is immunotherapy effective (or not) in patients with MSI/MMRD tumors? Bull Cancer 106:105–113
7. Islam F, Gopalan V, Law S, Tang JC, Lam AK (2019) FAM134B promotes esophageal squamous cell carcinoma in vitro and its correlations with clinicopathologic features. Hum Pathol 87:1–10
8. Chai AW, Cheung AK, Dai W, Ko JM, Ip JC, Chan KW, Kwong DL, Ng WT, Lee AW, Ngan RK, Yau CC, Tung SY, Lee VH, Lam AK, Pillai S, Law S, Lung ML (2016) Metastasis-suppressing NID2, an epigenetically-silenced gene, in the pathogenesis of nasopharyngeal carcinoma and esophageal squamous cell carcinoma. Oncotarget 7:78859–78871
9. Yu VZ, Wong VC, Dai W, Ko JM, Lam AK, Chan KW, Samant RS, Lung HL, Shuen WH, Law S, Chan YP, Lee NP, Tong DK, Law TT, Lee VH, Lung ML (2015) Nuclear localization of DNAJB6 is associated with survival of patients with esophageal cancer and reduces AKT signaling and proliferation of cancer cells. Gastroenterology 149:1825–1836
10. Chan D, Tsoi MY, Liu CD, Chan SH, Law SY, Chan KW, Chan YP, Gopalan V, Lam AK, Tang JC (2013) Oncogene GAEC1 regulates CAPN10 expression which predicts survival in esophageal squamous cell carcinoma. World J Gastroenterol 19:2772–2780
11. Chan KW, Lee PY, Lam AK, Law S, Wong J, Srivastava G (2006) Clinical relevance of Fas expression in oesophageal squamous cell carcinoma. J Clin Pathol 59:101–104
12. Lam KY, Law S, Tin L, Tung PH, Wong J (1999) The clinicopathological significance of p21 and p53 expression in esophageal squamous cell carcinoma: an analysis of 153 patients. Am J Gastroenterol 94:2060–2068
13. Lam KY, L oke SL, Chen WZ, Cheung KN, Ma L (1995) Expression of p53 in oesophageal

squamous cell carcinoma in Hong Kong Chinese. Eur J Surg Oncol 21:242–247
14. Lam KY, Law S, Ma LT, Ong SK, Wong J (1997) Pre-operative chemotherapy for squamous cell carcinoma of the oesophagus: do histological assessment and p53 overexpression predict chemo-responsiveness? Eur J Cancer 33:1221–1225
15. Law AK, Lam KY, Lam FK, Wong TK, Poon JL, Chan FH (2003) Image analysis system for assessment of immunohistochemically stained proliferative marker (MIB-1) in oesophageal squamous cell carcinoma. Comput Methods Prog Biomed 70:37–45
16. Lam KY, Law SY, So MK, Fok M, Ma LT, Wong J (1996) Prognostic implication of proliferative markers MIB-1 and PC10 in esophageal squamous cell carcinoma. Cancer 77:7–13
17. Xu WW, Li B, Lam AK, Tsao SW, Law SY, Chan KW, Yuan QJ, Cheung AL (2015) Targeting VEGFR1- and VEGFR2-expressing non-tumor cells is essential for esophageal cancer therapy. Oncotarget 6:1790–1805
18. Ramos-Vara JA (2011) Principles and methods of immunohistochemistry. In: Drug safety evaluation. Humana Press, Totowa, New Jersey, pp 83–96
19. Kabiraj A, Gupta J, Khaitan T, Bhattacharya PT (2015) Principle and techniques of immunohistochemistry—a review. Int J Biol Med Res 6:5204–5210
20. Renshaw S (2006) Immunohistochemistry: methods express. Royal College of general practitioners. Scion Publishing, Banbury
21. Abcam. Sectioning of paraffin embedded tissues. https://docs.abcam.com/pdf/protocols/sectioning-of-paraffin-embedded-tissue.pdf
22. Hewitt SM, Baskin DG, Frevert CW, Stahl WL, Rosa-Molinar E (2014) Controls for immunohistochemistry: the Histochemical Society's standards of practice for validation of immunohistochemical assays. J Histochem Cytochem 62:693–697
23. Scalia CR, Boi G, Bolognesi MM, Riva L, Manzoni M, DeSmedt L, Bosisio FM, Ronchi S, Leone BE, Cattoretti G (2017) Antigen masking during fixation and embedding, dissected. J Histochem Cytochem 65:5–20
24. ThermoFisher Scientific, IHC Immunodetection (staining). https://www.thermofisher.com/au/en/home/life-science/protein-biology/protein-biology-learning-center/protein-biology-resource-library/pierce-protein-methods/ihc-immunodetection.html
25. Webster JD, Miller MA, DuSold D, Ramos-Vara J (2009) Effects of prolonged formalin fixation on diagnostic immunohistochemistry in domestic animals. J Histochem Cytochem 57:753–761

Chapter 22

Radiotherapy for Cervical Esophageal Squamous Cell Carcinoma

Dora L. W. Kwong, Wendy W. L. Chan, and Ka On Lam

Abstract

Cervical esophageal carcinoma (CEC) is rare, accounting for 2–10% of esophageal cancers and is mostly squamous cell carcinoma. Because of the anatomical proximity of CEC to larynx, surgical treatment would involve pharyngo-laryngo-esophagectomy (PLE) with inherent high mortality and morbidity. Laryngeal preservation is an important consideration, and definitive chemoradiotherapy is the recommended treatment. Treatment strategy of CEC can be more akin to treatment for head and neck cancers than to thoracic esophageal cancers. Since the exact location, extent of primary and nodal metastasis varies between patients, radiotherapy treatment needs to be individualized. The optimal radiation dose for CEC is uncertain, but retrospective data suggests that higher radiation dose of at least 60 Gy is associated with better local control and survival. Advanced radiotherapy technique, like intensity modulated radiotherapy, is usually required to achieve high dose to tumor while protecting normal tissues from excessive radiation.

Key words Cervical esophageal cancer, Laryngeal preservation, Chemoradiotherapy, Intensity modulated radiotherapy

1 Introduction

The cervical esophagus is the short segment of esophagus that lies in the neck. It starts immediately distal to hypopharynx, approximately 18 cm from incisor, and extends from cricopharynx to the thoracic inlet. Anatomically, the superior border starts at the lower border of the cricoid cartilage and inferior border lies at the level of the sternal notch. Anterior to the cervical esophagus is the airway which proximally is the larynx that lies directly anterior to the hypopharynx and the trachea distal to larynx. Ninety-five percent of cervical esophageal cancer (CEC) is squamous cell carcinoma and accounts for <5% of all esophageal cancers [1].

CEC can extend superiorly to involve hypopharynx and inferiorly to thoracic esophagus. In locally advanced disease, there can be infiltration to nearby anatomical structures like the cricoid, thyroid cartilage, or thyroid gland. Lymph node metastases are also

Alfred K. Lam (ed.), *Esophageal Squamous Cell Carcinoma: Methods and Protocols*, Methods in Molecular Biology, vol. 2129, https://doi.org/10.1007/978-1-0716-0377-2_22,

common, especially lymph nodes in supraclavicular fossa. Since smoking and alcohol are common etiological factors for head and neck cancers and esophageal cancers, synchronous tumors are not uncommon. As CEC lies near larynx or may extend to hypopharynx, conventional surgical treatment would involve PLE, with significant mortality and morbidity [2]. Thus, organ preservation is important consideration besides cancer control. Chemoradiotherapy is established treatment for laryngeal preservation in treatment of laryngeal and hypopharyngeal carcinoma, and similar strategy is applied in treatment of CEC. Depending on the exact location, size, and extent of tumor, the treatment of CEC can be more akin to treatment of head and neck cancers than for thoracic and distal esophageal cancers.

The optimal management of CEC has not been established [3]. There is no randomized trial comparing surgery to organ preserving approach like chemoradiotherapy or radiotherapy. In a single center retrospective review, Cao et al. compared treatment outcomes after primary radiotherapy (alone or with concurrent chemotherapy, $n = 161$) and primary surgery ($n = 63$) in CEC. There was no significant difference in 2-year local control (69.9% and 69.8%), regional control (79.5% and 69.8%), distant metastases free survival (74.3% and 62.5%), or overall survival rates (49.3% and 50.7%), respectively, between the two treatment groups [4]. In view of the similarities in outcomes, the authors recommended primary radiotherapy for larynx preservation, with surgery offered subsequently for patients who do not respond to radiotherapy.

International guidelines including National Comprehensive Cancer Network (NCCN: www.nccn.org) and European Society for Medical Oncology (ESMO: www.ESMO.org) also recommend definitive chemoradiotherapy as the standard treatment. However, since most reported results on radiotherapy or chemoradiotherapy for CEC are from retrospective single-institutional and population-level series, the optimal choice of chemotherapy, dose of radiation, and sequence of combination of chemotherapy and radiotherapy are uncertain. Thus, results from large randomized head and neck cancers trials on laryngeal preservation are often used as reference in treatment of CEC.

2 Materials

2.1 Definitive Chemoradiotherapy

The RTOG 85-01 study is a randomized, phase 3 trial comparing definitive chemoradiotherapy with radiotherapy alone for the treatment of thoracic esophageal cancer [5, 6]. The chemoradiotherapy arm received 50 Gy in 25 fractions with 2 cycles of cisplatin and 5 fluorouracil (5FU) concurrent with radiotherapy and 2 more cycles after completing radiotherapy (*see* **Note 1a**). The radiotherapy alone arm received 64 Gy in 32 fractions. A total of 129 patients were enrolled in the randomized trial, and the trial was stopped early since early results showed benefit of chemoradiotherapy over radiotherapy alone. A long-term follow-up report included another 73 patients prospectively recruited after completion of the randomized trial and treated with chemoradiotherapy alone. Among 107 patients with squamous cell carcinoma, the 5-year overall survival with chemoradiotherapy was 21% compared with 0% in patients treated with radiotherapy alone. Although this study did not include patients with CEC, results from this study formed the basis for definitive chemoradiotherapy as non-surgical treatment for esophageal cancers.

The optimal radiation dose required for treatment of CEC is less certain. Using the same combined chemotherapy approach as in RTOG 85-01 study, the RTOG 94-05/INT 0123 trial tested if dose escalation from 50.4 Gy to 64.8 Gy improves local control or survival. The higher dose conferred no significant advantage [6].

As CECs grow aggressively in an area of abundant lymphatic drainage and frequently extend toward the hypopharynx, these tumors are sometimes treated with schedules as for locally advanced head and neck squamous cell carcinoma. For hypopharyngeal squamous cell carcinoma or other locally advanced head and neck cancers, the standard radiotherapy dose is 70 Gy in 35 fractions to primary tumor and involved nodes with concurrent cisplatin 100 mg/m^2 on day 1, 22, and 43 of radiotherapy (*see* **Note 1b**). Similar approach has been used in treatment of CEC [7]. With advancement in radiotherapy technique, high radiation dose to tumor is achievable, and since definitive chemoradiotherapy is often the only sole curative treatment option, CEC are often treated to a higher dose up to 60–70 Gy [8]. To increase radiation to tumor to above 60 Gy, conformal radiotherapy like intensity modulated radiotherapy is often necessary. The advantage of higher dose of radiation is supported by retrospective data which showed that radiation dose of 60 Gy or more with concurrent chemotherapy improved loco-regional control with no significant increase in late toxicities including swallowing dysfunction, esophageal stenosis, or tracheal-esophageal fistula [9, 10]. Although effective, this high dose may not be well tolerated especially for long esophageal irradiation. Reduced field to boost gross disease after 50 Gy should be considered.

Table 1 summarizes results of contemporary reported series using definitive chemoradiotherapy for CEC [10–19]. With modern radiotherapy, the 3 years loco-regional control rates ranged from 35.3% to 70.4% and overall survival ranged from 39.3% to 58.4%, with a tendency of better outcome with higher radiation dose and use of intensity modulated radiotherapy.

Most regimes include concurrent chemotherapy during radiotherapy. The most commonly used chemotherapeutic agents include platinum group like cisplatin, nedaplatin, or oxaliplatin.

Table 1
Contemporary series on outcome with definitive chemoradiotherapy with high dose radiation (≥60 Gy)

Authors/ref. number	Year	Patient number	RT dose	CT	Locoregional control/ PFS (%)	Overall survival (%)
Zhang [11]	2015	102	50–70 Gy	P+D/F	35.3 (3 year LRC)	39.3
Cao [12]	2016	64	60–70 Gy	P	74.5 (2 year LC)	42.5
McDowell [13]	2017	Ph1: 21 Ph2: 23 Ph3: 37	54 Gy ≥60 Gy ≥60 Gy	F+P/M P P	43 (2 year LRC) 57 (2 year LRC) 68 (2 year LRC)	33 43 53
Li [14]	2017	92	60 Gy	D+N/S1 +N	42.1 (3 year PFS)	49.8
Zhao [15]	2017	86	50–70 Gy	F+P/C/ S1	57.9 (3 year LRC)	53.6
Kumabe [16]	2017	37	60–70 Gy	PF	19.9 (10 year PFS) 30.2 (10 year LFS)	35.6
Ito [17]	2017	80	60–70 Gy	PF	60.6 (3 year LRC) 37 (3 year PFS)	66.6
Kim [10]	2018	35 44	<59.4 Gy ≥59.4 Gy	P+S1/ F/P	45.3 (3 year LRC) 70.4 (3 year LRC)	49.1 58.4
Okamoto [18]	2018	11	60–70 Gy	DPF	64 (2 year PFS)	72
Sakanaka [19]	2018	30	60 Gy (median)	F+P/N	43.7 (5 year LRC)	48.3

RT radiotherapy, *Ph* phase, *CT* chemotherapy, *P* cisplatin, *F* 5-fluorouracil, *M* mitomycin, *N* nedaplatin, *S1* TS1, *D* docetaxel, *C* capecitabine, *LRC* locoregional control, *PFS* progression free survival, *LFS* laryngectomy free survival

Fluoropyrimidine like 5-fluorouracil infusion or oral capecitabine or TS1 (Tegafur/gimeracil/oteracil) and taxane like docetaxel or paclitaxel may be used alone or in combination with platinum agents.

2.2 Chemoselection

Chemoselection is a treatment approach that promotes laryngeal preservation in laryngeal cancer cases [20]. Neoadjuvant or induction chemotherapy is used for selecting patients for definitive chemoradiotherapy for laryngeal preservation in locally advanced head and neck squamous cell carcinoma. It has been shown that response to neoadjuvant chemotherapy predicts for increased chance of laryngectomy free survival after radiotherapy. Chemoselection is a strategy that involves assigning the appropriate radical treatment according to the primary tumor's response to neoadjuvant chemotherapy. Surgery is performed for poor responders to neoadjuvant chemotherapy, while radiotherapy is performed on good responders to neoadjuvant chemotherapy. Similar approach has been tried in CEC.

Suzuki et al. reported 20 patients with CEC treated with concurrent chemoradiotherapy [21]. Fourteen of the patients also received multiagent neoadjuvant chemotherapy before radiotherapy. Response to neoadjuvant chemotherapy (complete or partial response) was found to be the only significant factor predicting better progression free survival. According to response to neoadjuvant chemotherapy, ten good responders (complete or partial response) showed 2-year survival rate of 80%, whereas that for poor responders (stable and progressive disease) was 0% ($p = 0.006$). In another retrospective study, Nakata et al. compared chemoselection ($n = 32$) and definitive radiotherapy ($n = 10$) in patients with CEC [22]. The 2-year loco-regional control rates for the chemoselection and primary radiotherapy groups were 68% and 25%, respectively ($p = 0.045$) and the overall survival was 65.1% and 40%, respectively ($p = 0.017$). The authors concluded that chemoselection achieved favorable results and can be applied as a treatment strategy for CEC.

Neoadjuvant chemotherapy usually involves combination chemotherapy that includes platinum and fluoropyrimidine combination or with addition of taxane [23] (*see* **Note 2**). Response evaluation was performed after 2–3 cycles of chemotherapy, and >30% decrease in endoscopic or CT-determined major primary tumor axis is considered as good response.

2.3 Salvage Pharyngolaryngectomy with Total Esophagectomy Following Definitive Chemoradiotherapy

For cases who failed to achieve complete remission or have locoregional recurrence after high-dose definitive chemoradiotherapy, salvage surgery may still be an option. However, salvage surgery is generally associated with high morbidity and mortality. Niwa et al. reported nine patients who underwent salvage total pharyngolaryngectomy and total esophagectomy; the mortality and morbidity rates were 22% and 89%, respectively [24]. Four patients (44%) developed tracheal necrosis, which in two patients eventually led to lethal hemorrhage. Thus, salvage surgery is considered a highly demanding surgical procedure that should be carefully planned and conducted in selected centers of excellence. Measures must be taken to preserve the tracheal blood supply.

2.4 Adjuvant Radiotherapy or Chemoradiotherapy After Pharyngo-Laryngo-Esophagectomy

For cases who had advanced disease with involvement of the larynx at diagnosis, laryngeal preservation may not be possible. Resectable cases should have upfront surgery with PLE with or without neck dissection. These cases would require post-operative adjuvant radiotherapy or chemoradiotherapy (*see* **Note 3**). Treatment is like adjuvant radiotherapy or chemoradiotherapy for laryngeal or hypopharyngeal carcinoma. Adjuvant radiotherapy will be 60 Gy/ 30 fractions if resection margin is clear. If resection margin is positive, the residual disease area may receive up to 66 Gy/33 fractions. Concurrent chemoradiotherapy is indicated for positive resection margin or evidence of extracapsular spread in nodal disease [25].

3 Methods

3.1 Procedures of Radiotherapy

3.1.1 Patient and Simulation

Patient will lie in supine position, with head rest and arms down by the sides. A thermoplastic mask which covers from the vertex to the shoulders is made for immobilization. Planning CT scan will be taken with patient in immobilization and in treatment position. For intensity modulated radiotherapy (IMRT), slice thickness of 2–3 mm is required.

3.1.2 Target Volumes

Gross tumor volume (GTV) is defined as all known gross disease as defined by imaging and from clinical and endoscopic information. Image fusion of the diagnostic CT scan, MRI, or PET/CT scan with the planning CT will help localization of the primary tumor (GTV-P) and any involved lymph nodes (GTV-N) (Fig. 1).

Clinical target volume (CTV) includes margins to cover the subclinical involvement around the GTV. To limit the highest dose area to the primary, the CTV-P is created by adding 0–5 mm from the GTV-P. The primary high-risk CTV (CTV-P-HR) is created by adding a 2–3 cm margin in the craniocaudal direction and a 0.5–1 cm margin in the radial direction of the GTV-P. The margin should not cross uninvolved anatomical borders like the vertebrae. The high-risk nodal CTV (CTV-N1) is created by adding a 0.5 cm margin to grossly enlarged lymph nodes. Elective nodal irradiation should extend at least one echelon nodal level beyond the enlarged nodes and commonly include levels III, IV, VI in neck and may extend to paraesophageal and paratracheal lymph nodes of the upper mediastinum down to the carina (CTV-N2).

The combined volumes of CTV-P and CTV-N will be the final CTV for formulation of the planning target volume (PTV). PTV will provide a margin around the CTV to compensate for variations in daily treatment setup. With use of IMRT, PTV is created by adding a 5 mm margin to the CTV.

3.1.3 Dose Prescription

As discussed above, a broad range of radiation dose can be used for the primary, from 50 to 70 Gy. Although higher dose was associated with better local control, the exact dose used for individual patient may vary with the extent of the primary. In general, high dose (≥60 Gy) should be limited to small area because of risk of esophageal perforation or development of tracheal-esophageal fistula. For large primary tumor, the total dose that can be given would be less. Dose per fraction should not be greater than 2 Gy unless it is for palliative purpose. With the complicated anatomy in neck, IMRT is recommended to deliver high dose to tumor without exceeding tolerance of surrounding organs at risk (OARs).

For definitive chemoradiotherapy, PTV-P can be treated to 66–70 Gy in 33–35 fractions, 5 fractions per week over 6.5–7 weeks. The PTV-P-HR is prescribed 60 Gy. PTV-N1 is

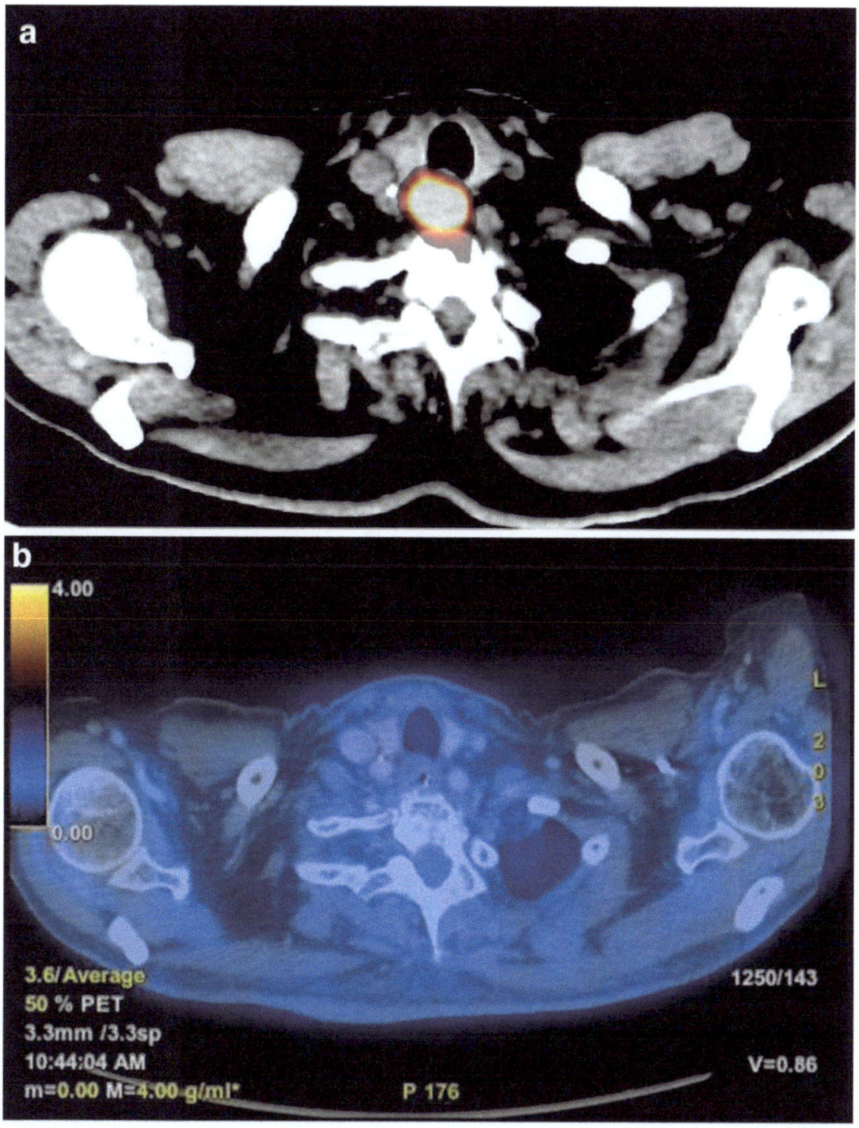

Fig. 1 (**a**) Fusion image of PET with planning CT to show the FDG avid primary tumor (**b**) PET scan 3 months after chemoradiotherapy showed no FDG uptake in esophagus

prescribed 70 Gy. Elective nodal irradiation (PTV-N2) is prescribed 50–54 Gy. IMRT will allow simultaneous irradiation of all targets (Fig. 2). The OARs include the spinal cord, thyroid, brachial plexus, heart, and lung. In the adjuvant setting, the esophagus may be reconstructed by a gastric or small bowel conduit; this conduit should be considered as OAR also and their tolerance should not be exceeded [26] (Table 2).

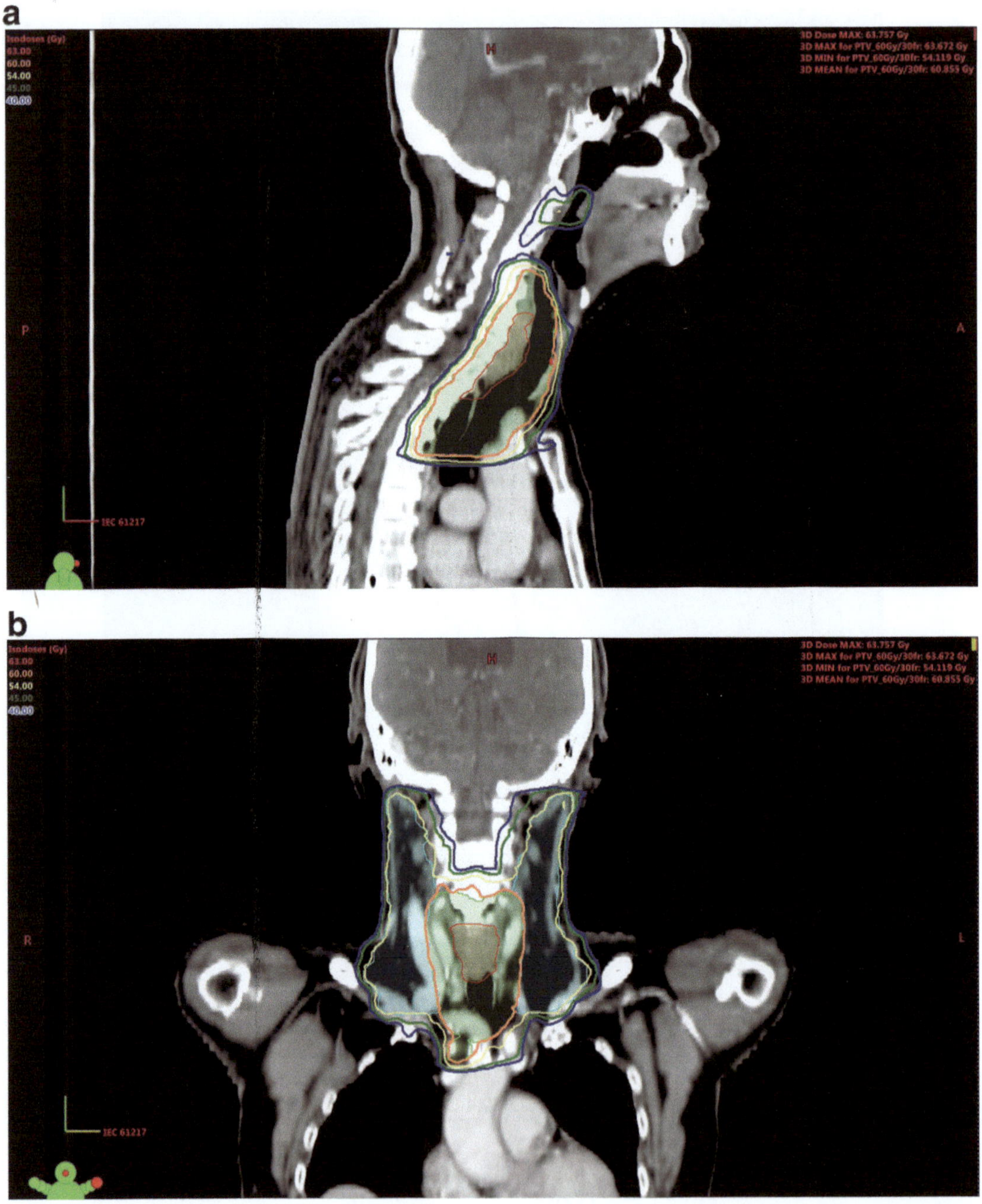

Fig. 2 Sagittal (**a**) and coronal (**b**) view of radiation dose distribution for a case of cervical esophageal squamous cell carcinoma treated with definitive chemoradiotherapy using IMRT. Filled red area: gross tumor volume (GTV); filled green area: high risk primary tumor volume (PTV-P-HR), prescribed to 60 Gy (orange isodose line); filled blue area: prophylactic nodal irradiation (PTV-N2), prescribed to 54 Gy (yellow isodose line). Spinal cord dose was kept below 45 Gy (45 Gy: green isodose line; 40 Gy: blue isodose line)

Table 2
Dose constraint for organs at risk (OAR)

OAR	Goal
Spinal cord	$D_{max} \leq 45$ Gy
Brachial plexus	$D_{max} \leq 60$ Gy
Intrathoracic stomach	$D_{max} \leq 60$ Gy
Thyroid	V45 < 50%
Bilateral lung	V20 < 30%
Heart	V30 < 40% V40 < 30%

D_{max} maximum dose, *V20, V30, V40, V45* volume that received at least 20 Gy, 30 Gy, 40 Gy, 45 Gy, respectively

3.1.4 Radiotherapy Planning and Treatment

The complex anatomy of the head and neck would require at least 3-dimensional conformal radiotherapy (3DCRT) and IMRT is preferable. Intensity modulation can be achieved by multiple fields (5–9 fields) or volumetric modulated arc radiotherapy (VMAT) or by tomotherapy. Boost fields are required for 3DCRT but IMRT can achieve simultaneous boost. The planning goal is to give at least 95% of PTV the prescribed dose and keep the maximal dose in PTV to no more than 107% of prescribed dose while respecting the OAR constraints.

Mucositis and skin reaction are common during radiotherapy, and patient should be monitored closely for nutritional status and weight loss during radiotherapy. Cone beam CT can be performed weekly to monitor accuracy of setup. Remolding and re-planning may be required if there is significant weight loss and contour change.

4 Notes

1. Options of chemoradiotherapy.
   (a) Definitive chemoradiotherapy for esophageal cancers (RTOG 8501):

   RT dose fractionation: 50 Gy in 25 fractions over 5 weeks.

   Chemotherapy: cisplatin 75 mg/m^2 IV day 1 on weeks 1, 5, 8, and 11. 5FU 1000 mg/m^2/day continuous IV infusion for 4 days on weeks 1, 5, 8, and 11.

   (b) Definitive chemoradiotherapy for locally advanced head and neck cancers:

   RT dose fractionation: 70 Gy in 35 fractions over 7 weeks.

Chemotherapy: cisplatin 100 mg/m^2 IV on day 1, 22, and 43 of RT.

For patients who cannot tolerate cisplatin, alternative choice: weekly paclitaxel (50 mg/m^2) and carboplatin (AUC = 2) concurrent with RT.

2. Options of neoadjuvant chemotherapy for chemoselection:
   (a) TPF:

   Docetaxel 75 mg/m^2 IV day 1.

   Cisplatin 75 mg/m^2 IV day 1.

   5FU 1000 mg/m^2 continuous IV infusion, days 1–5.

   Prophylactic GCSF support is recommended.

   (b) PF:

   Cisplatin 100 mg/m^2 IV day 1.

   5FU 1000 mg/m^2 continuous IV infusion, days 1–5.
3. Adjuvant chemoradiotherapy after PLE:

   RT dose fractionation: 60 Gy in 30 fractions, additional 6 Gy boost may be given to site of positive resection margin; chemotherapy: cisplatin 100 mg/m^2 IV on day 1, 22, and 43 of RT.

References

1. Grass GD, Cooper SL, Armeson K, Garrett-Mayer E, Sharma A (2015) Cervical esophageal cancer: a population-based study. Head Neck 37:808–814
2. Daiko H, Hayashi R, Saikawa M, Sakuraba M, Yamazaki M, Miyazaki M, Ugumori T, Asai M, Oyama W, Ebihara S (2007) Surgical management of carcinoma of the cervical esophagus. J Surg Oncol 96:166–172
3. Hoeben A, Polak J, Van De Voorde L, Hoebers F, Grabsch HI, de Vos-Geelen J (2016) Cervical esophageal cancer: a gap in cancer knowledge. Ann Oncol 27:1664–1674
4. Cao CN, Luo JW, Gao L, Xu GZ, Yi JL, Huang XD, Li SY, Xiao JP, Liu SY, Xu ZG, Tang PZ (2014) Primary radiotherapy compared with primary surgery in cervical esophageal cancer. JAMA Otolaryngol Head Neck Surg 140:918–926
5. Cooper JS, Guo MD, Herskovic A, Macdonald JS, Martenson JA Jr, Al-Sarraf M, Byhardt R, Russell AH, Beitler JJ, Spencer S, Asbell SO, Graham MV, Leichman LL (1999) Chemoradiotherapy of locally advanced esophageal cancer: long-term follow-up of a prospective randomized trial (RTOG 85-01). Radiation Therapy Oncology Group. JAMA 281:1623–1627
6. Kachnic LA, Winter K, Wasserman T, Kelsen D, Ginsberg R, Pisansky TM, Martenson J, Komaki R, Okawara G, Rosenthal SA, Willett CG, Minsky BD (2001) Longitudinal quality-of-life analysis of RTOG 94-05 (Int 0123):a phase III trial of definitive chemoradiotherapy for esophageal cancer. Gastrointest Cancer Res 4:45–52
7. Huang SH, Lockwood G, Brierley J, Cummings B, Kim J, Wong R, Bayley A, Ringash J (2008) Effect of concurrent high-dose cisplatin chemotherapy and conformal radiotherapy on cervical esophageal cancer survival. Int J Radiat Oncol Biol Phys 71:735–740
8. Song T, Liang X, Fang M, Wu S (2015) High-dose versus conventional-dose irradiation in cisplatin-based definitive concurrent chemoradiotherapy for esophageal cancer: a systematic review and pooled analysis. Expert Rev Anticancer Ther 15:1157–1169
9. Chen Y, Zhu HP, Wang T, Sun CJ, Ge XL, Min LF, Zhang XW, Jia QQ, Yu J, Yang JQ, Allgayer H, Abba ML, Zhang XZ, Sun XC

(2017) What is the optimal radiation dose for non-operable esophageal cancer? Dissecting the evidence in a meta-analysis. Oncotarget 8:89095–89107

10. Kim TH, Lee IJ, Kim JH, Lee CG, Lee YC, Kim JW (2019) High-dose versus standard-dose radiation therapy for cervical esophageal cancer: retrospective single-institution study. Head Neck 41:146–153
11. Zhang P, Xi M, Zhao L, Qiu B, Liu H, Hu YH, Liu MZ (2015) Clinical efficacy and failure pattern in patients with cervical esophageal cancer treated with definitive chemoradiotherapy. Radiother Oncol 116:257–261
12. Cao CN, Luo JW, Gao L, Xu GZ, Yi JL, Huang XD, Wang K, Zhang SP, Qu Y, Li SY, Xiao JP, Zhang Z (2016) Intensity-modulated radiotherapy for cervical esophageal squamous cell carcinoma: clinical outcomes and patterns of failure. Eur Arch Otorhinolaryngol 273:741–747
13. McDowell LJ, Huang SH, Xu W, Che J, Wong RKS, Brierley J, Kim J, Cummings B, Waldron J, Bayley A, Hansen A, Witterick I, Ringash J (2017) Effect of intensity modulated radiation therapy with concurrent chemotherapy on survival for patients with cervical esophageal carcinoma. Int J Radiat Oncol Biol Phys 98:186–195
14. Li HX, Liu J, Cheng Y, Liu MN, Fang WT, Lv CX (2018) Concurrent chemoradiotherapy for cervical esophageal squamous cell carcinoma: treatment results from a prospective observational study. Dis Esophagus 31:1–6
15. Zhao L, Zhou Y, Mu Y, Chai G, Xiao F, Tan L, Lin SH, Shi M (2017) Patterns of failure and clinical outcomes of definitive radiotherapy for cervical esophageal cancer. Oncotarget 8:21852–21860
16. Kumabe A, Zenda S, Motegi A, Onozawa M, Nakamura N, Kojima T, Daiko H, Shigematsu N, Akimoto T (2017) Long-term clinical results of concurrent chemoradiotherapy for patients with cervical esophageal squamous cell carcinoma. Anticancer Res 37:5039–5044
17. Ito M, Kodaira T, Tachibana H, Tomita N, Makita C, Koide Y, Kato D, Abe T, Muro K, Tajika M, Niwa Y, Hasegawa Y (2017) Clinical results of definitive chemoradiotherapy for cervical esophageal cancer: comparison of failure pattern and toxicities between intensity-modulated radiotherapy and 3-dimensional conformal radiotherapy. Head Neck 39:2406–2415
18. Okamoto H, Taniyama Y, Sakurai T, Heishi T, Teshima J, Sato C, Maruyama S, Ito K, Onodera Y, Konno-Kumagai T, Ishida H, Kamei T (2018) Definitive chemoradiotherapy with docetaxel, cisplatin, and 5-fluorouracil (DCF-R) for advanced cervical esophageal cancer. Esophagus 15:281–285
19. Sakanaka K, Ishida Y, Fujii K, Itasaka S, Miyamoto S, Horimatsu T, Muto M, Mizowaki T (2018) Long-term outcome of definitive radiotherapy for cervical esophageal squamous cell carcinoma. Radiat Oncol 13:7
20. Spector ME, Rosko AJ, Swiecicki PL, Chad Brenner J, Birkeland AC (2018) From VA larynx to the future of chemoselection: defining the role of induction chemotherapy in larynx cancer. Oral Oncol 86:200–205
21. Suzuki G, Yamazaki H, Ogo E, Abe T, Eto H, Muraki K, Hattori C, Umeno H, Nakashima T, Tanaka T, Nakamura S, Yoshida K (2014) Multimodal approach for cervical esophageal carcinoma: role of neoadjuvant chemotherapy. Anticancer Res 34:1989–1992
22. Nakata Y, Hanai N, Nishikawa D, Suzuki H, Koide Y, Fukuda Y, Nomura M, Kodaira T, Shimizu T, Hasegawa Y (2017) Comparison between chemoselection and definitive radiotherapy in patients with cervical esophageal squamous cell carcinoma. Int J Clin Oncol 22:1034–1041
23. Blanchard P, Bourhis J, Lacas B, Posner MR, Vermorken JB, Cruz Hernandez JJ, Bourredjem A, Calais G, Paccagnella A, Hitt R, Pignon JP, Meta-Analysis of Chemotherapy in Head and Neck Cancer, Induction Project, Collaborative Group (2013) Taxane-cisplatin-fluorouracil as induction chemotherapy in locally advanced head and neck cancers: an individual patient data meta-analysis of the meta-analysis of chemotherapy in head and neck cancer group. J Clin Oncol 31:2854–2860
24. Niwa Y, Koike M, Fujimoto Y, Oya H, Iwata N, Nishio N, Hiramatsu M, Kanda M, Kobayashi D, Tanaka C, Yamada S, Fujii T, Nakayama G, Sugimoto H, Nomoto S, Fujiwara M, Kodera Y (2016) Salvage pharyngolaryngectomy with total esophagectomy following definitive chemoradiotherapy. Dis Esophagus 29:598–602
25. Expert Panel on Radiation Oncology-Head and Neck, Salama JK, Saba N, Quon H, Garg MK, Lawson J, MW MD, Ridge JA, Smith RV, Yeung AR, Yom SS, Beitler JJ (2011) ACR appropriateness criteria® adjuvant therapy for resected squamous cell carcinoma of the head and neck. Oral Oncol 47:554–559
26. Liu Q, Cai XW, Fu XL, Chen JC, Xiang JQ (2015) Tolerance and dose-volume relationship of intrathoracic stomach irradiation after esophagectomy for patients with thoracic esophageal squamous cell carcinoma. Oncotarget 6:32220–32227

Chapter 23

Radiotherapy for Thoracic Esophageal Squamous Cell Carcinoma

Wendy W. L. Chan, Ka On Lam, and Dora L. W. Kwong

Abstract

Esophageal squamous cell carcinoma (ESCC) is an aggressive disease. Many patients have locally advanced disease or already have distant metastasis at presentation. Radiotherapy plays an important role in the treatment of esophageal squamous cell carcinoma. Neoadjuvant chemoradiotherapy improves the survival and surgical outcome compared to surgery alone. Definitive radiotherapy (RT) with or without chemotherapy is used in patients who decline surgery or are medically inoperable. Palliative radiotherapy using external beam radiotherapy or intraluminal brachytherapy is effective for dysphagia and pain control.d

Key words Esophageal cancer, Radiotherapy, Brachytherapy, Dysphagia

1 Introduction

Esophageal cancer is the eighth most common cancer and the sixth leading cause of cancer-related mortality in the world. Surgery is a standard of treatment in esophageal cancer. However, many of the patients with esophageal cancer are locally advanced. Radiotherapy plays a key role in treatment, often in combination with chemotherapy and surgery. Neoadjuvant chemoradiotherapy can downstage the disease and facilitate operation. For patients with unresectable disease or who are medically not fit for surgery, radical chemoradiotherapy improves survival over radiotherapy alone. For patients with dysphagia or bleeding, palliative radiotherapy can be used to relieve symptoms.

1.1 Landmarks of ESCC

The location of the primary ESCC tumor is defined by the position of the upper end of the cancer in the esophagus. It is measured from the incisors to the proximal edge of the tumor at endoscopy. The sternal notch is usually at 18 cm, carina at 25 cm, and esophagogastric junction at 40 cm. Esophageal cancer is divided into three portions: cervical, intrathoracic, and abdominal. The intrathoracic

Alfred K. Lam (ed.), *Esophageal Squamous Cell Carcinoma: Methods and Protocols*, Methods in Molecular Biology, vol. 2129,
https://doi.org/10.1007/978-1-0716-0377-2_23,

Table 1
Primary site of esophageal cancer based on proximal edge of tumor

Anatomic name	Esophageal location	Anatomic boundaries	Distance from incisors to proximal edge of tumor
Cervical	Upper	Hypopharynx to sternal notch	15 to <20 cm
Thoracic	Upper	Sternal notch to azygos vein	20 to <25 cm
	Middle	Lower border of azygos vein to inferior pulmonary vein	25 to <30 cm
	Lower	Lower border of inferior pulmonary vein to esophagogastric junction	30 to <40 cm
Abdominal	Esophagogastric junction/cardia	Esophagogastric junction to 5 cm below esophagogastric junction	40–45 cm

portion is further divided into upper, middle, and lower thirds (Table 1). ESCCs occur most frequently in the middle-third and least commonly in the upper-third.

1.2 Local Spread and Lymphatic Spread of ESCC

Most esophageal cancers are locally advanced at presentation because there is no peri-esophageal serosa to inhibit their growth. They can infiltrate into adjacent structures, most frequently into the trachea, aorta, pleura, diaphragm, vertebrae, and recurrent laryngeal nerves. It also spreads longitudinally along the submucosal lymphatics to form skip lesions as much as 80 mm from the primary tumor, and this occurs in up to a third of cases.

The extensive, longitudinal interconnecting lymphatic system not only accounts for the early lymph node metastasis but also facilitates the potential risk of lymphatic involvement longitudinally throughout the entire length of the esophagus rather than just segmental nodal involvement. A meta-analysis involving 18,415 patients from 45 observational studies evaluated the rate of lymph node involvement in thoracic esophageal cancers [1]. It revealed that the incidences of lymph node involvement in the cervical, upper-mediastinal, mid-mediastinal, lower-mediastinal, and abdominal levels were 30.7, 42.0, 12.9, 2.6, and 9% for upper thoracic esophageal cancers; 16.8, 21.1, 28.1, 7.8, and 21.4% for middle thoracic esophageal cancers; and 11.0, 10.5, 19.6, 23.0, and 39.9% for lower thoracic esophageal cancers, respectively. These data indicated that esophageal cancer has an unpredictable pattern of lymphatic spread.

In theory, the clinical target volume (CTV) should cover the gross lesion and the uninvolved lymph nodes at risk of microscopic disease. Nevertheless, the radiotherapy field would be too extensive to encompass all cervical, mediastinal, and upper abdominal lymph nodes because of normal tissue tolerance. In practice, only the lymph node regions with higher risk are included. For example, when treating the upper esophageal cancers, the bilateral supraclavicular and upper/middle mediastinal lymph nodes are irradiated but not the lower para-esophageal lymph nodes.

1.3 Indications for Radiotherapy

Surgery is the mainstay of curative treatment for most patients with esophageal cancer who are medically fit and whose diseases are resectable. However, only 40% of patients survive for 2 years [2]. Radiotherapy is an effective treatment for ESCC. Neoadjuvant chemoradiotherapy (CRT) leads to a survival benefit compared to surgery alone. Definitive radiotherapy (RT) with or without chemotherapy has also been used in patients who decline surgery or are medically inoperable. Many patients with ESCC are elderly, have poor performance status, or have distant metastasis at presentation. Palliative radiotherapy is effective for dysphagia and pain control.

1.3.1 Neoadjuvant Chemoradiotherapy

There is no clear evidence to show neoadjuvant radiotherapy alone improves the survival of patients with resectable esophageal cancer. A Cochrane quantitative meta-analysis including 1147 patients from five randomized controlled trials was conducted to assess the benefit of neoadjuvant radiotherapy compared to surgery alone. Many patients had squamous cell carcinoma. Neoadjuvant radiotherapy led to a relative reduction in the risk of death by 11% with a hazard ratio (HR) of 0.89 (95% confidence interval [CI] 0.78–1.01) and an absolute survival benefit of 3% at 2 years and 4% at 5 years [3]. This result is not statistically significant ($p = 0.062$), and the clinical effect is modest. Thus, neoadjuvant radiotherapy alone is not a standard treatment before radical esophagectomy.

Both neoadjuvant chemotherapy and neoadjuvant CRT can be used before surgery to downstage the tumor and increase the resectability. A recent meta-analysis including 866 patients compared neoadjuvant CRT with neoadjuvant chemotherapy [4]. The conclusions were in favor of neoadjuvant CRT, with improvement in survival (3-year survival rate: risk ratios [RR] 0.78, 95% CI 0.62–0.98, $p = 0.03$; 5-year survival rate: RR 0.69, 95% CI 0.50–0.96, $p = 0.03$), R_0 resection rate (RR 0.87, 95% CI 0.81–0.92, $p < 0.0001$), and pathological complete response (pCR) (RR 0.16, 95% CI 0.09–0.28, $p < 0.00001$). Another systematic review of 3640 participants by Courrech Staal et al. reported the use of neoadjuvant CRT (with chemotherapy predominantly using 5FU/cisplatin) attained R_0 resection rate of 88.4% and pCR rate of 25.8% [5]. Five-year survival rates ranged 16–59% in all patients and 3–62% in those with a pCR. The most common CRT-related toxicity was neutropenia. The in-hospital mortality rate after esophagectomy following CRT was 5.2%.

The most promising result was reported in the Chemoradiotherapy for Esophageal Cancer Followed by Surgery Study (CROSS) [6, 7]. This phase III randomized study randomized

366 patients with resectable esophageal cancer (T1N1M0 or T2-3N0-1M0) into neoadjuvant CRT ($n = 178$) or surgery alone ($n = 188$). The neoadjuvant CRT regimen consisted of radiotherapy 41.4 Gy in 23 fractions over 4.5 weeks concurrent with 5 weekly cycles of paclitaxel (50 mg/m^2) and carboplatin (AUC = 2). Surgery was performed 4–6 weeks after neoadjuvant CRT. In this study, 275 patients had adenocarcinoma and 84 patients had squamous cell carcinoma. Neoadjuvant CRT improved the R_0 resection rate compared with surgery alone (92%, 148/161 patients versus 69%, 111/161 patients; $p < 0.001$). pCR rate was 29% in the neoadjuvant CRT group. Neoadjuvant CRT also significantly prolonged the median overall survival (48.6 months versus 24.0 months, HR 0.68, 95% CI 0.53–0.88, $p = 0.003$). The improvement in survival was more pronounced in the ESCC compared with esophageal adenocarcinoma. Median overall survival for patients with ESCC was 81.6 months (95% CI 47.2–116.0) in the neoadjuvant CRT plus surgery group and 21.1 months (95% CI 15.4–26.7) in the surgery alone group (HR 0.48, 95% CI 0.28–0.83, $p = 0.008$). More importantly, the post-operative complication rates and post-operative mortality rates were not different between the two groups.

Another recently published phase III randomized controlled trial (NEOCRTEC5010) allocated 451 Chinese patients with ESCC, clinically staged as T1-4N1M0/T4N0M0, into neoadjuvant CRT plus surgery arm ($n = 224$) and surgery alone arm ($n = 227$) [8]. Patients in the neoadjuvant CRT arm received radiotherapy 40 Gy in 20 fractions over 4 weeks concurrent with vinorelbine and cisplatin. Compared with surgery alone, neoadjuvant CRT plus surgery improved the R_0 resection rate (98.4% versus 91.2%, $p = 0.002$), median overall survival (100.1 versus 66.5 months, HR 0.71, 95% CI 0.53–0.96, $p = 0.025$), and disease-free survival (100.1 versus 41.7 months, HR 0.58, 95% CI 0.43–0.78, $p < 0.001$).

Four to 6 weeks following completion of neoadjuvant CRT, patients are reassessed with esophagogastroduodenoscopy (OGD) and positron-emission tomography-computerized tomography scan (PET-CT) with intravenous contrast for response and respectability. Patients who achieve pCR after neoadjuvant CRT have a better prognosis. pCR rate is associated with age, smoking habit, tumor length, tumor grade, treatment time, radiation dose, and chemotherapy [9, 10] (*see* **Note 1**).

1.3.2 Definitive Chemoradiotherapy

Definitive CRT should be considered in patients who are medically inoperable or who decline surgery if their disease can be encompassed in a radical radiotherapy volume. In the landmark RTOG 85-01 study, concomitant CRT 50 Gy in 25 fractions over 5 weeks with two concurrent and two adjuvant cycles of cisplatin (75 mg/m^2

on day 1) and 5FU (1000 mg/m^2 over 4 h on day 1–4) showed superiority over radiotherapy alone (64 Gy in 32 fractions over 6.4 weeks) [11]. Most patients had ESCC. Patients treated with CRT had a significant improvement in both median survival (14 months vs. 9 months) and 5-year survival (27% versus 0%, $p < 0.0001$). Persistence of disease was the greatest cause of treatment failure in both arms. It was less common in the CRT arm (26%, $n = 34/130$) than the RT alone arm (37%, $n = 23/62$). This study demonstrated that CRT should be the standard non-surgical treatment for esophageal cancer (*see* **Note 2**).

The INT-0123 study repeated the RTOG-8501 study and compared high-dose (64.8 Gy) radiotherapy with standard-dose (50.4 Gy) radiotherapy concurrent with cisplatin/5FU [12]. The study failed to show superiority with high-dose radiotherapy (64.8 Gy). There was no significant difference in median survival (13.0 months versus 18.1 months), 2-year survival (31% versus 40%), or local/regional failure and local/regional persistence of disease (56% versus 52%) between the high-dose and standard-dose groups. The study was prematurely closed because of multiple deaths in the high-dose group (11 versus 2 treatment deaths). However, 7 of the 11 treatment-related deaths in the high-dose group occurred before the radiation dose reached 50.4 Gy, and the high-dose group also received a significantly lower dose of 5FU, which might have affected the outcomes in that group. An increasing number of evidences demonstrated the safety and efficacy of radiation doses ≥60 Gy. With modern radiation techniques, such as intensity-modulated radiotherapy (IMRT) or volumetric modulated arc therapy (VMAT), more conformal and higher radiation dose could be given with more organs-at-risk sparing. Simultaneous boost with small margins to the gross tumor volume (GTV) using IMRT can be considered, for example, 55 Gy in 25 fractions.

Radical radiotherapy alone may be reserved for patients who cannot tolerate chemotherapy or surgery. If the tumor is small and well localized (<5 cm in length), hypofractionated radiotherapy with dose 50–55 Gy in 20 fractions can be given [13]. With larger tumors, conventional fractionation with 60 Gy in 30 fractions is used for better tolerance but need balancing on the dose to the OARs (*see* **Note 3**).

1.3.3 Postoperative Radiotherapy

There is no clear evidence to prove the benefits of postoperative radiotherapy. A meta-analysis by Malthaner et al. failed to detect a survival benefit of postoperative radiotherapy (RR for death at 1 year, 1.23, 95% CI 0.95–1.59, $p = 0.11$) [14]. Postoperative radiotherapy is mainly reserved for patients with R1 (microscopic residual) and patients with circumferential margin with low nodal involvement (e.g., fewer than three lymph nodes involved). The radiation field is usually limited to site with residual disease and dose is up to bowel tolerance dose because of gastric pull-up or sometimes, intestinal interposition.

1.3.4 Palliative Radiotherapy

Both external beam radiotherapy (ERT) and intraluminal brachytherapy (ILT) are effective in improving malignant dysphagia.

External Beam Radiotherapy

ERT can palliate symptoms including dysphagia, chest pain, and bleeding. ERT can relieve dysphagia in 60–80% of cases, but the benefits are usually delayed with maximal response in around 4–6 weeks after treatment. Typical doses include 30 Gy in 10 daily fractions over 2 weeks and 35 Gy in 15 fractions over 3 weeks. Shorter fractionation schedules, for example, 20 Gy in 5 fractions over 1 week, can also be given but the effect may not be durable. ERT can be performed safely after stent insertion. Previous studies showed that post-stenting ERT effectively prolongs duration of dysphagia relief (7 months versus 3 months, $p = 0.002$) and improves overall survival (180 days versus 120 days, $p = 0.009$) compared with stenting alone without increasing the incidence of neither complications nor treatment-related mortality [15] (*see* **Note 4**).

Brachytherapy

ILT has the advantage over ERT by its ability to deliver a large radiation dose with great spatial precision, giving more sparing to the organs-at-risk as well as earlier tumor response. In addition, when compared to self-expanding metal stents, ILT also has fewer requirements for re-intervention, longer survival, and better quality of life [15].

Before ILT, endoscopic dilatation was undertaken to a maximum of 11 mm. A flexible applicator (e.g., Bonvoisin-Gérard Esophageal Applicator, Nucletron, Veenendaal, the Netherlands) with a diameter of 10 mm was passed down the esophagus. A single dose of 12 Gy or 8 Gy for two fractions using high dose rate (HDR) with radioisotope Iridium-192 is delivered at 10 mm from the source axis of the applicator. The standard active length of the application was the tumor length plus 2 cm extra at both ends of the tumor (Fig. 1). If ERT and 5FU-based chemotherapy are used with ILT, the recommended dose of ILT is HDR 10 Gy in 2 weekly fractions of 5 Gy each. ILT should follow external beam radiation therapy and should not be given concurrently with chemotherapy [16] (*see* **Note 5**).

2 Materials

2.1 Pre-treatment Investigations

1. Nutritional assessment.
2. Blood tests: complete blood count, liver and renal function test, hepatitis serology.

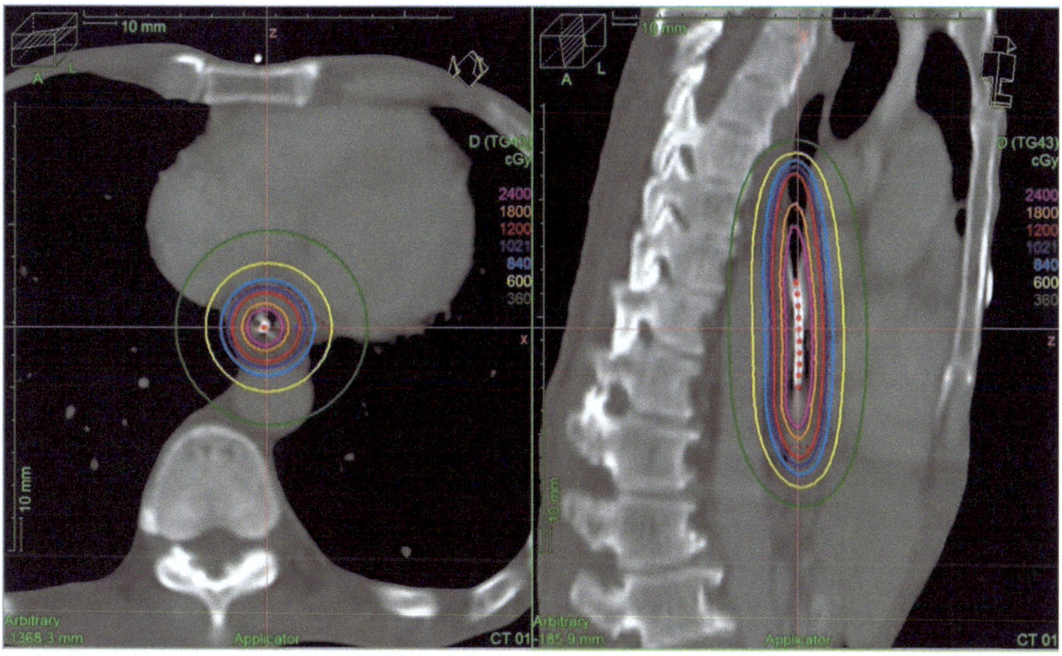

Fig. 1 Brachytherapy for esophageal squamous cell carcinoma (12 Gy in single fraction). Red dots: radioactive source; Purple line: 24 Gy isodose line; Orange line: 18 Gy isodose line, Red line: 12 Gy isodose line, Yellow line: 6 Gy isodose line

3. Endoscopic examination: OGD + endoscopic ultrasound (EUS), tumor biopsy.
4. Imaging: computed tomography (CT) of thorax, abdomen and pelvis, PET-CT with intravenous contrast is preferred for operable cases, ultrasound of neck.
5. Respiratory assessment: lung function test for operable cases and cases for radical radiotherapy.
6. Cardiac assessment (if operable cases): echocardiogram.

2.2 Planning and Treatment

1. Thermoplastic cast for IMRT and radiotherapy needs to cover supraclavicular lymph node.
2. Planning CT with intravenous contrast if renal function is fit.
3. Fusion with PET-CT with planning CT for radiotherapy planning.
4. Dose calculation after contouring the targets.
5. Treatment with radiotherapy machine (linear accelerator).

3 Methods

3.1 Procedures of Radiotherapy

3.1.1 Simulator

Palliative radiotherapy for esophageal cancer using anterior-posterior (AP) opposing fields can be planned on a simulator. Patients lie supine with arms by their sides as lateral or oblique beams are not used. The gross tumor volume (GTV) is localized with all diagnostic data from endoscopy and CT scan. Barium swallow during simulation can help to determine the longitudinal extent of the esophageal tumor. The field border is chosen to allow 3–4 cm superoinferior margin and 1.5–2 cm axial margin from the GTV.

3.1.2 CT Planning

Immobilization

Patients are treated in lying supine position, with arms above the head, ideally immobilized with a vacuum-formed polystyrene bag (e.g., Vacloc). For treatment of cervical or upper third of the esophagus, patients should be immobilized in a Perspex or thermoplastic shell fixed to the couch with cervical spine straight.

CT Scanning

Planning CT scan is done with patient immobilized in the treatment position. CT scan at a slice thickness of 3 mm is obtained from hyoid bone to the L2 vertebra, preferably with intravenous contrast. 4D-CT can be used for defining the internal target volume (ITV) expansion to accommodate target motion with respiration and ensure adequate coverage of the target volumes. In cases with large respiratory motion (excess of 5 mm), the use of modern techniques such as respiratory gating or abdominal compression could be considered. Planning CT with fusion of PET-CT images can help delineate tumor volumes more accurately.

Target Volume Definition

GTV-primary (GTV-P) is the site of the primary esophageal tumor. The superior and inferior extent of GTV-P should be defined with all information from endoscopy, EUS, diagnostic and planning CT, and PET-CT images. The GTV-P should encompass the greatest apparent extent of tumor superiorly and inferiorly from findings of all these investigations. The entire esophageal wall, including any disease that has extended through the wall, should be contoured as the GTV-P.

GTV-lymph node (GTV-N) includes all grossly involved lymph nodes. All enlarged mediastinal lymph nodes and all FDG-avid lymph nodes are included in the GTV-N.

CTV covers the subclinical involvement around the GTV (CTV-P) and the high-risk nodal sites (CTV-N).

CTV-P is produced by expanding the GTV-P superiorly and inferiorly by 3–4 cm along the axis of the esophagus. For very proximal tumors, the upper border should not extend above the level of cricoid cartilage unless it is involved. For distal esophageal tumors or esophagogastric junction tumors, a 2 cm margin along the gastric mucosa is given to avoid unacceptable large involvement of stomach or other abdominal organs. Radially, a 10 mm margin from the outer esophageal wall is to encompass the peri-esophageal lymph nodes. Structures such as the pericardial sac, vertebral body, pleura, and vessels are excluded from the CTV-P if there is no infiltration by the tumor. In cases where the tumor is located at close proximity with the heart or liver, the CTV expansion is limited to 5 mm. If robust motion management techniques such as respiratory gating or ITV approach are employed, the heart and liver can be entirely excluded.

CTV-N is expanded from the GTV-N with 1 cm margin isotropically. There is no consensus on elective nodal irradiation. In view of the early and extensive nodal involvement in esophageal cancer, many centers now recommend irradiating the high-risk nodal sites. For the cervical and upper ESCC, CTV-N includes bilateral supraclavicular, adjacent para-esophageal, upper, and middle mediastinal lymph nodes. For middle thoracic ESCC, CTV-N includes the adjacent para-esophageal, upper, and middle mediastinal lymph nodes. For lower thoracic ESCC, the middle and lower para-esophageal lymph nodes as well as the abdominal lymph nodes (left gastric and celiac nodes) should be included.

Planning target volume (PTV) is then expanded from both CTV-P and CTV-N by 1 cm superoinferiorly and 0.5 cm axially. These margins should be confirmed as appropriate for each individual departmental practice if the internal margin and setup errors have been measured. If respiratory gating or 4D-CT is used, the degree of respiratory motion can be incorporated into the PTV expansion.

Beam Arrangement (Fig. 2a, b)

For palliative radiotherapy to esophagus, mainly AP opposing fields are used. For 3D conformal radiotherapy (3D-CRT), thoracic esophageal volumes can be treated with three-field techniques (involving one anterior and two posterior oblique beams) or with four equispaced beams. Compared with AP opposing fields, these beam arrangements can decrease dose to the spinal cord but may cause higher dose to the lung.

More centers now use IMRT with 5–7 coplanar beams for neoadjuvant or radical radiotherapy for esophageal cancers. A meta-analysis concluded that IMRT, compared with 3D-CRT, significantly reduces the average percent volumes of lung and heart irradiated, improves overall survival, and shows no difference in radiation toxicity [17].

Dose Acceptance and Organs-at-Risks (OARs)

Isodose distribution and dose volume histogram (DVH) of RT planning should be examined to ensure adequate coverage of the targets and conforming dose limits to OARs. At least 95% of the PTV should receive the prescribed dose. The PTV minimum should be more than 95%, and the PTV maximum should not be

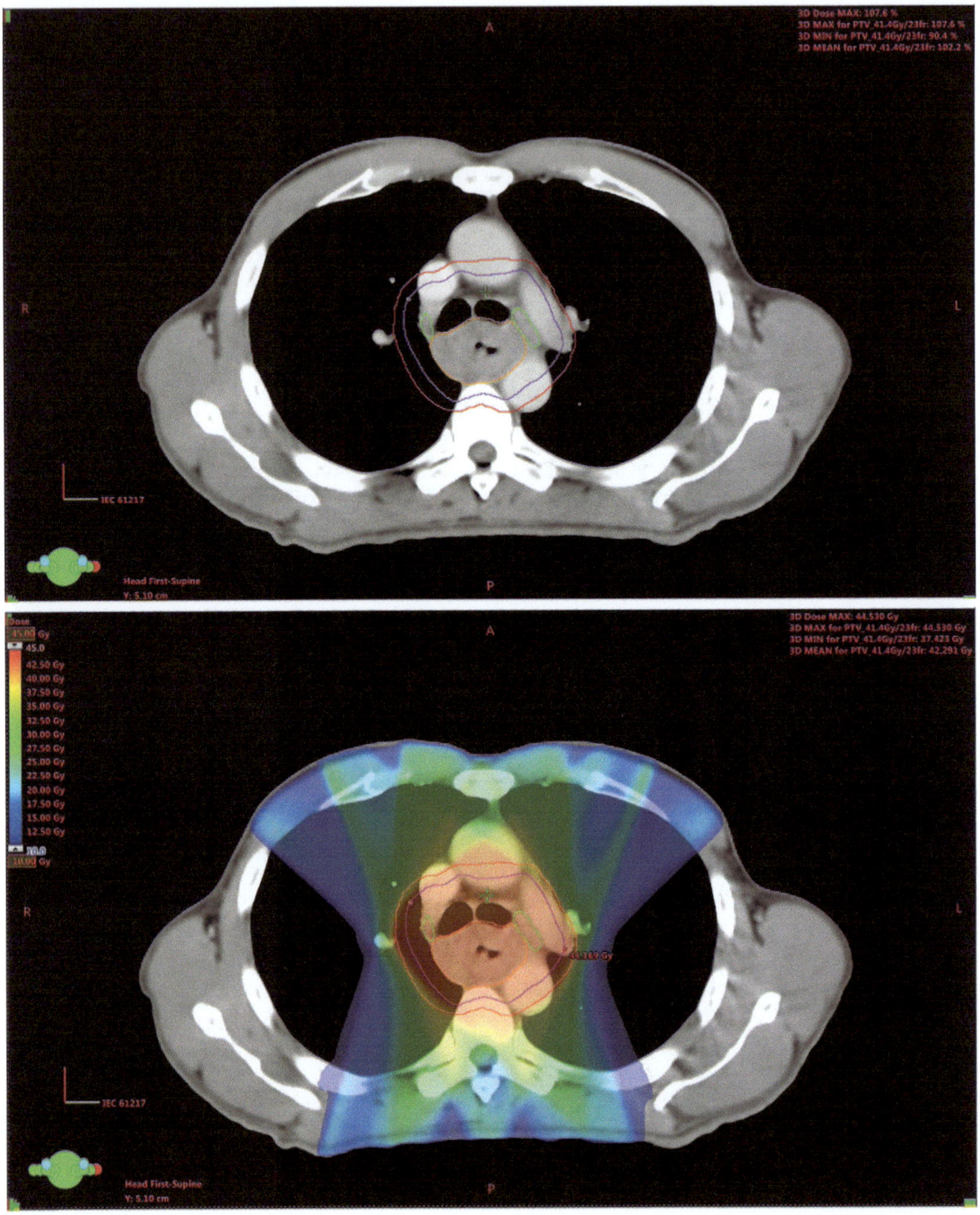

Fig. 2 Example of squamous cell carcinoma of upper esophagus for neoadjuvant chemoradiotherapy 41.4 Gy in 23 fractions concurrent with weekly paclitaxel-carboplatin. (**a**) Axial cut of planning CT, contouring of GTV-primary, GTV-lymph node, CTV, and PTV 41.4 Gy. Orange line: GTV-primary; Green line: GTV-lymph node; Purple line: CTV; Red line: PTV 41.4 Gy. (**b**) Isodose with colorwash with PTV receiving 41.4 Gy/23 fractions and sparing the dose to the lungs and spinal cord

Table 2
Tissue constraints

Region of interest/organ at risk	Dose constraint
PTV	V95%[a] > 99.0% of the prescribed dose
PTV minimum	PTV_{min} > 93% of the prescribed dose
D_{max} of PTV	<107% of the prescribed dose
GTV	GTV_{min} > 100% of the prescribed dose
Spinal cord	Max dose ≤ 45 Gy
Combined lungs	V20[b] ≤ 25%
Heart	V40[c] ≤ 30%
Liver	V30[d] < 60%, mean < 30–35 Gy
Individual kidney	V20[e] < 25%, mean < 17.5 Gy

[a]V95% = 95% PTV volume
[b]V20 = Volume of total lung receiving 20 Gy
[c]V40 = Volume of heart receiving 40 Gy
[d]V30 = Volume of liver receiving 30 Gy
[e]V20 = Volume of each kidney receiving 20 Gy

over 107% of the prescribed dose. Tissue constraints should be met and recorded for each patient plan. The dose volume constraints for OARs are as shown in Table 2.

4 Notes

1. Neoadjuvant chemoradiotherapy.
   CROSS:

Radiotherapy	41.4 Gy in 23 fractions over 4.5 weeks	
Chemotherapy	Paclitaxel 50 mg/m^2 Carboplatin AUC = 2	Weekly for 5 cycles, concurrent with RT

   NEOCRTEC5010:

Radiotherapy	40 Gy in 20 fractions over 4 weeks	
Chemotherapy	Vinorelbine 25 mg/m^2 on D1, D8 Cisplatin 75 mg/m^2 D1 or 25 mg/m^2 on D1–4	Every 3 weeks for 2 cycles, concurrent with RT

2. Definitive chemoradiotherapy.
   RTOG-8501

Radiotherapy	50 Gy in 25 fractions over 5 weeks	
Chemotherapy	Cisplatin 75 mg/ m^2 D1 5FU 1000 mg/ m^2 D1–4	Given at week 1, 5, 8, 11 (2 cycles concurrent with RT and 2 cycles starting 3 weeks after RT)

3. Definitive radiotherapy alone.

Radiotherapy	50–55 Gy in 20 fractions over 5 weeks 60 Gy in 30 fractions over 6 weeks

4. Palliative radiotherapy.

Radiotherapy	30 Gy in 10 fractions over 2 weeks 35 Gy in 15 fractions over 3 weeks 20 Gy in 5 fractions over 1 week

5. Palliative brachytherapy.

Brachytherapy	12 Gy in 1 fraction 16 Gy in 2 fractions
Brachytherapy should not be concurrent with ERT or chemotherapy	

References

1. Ding X, Zhang J, Li B, Wang Z, Huang W, Zhou T, Wei Y, Li H (2012) A meta-analysis of lymph node metastasis rate for patients with thoracic oesophageal cancer and its implication in delineation of clinical target volume for radiation therapy. Br J Radiol 85:e1110–e1119. https://doi.org/10.1259/bjr/12500248
2. Wouters MW, Gooiker GA, van Sandick JW, Tollenaar RA (2012) The volume-outcome relation in the surgical treatment of esophageal cancer: a systematic review and meta-analysis. Cancer 118:1754–1763. https://doi.org/10.1002/cncr.26383
3. Arnott SJ, Duncan W, Gignoux M, Hansen HS, Launois B, Nygaard K, Parmar MK, Rousell A, Spilopoulos G, Stewart G, Tierney JF, Wang M, Rhugang Z, Oeosphageal Cancer Collaborative Group (2005) Preoperative radiotherapy for esophageal carcinoma. Cochrane Database Syst Rev 4:CD001799
4. Zhao X, Ren Y, Hu Y, Cui N, Wang X, Cui Y (2018) Neoadjuvant chemotherapy versus neoadjuvant chemoradiotherapy for cancer of the esophagus or the gastroesophageal junction: a meta-analysis based on clinical trials. PLoS One 13:e0202185. https://doi.org/10.1371/journal.pone.0202185
5. Courrech Staal EF, Aleman BM, Boot H, van Velthuysen ML, van Tinteren H, van Sandick JW (2010) Systematic review of the benefits and risks of neoadjuvant chemoradiation for oesophageal cancer. Br J Surg 97:1482–1496. https://doi.org/10.1002/bjs.7175
6. van Hagen P, Hulshof MC, van Lanschot JJ, Steyerberg EW, van Berge Henegouwen MI, Wijnhoven BP, Richel DJ, Nieuwenhuijzen GA, Hospers GA, Bonenkamp JJ, Cuesta MA, Blaisse RJ, Busch OR, ten Kate FJ, Creemers GJ, Punt CJ, Plukker JT, Verheul HM, Spillenaar Bilgen EJ, van Dekken H, van der Sangen

MJ, Rozema T, Biermann K, Beukema JC, Piet AH, van Rij CM, Reinders JG, Tilanus HW, van der Gaast A, CROSS Group (2012) Preoperative chemoradiotherapy for esophageal or junctional cancer. N Engl J Med 366:2074–2084. https://doi.org/10.1056/NEJMoa1112088

7. Shapiro J, van Lanschot JJB, Hulshof MCCM, van Hagen P, van Berge Henegouwen MI, Wijnhoven BPL, van Laarhoven HWM, Nieuwenhuijzen GAP, Hospers GAP, Bonenkamp JJ, Cuesta MA, Blaisse RJB, Busch ORC, Ten Kate FJW, Creemers GM, Punt CJA, Plukker JTM, Verheul HMW, Bilgen EJS, van Dekken H, van der Sangen MJC, Rozema T, Biermann K, Beukema JC, Piet AHM, van Rij CM, Reinders JG, Tilanus HW, Steyerberg EW, van der Gaast A, CROSS study group (2015) Neoadjuvant chemoradiotherapy plus surgery versus surgery alone for oesophageal or junctional cancer (CROSS): long-term results of a randomised controlled trial. Lancet Oncol 16:1090–1098. https://doi.org/10.1016/S1470-2045(15)00040-6
8. Yang H, Liu H, Chen Y, Zhu C, Fang W, Yu Z, Mao W, Xiang J, Han Y, Chen Z, Yang H, Wang J, Pang Q, Zheng X, Yang H, Li T, Lordick F, D'Journo XB, Cerfolio RJ, Korst RJ, Novoa NM, Swanson SJ, Brunelli A, Ismail M, Fernando HC, Zhang X, Li Q, Wang G, Chen B, Mao T, Kong M, Guo X, Lin T, Liu M, Fu J, AME Thoracic Surgery Collaborative Group (2018) Neoadjuvant chemoradiotherapy followed by surgery versus surgery alone for locally advanced squamous cell carcinoma of the esophagus (NEOCRETEC5010): a phase III multicenter, randomized, open-label clinical trial. J Clin Oncol 36:2796–2803. https://doi.org/10.1200/JCO.2018.79.1483
9. Huang RW, Chao YK, Wen YW, Chang HK, Tseng CK, Chan SC, Liu YH (2014) Predictors of pathological complete response to neoadjuvant chemoradiotherapy for esophageal squamous cell carcinoma. World J Surg Oncol 12:170. https://doi.org/10.1186/1477-7819-12-170
10. Tan Z, Yang H, Wen J, Luo K, Liu Q, Hu Y, Zhang L, Liu M, Yun J, Fu J (2018) Clinical predictors of pathologically response after neoadjuvant chemoradiotherapy for esophageal squamous cell carcinoma: long term outcomes of a phase II study. J Thorac Dis 10:5254–5259. https://doi.org/10.21037/jtd.2018.08.88
11. Cooper JS, Guo MD, Herskovic A, Macdonald JS, Martenson JA Jr, Al-Sarraf M, Byhardt R, Russell AH, Beitler JJ, Spencer S, Asbell SO, Graham MV, Leichman LL (1999) Chemoradiotherapy of locally advanced esophageal cancer: long-term follow-up of a prospective randomized trial (RTOG 85-01). Radiation Therapy Oncology Group. JAMA 281:1623–1627
12. Minsky BD, Pajak TF, Ginsberg RJ, Pisansky TM, Martenson J, Komaki R, Okawara G, Rosenthal SA, Kelsen DP (2002) INT 0123 (Radiation Therapy Oncology Group 94-05) phase III trial of combined-modality therapy for esophageal cancer: high-dose versus standard-dose radiation therapy. J Clin Oncol 20:1167–1174
13. Royal College of Radiologists. Radiation Dose Fractionation, second edition (2017). https://www.rcr.ac.uk/system/files/publication/field_publication_files/bfco163_dose_fractionation_2nd_ed_march2017.pdf
14. Malthaner RA, Wong RK, Rumble RB, Zuraw L, Members of the Gastrointestinal Cancer Disease Site Group of Cancer Care Ontario's Program in Evidence-based Care (2004) Neoadjuvant or adjuvant therapy for resectable esophageal cancer: a systematic review and meta-analysis. BMC Med 2:35
15. Dai Y, Li C, Xie Y, Liu X, Zhang J, Zhou J, Pan X, Yang S (2014) Interventions for dysphagia in oesophageal cancer. Cochrane Database Syst Rev 10:CD005048. https://doi.org/10.1002/14651858.CD005048.pub4. Review
16. Gaspar LE, Nag S, Herskovic A, Mantravadi R, Speiser B (1997) American Brachytherapy Society (ABS) consensus guidelines for brachytherapy of esophageal caancer. Clinical Research Committee, American Brachytherapy Society, Philadelphia, PA. Int J Radiat Oncol Biol Phys 38:127–132
17. Xu D, Li G, Li H, Jia F (2017) Comparison of IMRT versus 3D-CRT in the treatment of esophagus cancer: a systematic review and meta-analysis. Medicine (Baltimore) 96:e7685. https://doi.org/10.1097/MD.0000000000007685

Chapter 24

Systemic Therapy for Esophageal Squamous Cell Carcinoma

Ka On Lam, Wendy W. L. Chan, Tsz Him So, and Dora L. W. Kwong

Abstract

With more understanding of the tumor biology, esophageal squamous cell carcinoma (ESCC) and adenocarcinoma are increasingly recognized as different disease entities and are managed with different treatment approaches. Most patients with ESCC need systemic treatment at some point of their disease course, but only until recently, the progress in systemic treatment has been relatively stagnant compared with its adenocarcinoma counterpart. Platinum-based regimens remain the standard of care, while taxanes have been increasingly used upfront and in later lines of treatment. The attempts to personalize treatment for ESCC with various target therapies have been futile. Immune checkpoint inhibitors are now coming into play with promising activity and potentials to combine with different treatment modalities. The current chapter overviews the systemic treatment for ESCC and highlights the recent development.

Key words Esophageal squamous cell carcinoma, Chemotherapy, Target therapy, Immune checkpoint inhibitor

1 Introduction

Locoregional disease of ESCC is best managed with surgical resection with or without perioperative treatment, and 5-year overall survival (OS) of the cancer is in the range of 20–60% [1]. There is a propensity of benefit with neoadjuvant treatment for ESCC. In addition, the prognosis of advanced, metastatic disease is dismal and 5-year OS is <5%. Thus, most of the patients would require systemic treatment at some point during the disease course. Platinum, fluoropyrimidine, and more recently taxanes are common agents used in both the curative and palliative settings. Advancement in the knowledge of tumor biology challenges the practice of treating ESCC. To identify therapeutically relevant genomic alterations, Wang et al. performed next-generation sequencing on 302 advanced esophageal carcinomas and found more genomic alterations per sample for ESCC (esophageal squamous cell carcinoma vs. esophageal adenocarcinoma = 7.4:5.6). ESCC and esophageal adenocarcinoma had different sets of clinically relevant genomic alterations: *KRAS* (23% vs. 6%) and *ERBB2* (*HER-2*)

Alfred K. Lam (ed.), *Esophageal Squamous Cell Carcinoma: Methods and Protocols*, Methods in Molecular Biology, vol. 2129, https://doi.org/10.1007/978-1-0716-0377-2_24, © Springer Science+Business Media, LLC, part of Springer Nature 2020

(23% vs. 3%) occurred more frequently in esophageal adenocarcinoma whereas *PIK3CA* (24% vs. 10%), *PTEN* (11% vs. 4%), and *NOTCH* (17% vs. 3%) were enriched in ESCC [2]. The Cancer Genome Atlas (TCGA) performed a comprehensive molecular analysis on 164 carcinomas of the esophagus that were derived from both Western and Eastern populations. Again, molecular alterations vary between ESCC and esophageal adenocarcinoma with amplifications of *CCND1*, *SOX2*, and *TP63* more commonly detected in the former and higher frequency of *ERBB2 (HER2)*, *VEGFA*, *GATA4*, and *GATA6* in the latter. As expected, ESCC resembled squamous cell carcinomas of other organs more than esophageal adenocarcinoma [3]. The results partially explained the futility of target therapies that are active in esophageal adenocarcinoma but not in ESCC. It also called for a more histology-specific approach in designing future clinical trials for esophageal cancer.

1.1 Chemotherapy

ESCC usually presents late, and most of the patients require treatment with chemotherapy at some points during the course of their disease. Platinum, fluoropyrimidine, and taxanes are commonly used in various settings.

1.1.1 Perioperative

Neoadjuvant treatment has long been adopted for the treatment of ESCC and may promote tumor downstaging, facilitate resection, and eradicate potential micrometastasis. The landmark study by the Medical Research Council Oesophageal Cancer Working Party (OE02) randomized 802 previously untreated patients (ESCC: 31%) to surgery with or without 2 cycles of neoadjuvant cisplatin and 5-fluorouracil (5FU) [4]. OS was better in the chemotherapy arm (16.8 vs. 13.3 months, hazard ratio [HR] 0.79; $p = 0.004$) while HRs for treatment effect were the same for ESCC and esophageal adenocarcinoma (HR 0.78). The study result echoed in the Asian population when the JCOG9907 also reported superior 5-year OS with neoadjuvant over adjuvant cisplatin and 5FU (55% vs. 43%, HR 0.73; $p = 0.04$) [5]. Nevertheless, the clinical outcomes were still far from satisfactory, and attempts are being made to intensify the chemotherapy regimen (*see* **Note 1**). The ongoing JCOG1109 NEXT study (UMIN000009482) is a multicenter, randomized 3-arm study that compares neoadjuvant cisplatin +5FU versus cisplatin +5FU + radiotherapy versus docetaxel + cisplatin +5FU [6]. The study addresses whether intensifying the chemotherapy with a triplet regimen or with the addition of radiotherapy would improve clinical outcomes.

ESCC is sensitive to radiotherapy, and remarkable success has been achieved with the addition of concurrent radiotherapy to neoadjuvant chemotherapy. The Australasian Gastrointestinal Trials Group reported the updated meta-analysis in 2011 that included 4188 patients with about 3500 events from over 20 randomized trials. The HRs for all-cause mortality for neoadjuvant chemoradiotherapy and chemotherapy in ESCC were 0.80 and 0.92, respectively [7]. While the strategy with neoadjuvant chemoradiotherapy is commonly adopted, there has not been a standard regimen until recently. The CROSS study investigated the efficacy of weekly carboplatin + paclitaxel and concurrent radiotherapy in 368 patients (ESCC: 23%) with esophageal cancer [8]. The result was one of the most encouraging with neoadjuvant chemoradiotherapy: pathological complete response rate of 29% and OS of 49 months. Indeed, the long-term follow-up report suggested a highly promising outcome for ESCC (median OS 81.6 with neoadjuvant chemoradiotherapy vs. 21.1 months with surgery alone, HR 0.48; $p = 0.008$) [9]. The phase III randomized NEOCRTEC 5010 also reported similar outcomes with a neoadjuvant chemoradiotherapy regimen of vinorelbine and cisplatin [10]. The study regimen improved all study endpoints compared with surgery alone including R0 resection rate (98.4% vs. 91.2%; $p = 0.002$), OS (100.1 vs. 66.5 months, HR 0.71; $p = 0.025$) without increasing postoperative complications (*see* **Note 2**).

Compared to neoadjuvant approach, the evidence for adjuvant therapy is less convincing. Results of meta-analysis suggested a potential benefit of adjuvant chemotherapy over surgery alone in stage III or IV disease (RR = 0.43; $p = 0.00001$) but not stage I or II disease (RR = 1.12; $p = 0.68$) in terms of 3-year OS. The 5-year disease free survival was also in favor of adjuvant chemotherapy (RR = 0.79; $p = 0.04$) in those with positive lymph nodes [11]. Similarly, meta-analysis of adjuvant radiotherapy with or without chemotherapy suggested a potential benefit in terms of disease free survival but not OS [12] The meta-analysis results are hypothesis generating and future well-designed prospective study is warranted. At present, adjuvant therapy is not recommended in any of the international guidelines [13, 14] (*see* **Note 3**).

1.1.2 Palliative

The combination regimen of cisplatin and 5FU has been the standard of care for advanced ESCC over the past two decades [15–17]. In daily practice, many of the patients are not candidate for this regimen due to poor general condition, inadequate organ function, or comorbidities (*see* **Note 4**). Oxaliplatin, capecitabine, and S-1 are reasonable alternatives with better toxicity profile [18–20]. Taxanes may also have better tolerance and less dependent on renal function, which are often compromised in patients with ESCC due to various reasons [21–23]. In a phase II single-arm study of docetaxel reported by Muro et al., the response rate was 20% and the median OS was 8.1 months [24]. Combining docetaxel with cisplatin and 5FU was also feasible with high efficacy in early phase study. The JCOG1314 MIRACLE (UMIN000015107) study has been commenced in 2014 to confirm the superiority of 2-weekly docetaxel added to cisplatin and 5FU in a phase III randomized setting in Japan.

1.2 Target Therapy

Unlike esophageal adenocarcinoma, data to support target therapy for ESCC is scarce despite the latter having more genomic alterations per sample [2]. Mutation in *TP53* has been proposed as key factor in the carcinogenesis of ESCC as results from various whole-genome or whole-exome analyses have demonstrated a high frequency of somatic mutation in *TP53* (59–93%) [25–28]. In addition, various genes that involved in cell cycle regulations (*CCND1*, *CDKN2A*, *CDK4/6*, *MDM2*, *RB1*, *NFE2L2*, *CHEK1*, and *CHEK2*) or differentiation (*NOTCH1* and *NOTCH3*) were also altered in ESCC. The TCGA also reported alterations of *PIK3CA*, *PTEN*, or *PIK3R1* in 24% of tumors [3]. Nevertheless, most of these genetic alterations have not been identified as convincingly druggable targets and their discoveries have not yet been translated into clinical benefits so far.

1.2.1 Epidermal Growth Factor Receptor (EGFR)

Overexpression, rather than mutation, of EGFR is frequently found in ESCC and is associated with worse clinical outcomes. Moreover, nearly 80% of ESCC have downstream signaling pathway alterations involving *RAS* and *AKT* [25]. As such, targeting the EGFR signaling pathway is of potential therapeutic value.

Cetuximab, a chimeric monoclonal antibody against EGFR, was first studied in a randomized phase II study [17]. Addition of cetuximab to cisplatin and 5FU in first-line treatment improved overall response rate (ORR) (19% vs. 13%), progression free survival (PFS) (5.9 vs. 3.6 months), and OS (9.5 vs. 5.5 months). Nimotuzumab, a humanized anti-EGFR monoclonal antibody, combined with cisplatin and paclitaxel also showed efficacy and feasibility in a phase II study [29]. However, subsequent phase III POWER study that evaluated the addition of panitumumab, a fully human anti-EGFR monoclonal antibody, to cisplatin and 5FU was terminated after interim analysis for futility [30]. Overall, 71% of patients with panitumumab-chemotherapy vs. 51% of patients on chemotherapy alone had serious adverse events. Another phase 2/3 multicenter, randomized SCOPE1 study evaluated the role of cetuximab in chemoradiotherapy of esophageal cancer [31]. The primary endpoint was the treatment failure-free rate at week 24 for phase II and OS for phase III. The study was terminated due to futility at the interim analysis without continuation to phase III. The addition of cetuximab to chemoradiotherapy resulted in worse treatment failure-free rate at week 24 (66.4% vs. 76.9%), shorter median OS (22.1 vs. 25.4 months, HR 1.53; $p = 0.035$), and more treatment-related toxicities. The study enrolled both ESCC and esophageal adenocarcinoma, and detrimental effect of cetuximab was independent of histology type. Nevertheless, the study is still of reference value for ESCC as it represented 71% of patients in the cetuximab plus chemoradiotherapy arm. Lack of patient selection and absence of a valid predictive maker should be one of the underlying reasons for futility.

The COG study investigated the efficacy of gefitinib in chemotherapy-pretreated patients with esophageal cancer [32]. Gefitinib marginally prolonged the PFS (1.57 vs. 1.17 months, HR 0.80; $p = 0.02$) but not OS (3.73 vs. 3.67 months, HR 0.90; $p = 0.29$) over placebo. Gefitinib also improved patient-reported outcomes such as odynophagia in this advance setting. The outcomes were not different between ESCC and esophageal adenocarcinoma, but only 22% of patients were ESCC in the study arm. The subsequent companion biomarker study of COG (TRANS-COG) proposed that *EGFR* copy number gain might predict improved treatment outcomes with gefitinib [33]. *EGFR* copy number gain occurred in 15.6% of patients, and there was no significant correlation with any clinical features. At present, anti-EGFR monoclonal antibody cannot be recommended outside clinical trial setting. Further well-designed and biomarker-driven clinical trials are eagerly awaited.

1.2.2 Immune Checkpoint Inhibitor

Recognizing tumor cells and their eventual elimination from the body are crucial functions of our immune system. However, tumor cells are notorious for immune evasion that leads to the phenomenon of "immune escape" and development of cancer [34]. Programmed-death-1(PD-1) is a 55 kD type I transmembrane protein primarily expressed on activated T cells, B cells, myeloid cells, and antigen-presenting cells [35]. Binding of PD-1 to its ligands, PD-L1 and PD-L2, downregulates T-cell activation in both murine and human systems, leading to suppression of immune surveillance and cancer development [36–39]. Pembrolizumab and nivolumab are examples of monoclonal antibody against the PD-1 molecule, while atezolizumab, durvalumab, and avelumab are anti-PD-L1 monoclonal antibodies. These drugs have shown promising results in various cancers including melanoma [40, 41], renal cell carcinoma [42, 43], and non-small cell lung carcinoma [44–47]. PD-L1 or PD-L2 expression occurred in around half of ESCC patients [48]. They are also indicated for microsatellite instability high or mismatch repair protein deficient tumors, but these are uncommon in ESCC [3, 49]. The association of PD-L1 expression with worse clinical outcomes supports the rationale that blocking the interaction between PD-1 and its ligands might improve survival in ESCC. In the multi-cohort phase I KEYNOTE-028 study, pembrolizumab monotherapy demonstrated promising antitumor activity and manageable safety profile in patients having heavily pre-treated esophageal carcinoma with PD-L1 $\geq$ 1% [50]. Thirty-seven (41%) of 90 patients had PD-L1 positive tumor, and response was assessed in 23 of them. The ORR was 30.4%, and stable disease was observed in another 13.0% with a median duration of response of 40.0 weeks. Among the 18 patients with ESCC, the ORR was 27.8%. Based on these results, the subsequent phase II, single-arm KEYNOTE-180 study evaluated the activity of pembrolizumab monotherapy in patients with advanced, metastatic esophageal carcinoma who have failed two or more lines of therapy [51]. PD-L1 expression, defined as a combined positive score (CPS) of 10 or higher assessed by immunohistochemistry, was reported in 47.9%, and 52.1% of the 121 enrolled patients had ESCC. The ORR of the entire cohort was 9.9%, and numerically higher response rate was observed in those tumors with PD-L1 expression (ORR 13.8%) and ESCC (ORR 14.3%). The results were echoed in the phase II, single-arm ONO-4538-07 study in which nivolumab monotherapy was given in Japanese patients with ESCC refractory or intolerant to standard treatments [52]. PD-L1 expression was not required for study entry. Among the 64 evaluable patients, the ORR by Central Review was 17.2% and the responses were durable. Similar to pembrolizumab, nivolumab had a tolerable safety profile in patients with pre-treated ESCC, and there were no treatment-related deaths. The results of the phase III randomized KEYNOTE-181 study were presented at the American Society of Clinical Oncology Gastrointestinal Cancers Symposium 2019 [53]. The primary objectives were OS in patients with PD-L1 CPS $\geq$ 10, ESCC and in the total population. Compared with investigator's choice of chemotherapy (paclitaxel, docetaxel, and irinotecan), pembrolizumab monotherapy significantly improved OS in PD-L1 CPS $\geq$ 10 (9.2 vs. 6.7 months, HR 0.69; $p = 0.0074$) and ESCC (8.2 vs. 7.1 months, HR 0.78; $p = 0.0095$) but not in the total population (7.1 vs. 7.1 months, HR 0.89; $p = 0.0560$). In addition, the ORRs were significantly higher with pembrolizumab than chemotherapy. It reached 21.5% in PD-L1 CPS $\geq$ 10 (vs. 6.1% with chemotherapy; $p = 0.0006$), 16.7% in ESCC (vs. 7.4% with chemotherapy; $p = 0.0022$), and 13.1% in total population (vs. 6.7% with chemotherapy; $p = 0.0037$) (*see* **Note 5**).

While these reported studies have established the role of anti-PD1 monoclonal antibody in pre-treated ESCC, several questions remain unanswered. First, a more standardized method for assessment of PD-L1 expression and thus more precision selection is preferred. Currently, the eligibility of pembrolizumab and nivolumab studies was different with regard to PD-L1 status and definition of PD-L1 positivity (Table 1). It appeared that higher PD-L1 expression was associated with improved treatment outcomes, but negative PD-L1 did not necessarily equate to futility with anti-PD1 treatment. Second, the jury is still out for the optimal combination strategy. Pre-clinical and clinical data suggest that the combination of PD-1 and CTLA-4 receptor blockade may improve antitumor activity. In vitro combinations of nivolumab plus ipilimumab increase IFN-Y production over either agent alone. In a murine melanoma vaccine model, blockade with either CTLA-4 or PD-1

Table 1
Summary of landmark clinical trials of immune checkpoint inhibitors in esophageal squamous cell carcinoma (ESCC)

Study	Phase	N[a]	CPI	Definition of PD-L1 positivity	ORR (%)	PFS (months)	OS (months)
Published							
KEYNOTE-028	IB	18	Pem	≥1%[b]	27.8	1.8	7.0
KEYNOTE-180	II	63	Pem	CPS[c] ≥ 10	14.3	2.1	6.8
ONO-4538-07	II	65	Nivo	NA[d]	17.2	1.5	10.8
KEYNOTE-181	III	198	Pem	CPS[c] ≥ 10	16.7	2.2	8.2
Ongoing							
CHECKMATE-648	III	939[e]	Nivo + Ipi vs. CT + Nivo vs. CT alone	≥1%[b]	–	–	–
KEYNOTE-590	III	700[e]	CT + Pem vs. CT alone	CPS[c] ≥ 10	–	–	–

CPI checkpoint inhibitor, *ORR* objective response rate, *PFS* progression free survival, *OS* overall survival, *Pem* pembrolizumab, *Nivo* nivolumab, *Ipi* ipilimumab, *CT* chemotherapy, *CPS* combined positive score

[a]Number of ESCC only

[b]Percentage of scorable cells with membranous staining or the presence of a distinctive interface pattern in both neoplastic cells and contiguous mononuclear inflammatory cells

[c]CPS: defined as number of PD-L1 positive cells (tumor cells, macrophages, lymphocytes)/total number of tumor cells × 100

[d]Evaluable PD-L1 status required for study eligibility

[e]Target accrual number of all study arms

antibodies increased the proportion of CTLA-4- and PD-1-expressing CD4/CD8 tumor-infiltrating T effector cells, and dual blockade increased tumor infiltration of T effector cells with a decrease of intratumoral T regulatory cells, as compared to either agent alone [54]. On the other hand, chemotherapy causes tumor cell death and results in the release of tumor antigen delivery to antigen-presenting cells, which may enhance treatment efficacy with immune checkpoint inhibitors. The ongoing CHECKMATE-648 study (NCT03143153) and KEYNOTE-590 study (NCT03189719) may provide further insights. While both are global randomized controlled studies evaluating chemotherapy + anti-PD-1 monoclonal antibody in the first-line setting, the former also includes a third combination arm of anti-PD-1 and anti-CTLA-4 therapy. These studies have not yet completed accrual, but results are potentially practice changing (*see* **Note 6**).

1.2.3 Other Target Therapy

Other signaling pathways targeting *VEGF*, *HER2*, *mTOR*, *HGF*, and *COX-2* have been studied mostly in pre-clinical model or small-scale early phase clinical trials, but so far no significant therapeutic value has been demonstrated [55]. BKM120 is an oral pan-class I PI3K inhibitor and showed disease control rate of 51.2% in a phase II study involving 42 patients with ESCC [56]. The above results highlighted the difficulty in establishing a new standard of care in ESCC.

To conclude, systemic therapy remains an important component for the management of ESCC. However, there has been little progress with regard to chemotherapy and target therapy in the last decades. There is an unmet need for well-designed, biomarker-driven clinical trials dedicated to ESCC. Immune checkpoint inhibitors showed promising results and strategies to optimize their applications are ongoing.

2 Materials

2.1 Therapeutic Agents

1. Platinum: cisplatin, carboplatin, oxaliplatin.
2. Fluoropyrimidine: 5FU, capecitabine, S-1.
3. Taxanes: paclitaxel, docetaxel.
4. Immune checkpoint inhibitors: pembrolizumab.

2.2 Investigations

2.2.1 Pre-treatment Investigations

1. Nutritional assessment.
2. Blood tests: complete blood count, liver and renal function tests, hepatitis B serology; thyroid function test and serum cortisol if planned for immune checkpoint inhibitor.
3. Imaging: computed tomography of thorax, abdomen, and pelvis. Positron emission tomography is optional.
4. Endoscopic examination: tumour biopsy with esophagogastroduodenoscopy + endoscopic ultrasound. Assessment of bilateral vocal cords.
5. Cardiac assessment (if operable disease): echocardiogram.
6. Respiratory assessment (if operable disease or for radical chemoradiotherapy): lung function test.
7. Immunohistochemistry for PD-L1 and mismatch repair proteins (may include polymerase chain reaction for microsatellite instability) (for immune checkpoint inhibitor).

2.2.2 On-Treatment Investigations

1. Blood tests: complete blood count, liver and renal function tests; regular thyroid function test and serum cortisol if on immune checkpoint inhibitor.
2. Imaging: computed tomography of thorax, abdomen, and pelvis. Positron emission tomography is optional.

3 Methods

3.1 Neoadjuvant

1. CROSS: paclitaxel 50 mg/m^2 and carboplatin AUC 2 weekly for 5 weeks during concurrent radiotherapy.
2. MRC OE02: cisplatin 80 mg/m^2 day 1 + 5FU 1000 mg/m^2 days 1–4 every 3 weeks for 2 cycles.

3.2 Palliative

3.2.1 First Line

1. PF: cisplatin 80 mg/m^2 day 1 + 5FU 800 mg/m^2 days 1–5, every 3–4 weeks.

3.2.2 Second Line

1. Docetaxel: 60–75 mg/m^2 day 1 every 3 weeks.
2. Paclitaxel: 80 mg/m^2 day 1, 8, and 15 every 4 weeks.
3. Pembrolizumab: 200 mg day 1 every 3 weeks (if microsatellite instability-high or deficient mismatch repair protein).

3.2.3 Third Line or beyond

1. Pembrolizumab: 200 mg day 1 every 3 weeks.

4 Notes

1. Preoperative chemotherapy alone is less commonly practiced nowadays, but it can be considered in those patients who have received prior radiotherapy or other contraindications to radiotherapy.
2. Preoperative chemoradiotherapy should be considered in all eligible patients with locoregionally advanced esophageal squamous cell carcinoma.
3. There is a paucity of data supporting adjuvant treatment, either chemotherapy or target therapy, for resected squamous cell carcinoma. This must be judged on a case-by-case basis, taking into account the stage, lymph node, and resection margin status.
4. Patients with advanced ESCC are often old with compromised nutritional status and organ functions. Comprehensive nutritional counseling and assessment as well as close monitoring of organ functions are essential in those receiving palliative chemotherapy. Consideration should be given to less toxic regimens with monotherapy or carboplatin/oxaliplatin instead of cisplatin in selected cases.
5. Checking of the PD-L1, microsatellite instability status or mismatch repair protein facilitates patient selection for treatment with immune checkpoint inhibitor.

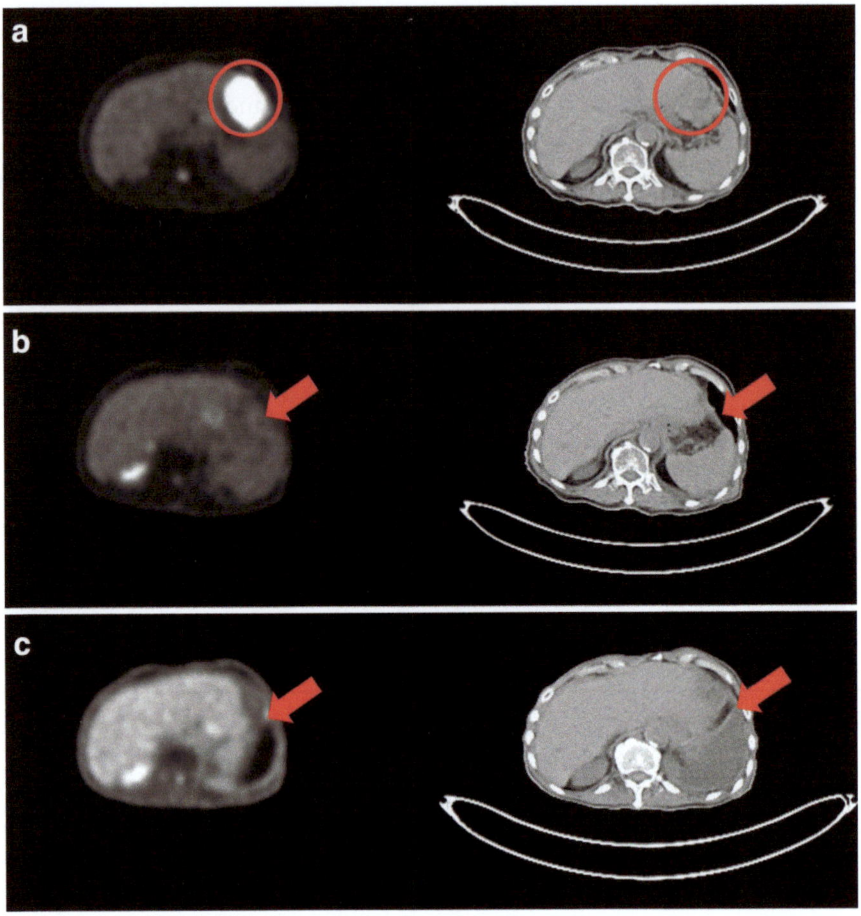

Fig. 1 Complete response of a metastatic carcinoma in abdominal lymph node lateral to segment II of liver in a patient treated with anti-PD1 monoclonal antibody [left, PET image; right, plain CT image]. (**a**) The metastatic carcinoma in a lymph node at pre-treatment scan [circled in RED]; (**b**) complete response after 4 months of treatment [RED arrow]; (**c**) durable complete response after 14 months of treatment [RED arrow]

6. Immune checkpoint inhibitor is active in heavily pre-treated patients but the time to response is usually longer (≥8 weeks) compared with chemotherapy (Fig. 1). Clinical trials are evaluating its role in the adjuvant and first-line setting.

References

1. Rice TW, Gress DM, Patil DT et al (2017) Cancer of the esophagus and esophagogastric junction-major changes in the American Joint Committee on Cancer eighth edition cancer staging manual. CA Cancer J Clin 67:304–317
2. Wang K, Johnson A, Ali SM et al (2015) Comprehensive genomic profiling of advanced esophageal squamous cell carcinomas and esophageal adenocarcinomas reveals similarities and differences. Oncologist 20:1132–1139
3. Cancer Genome Atlas Research Network and others (2017) Integrated genomic characterization of esophageal carcinoma. Nature 541:169–175
4. Medical Research Council Oesophageal Cancer Working Group (2002) Surgical resection with or without preoperative chemotherapy in

oesophageal cancer: a randomised controlled trial. Lancet 359:1727–1733

5. Ando N, Kato H, Igaki H et al (2012) A randomized trial comparing postoperative adjuvant chemotherapy with cisplatin and 5-fluorouracil versus preoperative chemotherapy for localized advanced squamous cell carcinoma of the thoracic esophagus (JCOG9907). Ann Surg Oncol 19:68–74
6. Kato K, Igaki H, Ito Y et al (2013) Next study (JCOG1109): a three-arm randomized phase III study comparing preoperative CDDP+5-FU(CF) versus docetaxel+CF versus CF-radiation followed by esophagectomy with D2-3 lymphadenectomy for locally advanced esophageal squamous cell cancer. J Clin Oncol 31(15_suppl):TPS4152-TPS4152
7. Sjoquist KM, Burmeister BH, Smithers BM et al (2011) Survival after neoadjuvant chemotherapy or chemoradiotherapy for resectable oesophageal carcinoma: an updated meta-analysis. Lancet Oncol 12:681–692
8. van Hagen P, Hulshof MC, van Lanschot JJ et al (2012) Preoperative chemoradiotherapy for esophageal or junctional cancer. N Engl J Med 366:2074–2084
9. Shapiro J, van Lanschot JJB, Hulshof MCCM et al (2015) Neoadjuvant chemoradiotherapy plus surgery versus surgery alone for oesophageal or junctional cancer (CROSS): long-term results of a randomised controlled trial. Lancet Oncol 16:1090–1098
10. Yang H, Liu H, Chen Y et al (2018) Neoadjuvant chemoradiotherapy followed by surgery versus surgery alone for locally advanced squamous cell carcinoma of the esophagus (NEOCRTEC5010): a phase III multicenter, randomized, open-label clinical trial. J Clin Oncol 36:2796–2803
11. Zhang SS, Yang H, Xie X et al (2014) Adjuvant chemotherapy versus surgery alone for esophageal squamous cell carcinoma: a meta-analysis of randomized controlled trials and nonrandomized studies. Dis Esophagus 27:574–584
12. Pasquali S, Yim G, Vohra RS et al (2017) Survival after neoadjuvant and adjuvant treatments compared to surgery alone for resectable esophageal carcinoma: a network meta-analysis. Ann Surg 265:481–491
13. NCCN Guidelines on Esophageal and Esophagogastric Junction Cancers. Version 2.2018
14. Lordick F, Mariette C, Haustermans K, Obermannová R, Arnold D (2016) Oesophageal cancer: ESMO clinical practice guidelines for diagnosis, treatment and follow-up. Ann Oncol 27:v50–v57
15. Bleiberg H, Conroy T, Paillot B et al (1997) Randomised phase II study of cisplatin and 5-fluorouracil (5-Fu) versus cisplatin alone in advanced squamous cell oesophageal cancer. Eur J Cancer 33:1216–1220
16. Levard H, Pouliquen X, Hay JM et al (1998) 5-fluorouracil and cisplatin as palliative treatment of advanced oesophageal squamouscell carcinoma. A multicentre randomised controlled trial. The French Associations for Surgical Research. Eur J Surg 164:849–857
17. Lorenzen S, Schuster T, Porschen R et al (2009) Cetuximab plus cisplatin-5-fluorouracil versus cisplatin-5-fluorouracil alone in first-line metastatic squamous cell carcinoma of the esophagus: a randomized phase II study of the Arbeitsgemeinschaft Internistische Onkologie. Ann Oncol 20:1667–1673
18. Qin TJ, An GL, Zhao XH et al (2009) Combined treatment of oxaliplatin and capecitabine in patients with metastatic esophageal squamous cell cancer. World J Gastroenterol 15:871–876
19. Wang J, Chang J, Yu H et al (2013) A phase II study of oxaliplatin in combination with leucovorin and fluorouracil as first-line chemotherapy in patients with metastatic squamous cell carcinoma of esophagus. Cancer Chemother Pharmacol 71:905–911
20. Akutsu Y, Kono T, Uesato M et al (2013) S-1 monotherapy as second- or third-line chemotherapy for unresectable and recurrent esophageal squamous cell carcinoma. Oncologia 84:305–310
21. Zhang X, Shen L, Li J et al (2008) A phase II trial of paclitaxel and cisplatin in patients with advanced squamous-cell carcinoma of the esophagus. Am J Clin Oncol 31:29–33
22. Huang J, Zhou Y, Zhang H et al (2013) A phase II study of biweekly paclitaxel and cisplatin chemotherapy for recurrent or metastatic esophageal squamous cell carcinoma: ERCC1 expression predicts response to chemotherapy. Med Oncol 30:343
23. Liu Y, Ren Z, Yuan L et al (2016) Paclitaxel plus cisplatin vs. 5-fluorouracil plus cisplatin as first-line treatment for patients with advanced squamous cell esophageal cancer. Am J Cancer Res 6:2345–2350
24. Muro K, Hamaguchi T, Ohtsu A et al (2004) A phase II study of single-agent docetaxel in patients with metastatic esophageal cancer. Ann Oncol 15:955–959
25. Song Y, Li L, Ou Y et al (2014) Identification of genomic alterations in oesophageal squamous cell cancer. Nature 509:91–95

26. Lin DC, Hao JJ, Nagata Y et al (2014) Genomic and molecular characterization of esophageal squamous cell carcinoma. Nat Genet 46:467–473
27. Gao YB, Chen ZL, Li JG et al (2014) Genetic landscape of esophageal squamous cell carcinoma. Nat Genet 46:1097–1102
28. Zhang L, Zhou Y, Cheng C et al (2015) Genomic analyses reveal mutational signatures and frequently altered genes in esophageal squamous cell carcinoma. Am J Hum Genet 96:597–611
29. Zhang X, Jia J, Lu M et al (2017) Nimotuzumab plus paclitaxel and cisplatin as 1st line treatment for unresectable esophageal squamous cell carcinoma: Longterm follow-up of survival in a phase II study. J Clin Oncol 35 (15_suppl):e15573
30. Moehler MH, Thuss-Patience PC, Brenner B et al (2017) Cisplatin/5-FU (CF) +/− panitumumab (P) for patients (pts) with non-resectable, advanced, or metastatic esophageal squamous cell cancer (ESCC): an open-label, randomized AIO/TTD/BDGO/EORTC phase III trial (POWER). J Clin Oncol 35(15_suppl):4011–4011
31. Crosby T, Hurt CN, Falk S et al (2013) Chemoradiotherapy with or without cetuximab in patients with oesophageal cancer (SCOPE1): a multicentre, phase 2/3 randomised trial. Lancet Oncol 14:627–637
32. Dutton SJ, Ferry DR, Blazeby JM et al (2014) Gefitinib for oesophageal cancer progressing after chemotherapy (COG): a phase 3, multicentre, double-blind, placebocontrolled randomised trial. Lancet Oncol 15:894–904
33. Petty RD, Dahle-Smith A, Miedzybrodzka Z et al (2014) Epidermal growth factor receptor copy number gain (EGFR CNG) and response to gefitinib in esophageal cancer (EC): results of a biomarker analysis of a phase III trial of gefitinib versus placebo (TRANS-COG). J Clin Oncol 32(15_suppl):4016
34. Swann JB, Smyth MJ (2007) Immune surveillance of tumors. J Clin Invest 17:1137–1146
35. Keir ME, Butte MJ, Freeman GJ, Sharpe AH (2008) PD-1 and its ligands in tolerance and immunity. Annu Rev Immunol 26:677–704
36. Freeman GJ, Long AJ, Iwai Y et al (2000) Engagement of the PD-1 immunoinhibitory receptor by a novel B7 family member leads to negative regulation of lymphocyte activation. J Exp Med 192:1027–1034
37. Latchman Y, Wood CR, Chernova T et al (2001) PD-L2 is a second ligand for PD-1 and inhibits T cell activation. Nat Immunol 2:261–268
38. Carter LL, Fouser LA, Jussif J et al (2002) PD-1: PD-L1 inhibitory pathway affects both CD4+ and CD8+ T cells and is overcome by IL-1. Eur J Immunol 32:634–643
39. Barber DL, Wherry EJ, Masopust D et al (2006) Restoring function in exhausted CD8 T cells during chronic viral infection. Nature 439:682–687
40. Larkin J, Chiarion-Sileni V, Gonzalez R et al (2015) Combined Nivolumab and Ipilimumab or Monotherapy in untreated melanoma. N Engl J Med 373:23–34
41. Robert C, Long GV, Brady B et al (2015) Nivolumab in previously untreated melanoma without BRAF mutation. N Engl J Med 372:320–330
42. Motzer RJ, Tannir NM, McDermott DF et al (2018) Nivolumab plus Ipilimumab versus Sunitinib in advanced renal-cell carcinoma. N Engl J Med 378:1277–1290
43. Motzer RJ, Escudier B, McDermott DF et al (2015) Nivolumab versus everolimus in advanced renal-cell carcinoma. N Engl J Med 373:1803–1813
44. Paz-Ares L, Luft A, Vicente D et al (2018) Pembrolizumab plus chemotherapy for squamous non-small-cell lung cancer. N Engl J Med 379:2040–2051
45. Gandhi L, Rodríguez-Abreu D, Gadgeel S et al (2018) Pembrolizumab plus chemotherapy in metastatic non-small-cell lung cancer. N Engl J Med 378:2078–2092
46. Borghaei H, Paz-Ares L, Horn L et al (2015) Nivolumab versus docetaxel in advanced non-squamous non-small-cell lung cancer. N Engl J Med 373:1627–1639
47. Antonia SJ, Villegas A, Daniel D et al (2018) Overall survival with durvalumab after Chemoradiotherapy in stage III NSCLC. N Engl J Med 379:2342–2350
48. Ohigashi Y, Sho M, Yamada Y et al (2005) Clinical significance of programmed death-1 ligand-1 and programmed death-1 ligand-2 expression in human esophageal cancer. Clin Cancer Res 11:2947–2953
49. Le DT, Uram JN, Wang H et al (2015) PD-1 blockade in tumors with mismatch-repair deficiency. N Engl J Med 372:2509–2520
50. Doi T, Piha-Paul SA, Jalal SI et al (2018) Safety and antitumor activity of the anti–programmed death-1 antibody pembrolizumab in patients with advanced esophageal carcinoma. J Clin Oncol 36:61–67
51. Shah MA, Kojima T, Hochhauser D et al (2019) Efficacy and safety of pembrolizumab for heavily pretreated patients with advanced, metastatic adenocarcinoma or squamous cell

carcinoma of the esophagus: The phase 2 KEYNOTE-180 Study. JAMA Oncol 5 (4):546–550. https://doi.org/10.1001/jamaoncol.2018.5441

52. Kudo T, Hamamoto Y, Kato K et al (2017) Nivolumab treatment for oesophageal squamous-cell carcinoma: an open-label, multicentre, phase 2 trial. Lancet Oncol 18:631–639
53. Kojima T, Muro K, Francois E et al (2019) Pembrolizumab versus chemotherapy as second-line therapy for advanced esophageal cancer: Phase III KEYNOTE-181 study. J Clin Oncol 37(suppl 4).; abstr 2
54. Curran MA, Montalvo W, Yagita H et al (2010) PD-1 and CTLA-4 combination blockade expands infiltrating T cells and reduces regulatory T and myeloid cells within B16 melanoma tumors. Proc Natl Acad Sci U S A 107:4275–4280
55. Digklia A, Voutsadakis IA (2013) Targeted treatments for metastatic esophageal squamous cell cancer. World J Gastrointest Oncol 5:88–96
56. Kato K, Doi T, Kojima T et al (2017) Phase II study of BKM120 in patients with advanced esophageal squamous cell carcinoma (EPOC1303). J Clin Oncol 35 (15_suppl):4069–4069

Chapter 25

Surgical Protocols for Squamous Cell Cancer of the Esophagus

María Carmen Fernández Moreno and Simon Law

Abstract

Surgery is the mainstay treatment for esophageal squamous cell carcinoma (ESCC). A major development in surgical therapy for esophageal cancer in the past two or three decades has been the marked reduction in surgical mortality rates as a result of improvement in staging technologies, patient selection, perioperative support systems, and surgical experience. Minimally invasive techniques are also becoming widely adopted. Protocol for surgical management of squamous cell cancer of the esophagus is described herein.

Key words Esophageal squamous cell carcinoma, Surgery, Esophagectomy, Lymphadenectomy, Complications, Morbidities, Minimally invasive esophagectomy

1 Introduction

1.1 Depth of Invasion for ESCC and Relation to Incidence of Nodal Metastases

Superficial esophageal cancers, whose invasion is limited to the mucosa or the submucosa, are categorized as in-situ cancer (Tis) and T1 tumor. T1 cancers are divided into T1a and T1b subcategories, depending on the depth of invasion. T1a cancers are further subclassified into: M1 or EP, intraepithelial cancer; M2 or LPM, cancer with invasion into the lamina propria mucosae; and M3 or MM, cancer reaching the muscularis mucosae. T1b tumors are divided into three categories: SM1, cancer with invasion into the superficial one third of the submucosa; SM2, cancer with invasion into the middle third of the submucosa; and SM3, cancer with invasion into the lower third of submucosa [1]. Advanced tumors include those whose invasion extends into or beyond the muscularis propria irrespective of the presence of regional lymph node metastases (T2–T4 tumors).

For lesions involving muscularis mucosa only, the rate of lymph node metastasis is about 9.3%, but when the depth of invasion reaches the submucosal layer, the rate of metastasis can be as high as 50%, and so endoscopic treatment may not be curative [1]. Endoscopic therapy is recommended for M1 and M2 lesions, while SM2

Alfred K. Lam (ed.), *Esophageal Squamous Cell Carcinoma: Methods and Protocols*, Methods in Molecular Biology, vol. 2129, https://doi.org/10.1007/978-1-0716-0377-2_25,

and SM3 tumors should not be resected endoscopically. For M3 and SM1 (up to 200 μm) cancers, endoscopic therapy is generally investigational and should be selected with care. Although circumferential lesions can be resected with endoscopic methods, the chance of resultant stricture is also high and has some bearing on the choice of therapy. Inaccuracies of preoperative diagnosis also dictate detailed pathological assessment of the resected specimens before the procedure can be regarded as curative. Additional therapies must be considered for cancers that do not meet the criteria for cure.

For relatively early disease (T1 disease not reaching the curative criteria for endoscopic treatment, T2 cancers with no nodal involvement), upfront esophagectomy is an option. For more advanced cancers, neoadjuvant therapy in the form of chemotherapy or chemoradiotherapy is often indicated. Definitive chemoradiation is used for patients who decline surgery, those deemed not to have enough physiological reserve to withstand an esophagectomy, or those with cervical esophageal tumor with intent of laryngeal preservation. In general, transthoracic approach with extended lymphadenectomy should be carried out. There is increasing evidence that extended nodal dissection for ESCC is not only important in improving staging of disease and prognostic but has therapeutic gain in enhancing survival [2–4].

2 Materials

Various surgical options exist for esophagectomy, which may depend on the location of tumor, the intended extent of lymphadenectomy, whether neoadjuvant therapies have been given or not, the organ used for esophageal substitution, route of reconstruction, and the preference of the surgeons. The following protocol refers to standard surgical resection of intrathoracic ESCC, and variations will be discussed in different sections.

2.1 Patient Selection

2.1.1 Disease Staging

Patients require accurate tumor staging to select the appropriate patients, maximize chance of complete (R0) resection, and select those for neoadjuvant therapies. All patients need preoperative staging and evaluation, including computed tomography (CT) scan of the chest and abdomen, upper gastrointestinal endoscopy and endoscopy coupled with endoscopic ultrasound (EUS), as well as bronchoscopy for patients with lesions situated at or above the carina to exclude airway involvement. Fluoroxyglucose-18 positron emission computed tomography (PET) has also become a standard imaging study. Percutaneous ultrasonography of the neck ± fine needle aspiration cytology of cervical lymph nodes is also useful.

2.1.2 Physiological Assessment

Radical surgery for esophageal carcinoma is an invasive procedure. Although recent advances in surgical techniques, anesthetic procedures, and perioperative management have led it to safer and more radical treatment, postoperative morbidities remain high [5]. Therefore, it is desirable that application of radical surgery be decided with due caution after evaluation of the patient conditions:

1. Performance status (PS): Performance status is a simple and useful index commonly used for comprehensive evaluation of the patient's general condition. Esophageal carcinoma patients with PS scores of 0–2 are generally considered as suitable candidates for radical surgery [6].
2. Pulmonary function tests: Pulmonary function test results are important indices for deciding the advisability of thoracotomy. Whether or not thoracotomy is indicated should be judged comprehensively, considering the results of spirometry, arterial blood gas analysis, chest radiography findings, CT findings, smoking history, and past medical history. Forced expiratory volume in 1 s (FEV1) % and diffuse capacity of the lungs for carbon monoxide (DLCO) have been reported to be independent predictive factors for postoperative respiratory complications [7].
3. Cardiac function tests: In principle, surgery is not indicated in patients with heart failure due to valvular disease or cardiomyopathy, severe arrhythmia, or myocardial infarction within 3 months prior to the onset. A resting or exercise electrocardiography (ECG) can be carried out for assessment. If any abnormality is found, the patient should be subjected to Holter ECG monitoring, echocardiography, cardiac catheterization, or exercise stress perfusion imaging.
4. Hepatic function tests: In cases of chronic hepatitis or hepatic cirrhosis, surgical treatment should be considered based on a comprehensive evaluation of blood counts and the results of blood coagulation tests, blood biochemistry tests, and hepatitis screening. Patients with significant cirrhosis should be carefully considered for surgery as results are generally poor.
5. Other considerations: Other diseases should be evaluated comprehensively such as mental disorders, acute-phase cerebrovascular disorder, depression, dementia to be referred for professional evaluation, etc.

2.2 Preoperative Preparations

Enhanced recovery after surgery (ERAS) programs have been employed successfully in many institutions and are shown to improve outcome. Major guidelines are published for its adoption [8–10]. The protocol used at the authors' institution is shown in Table 1. Many of the principles of ERAS are adopted.

Table 1
Proposed protocol of perioperative management for esophagectomy

Preoperative	
–Preoperative counseling	
–Nutritional assessment	Nasogastric tube feeding for those with significant stenosis of the esophagus, and oral supplement in those at risk of malnutrition
–Preoperative exercise	General and incentive spirometry + pre-habilitation program
–Stop smoking and alcohol intake	
–Chest physiotherapy	
–Carbohydrate loading on the day of surgery	No solid food 6 h before and fluid 2 h before surgery. Carbohydrate loading night before and finishes 2 h before surgery
–No need for bowel preparation unless colonic interposition is planned	
Intraoperative	
–Prophylactic antibiotics	
–Deep vein thrombosis prophylaxis	Mechanical ± pharmacological
–Judicious use of intraoperative fluids	
–Avoid hypothermia	
–Minimally invasive surgery if possible	
–Epidural analgesia	
Postoperative	
–Nutrition	POD1 carbohydrate drink, gradual advancement to soft diet by POD5 (if no vocal cord palsy and assessment by speech therapist shows no risk of aspiration) PPN/TPN (peripheral parenteral nutrition/total parenteral nutrition) in those at nutritional risk and oral intake insufficient
–Nasogastric tube	Removal on POD1 (if no vocal cord palsy and assessment by speech therapist shows no risk of aspiration)
–Analgesia	Epidural analgesia/patient-controlled analgesia/ multimodal analgesia
–Chest drain	Single closed small caliber drain (^{19}Fr Blake drain, which does not require underwater seal), removal POD 3–4 when output <200–300 ml per day
–Early mobilization	From POD1, supervised by physiotherapist
–Urinary catheter	Early removal as soon as close monitoring of urine output is not essential
–Intravenous fluid	Balanced intravenous fluid to avoid over- and under-hydration
–Deep vein thrombosis prophylaxis	

POD post-operation day

The following preoperative measures should be instituted:

1. Cessation of smoking and alcohol intake.
2. Incentive spirometry and chest physiotherapy ± pre-habilitation program.
3. Optimization of bronchodilator therapy in patients with asthma or significant chronic obstructive airway disease.

4. In patients with high-grade esophageal tumor stenosis, a fine-bore nasogastric tube can be placed for nutritional support while workup is performed and is preferable over parenteral nutrition, gastrostomy, or jejunostomy feeding. Oral nutritional supplementation is given [11].
5. Diabetic control should be optimized.
6. Immediate preoperative preparations include prophylactic antibiotics to be given at anesthesia induction and deep vein thrombosis prophylaxis. Bowel preparation is not necessary, unless a colonic interposition is intended.
7. Preoperative patient education and counseling.

3 Methods

The type of esophageal resection is dictated by the location of the tumor, the intended lymphadenectomy, the available choices for conduit, as well as by the surgeon's experience and preference.

3.1 Location of the Tumor and Implications

For intrathoracic ESCC, the standard approach will be a transthoracic esophagectomy with complete mediastinal lymphadenectomy. The esophageal anastomosis can be constructed in the right thoracic cavity (an Ivor Lewis or Lewis Tanner operation), or in the neck (three-phase/hole or McKeown esophagectomy). In general, the longer the proximal resection margin can be achieved, the less likely the margin will be involved and less recurrence at the anastomosis will occur. Therefore, for a lower third esophageal tumor, a choice generally exists for a cervical or intrathoracic anastomosis since there is ample proximal esophagus. For upper thoracic lesion, in order to gain enough margin, it is logical to place the anastomosis in the neck.

3.2 Lymphadenectomy

Nodal status is one of the most important prognostic factors in ESCC. Extended lymphadenectomy improves the staging accuracy, is prognostic, and evidences suggest that it improves survival. The National Comprehensive Cancer Network (NCCN) Guidelines for Oesophageal Cancers in the United States recommends that at least 15 lymph nodes should be removed for adequate nodal staging. The optimum number of nodes to be removed and examined after preoperative chemoradiation is unknown, although similar lymph node resection is generally recommended [2, 4].

3.2.1 Types of Lymphadenectomy

Lymphadenectomy is classified by the number of "fields" of nodal dissection; the three fields are cervical, mediastinal, and upper abdominal fields. Surgery should include at least a two-field (mediastinal and upper abdominal) lymphadenectomy. The third field (neck) is selectively carried out.

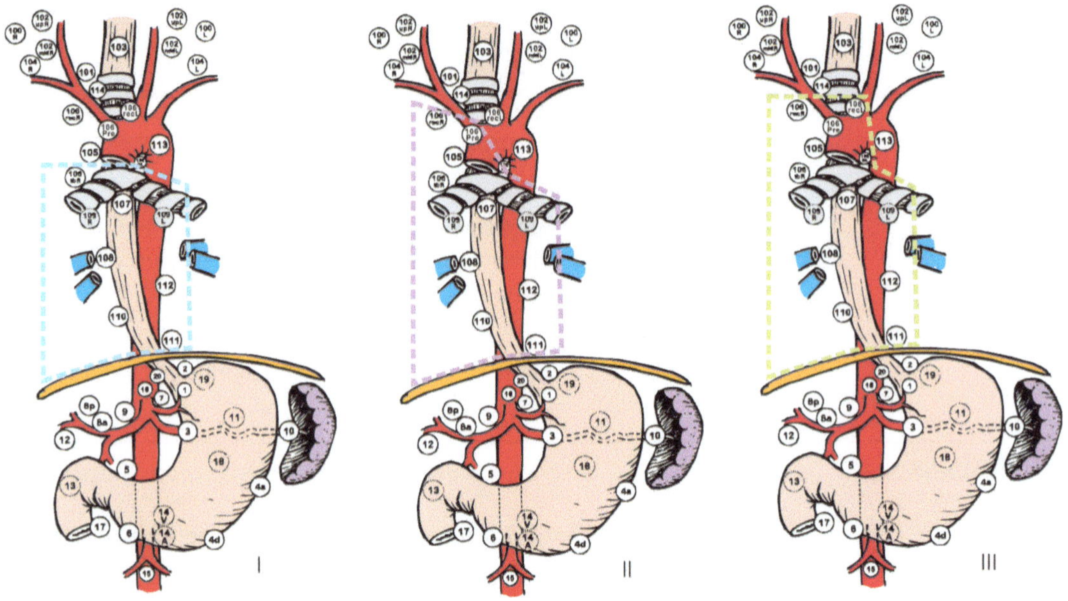

Fig. 1 Figure showing the various types of mediastinal lymphadenectomy. I: Standard, II: Extended, and III: Total mediastinal lymphadenectomy

There is little controversy with upper abdominal lymphadenectomy, which includes nodes along the celiac trunk, common hepatic and splenic arteries, as well as the lymph nodes along the lesser gastric curvature and in the lesser omentum. Morbidity and difficulties are low and is routinely carried out by most surgeons.

The additional second field of the mediastinum is further divided into (Fig. 1):

1. Standard: Lymphadenectomy of the posterior mediastinum, from the diaphragm up to the subcarinal area below the tracheal bifurcation.
2. Extended: Standard lymphadenectomy + right paratracheal region up to the nodes along the right recurrent laryngeal nerve and the brachiocephalic trunk.
3. Total: Adding to the extended dissection, the lymph nodes located in the left paratracheal region including lymph nodes alongside the left recurrent laryngeal nerve.

Three-field nodal dissection includes the first and second fields as well as a dissection in the neck to clear the brachiocephalic, deep lateral and external cervical nodes, and the right and left recurrent nerve lymphatic chains (deep anterior cervical nodes).

The most appropriate extent of lymphadenectomy remains a contentious issue, and in the context of multimodality treatment is even more complicated. In general, for ESCC, at least a total two-field lymphadenectomy should be performed. The concept of three-field lymphadenectomy, where bilateral cervical, complete mediastinal, and celiac trifurcation nodal dissection are carried out, has been championed mainly in Japan but is also routine in specialized centers in the East. It is important to state that the technique focuses on dissection along both recurrent laryngeal nerves; in that sense this should be treated as one entity extending from the infra-aortic area along the two recurrent laryngeal nerves to the neck. The high prevalence of nodal metastases and recurrence rates in this cervico-upper thoracic segment is the basis of such extended nodal dissection [12]. It is usually indicated for mid and upper third ESCC.

Three-field nodal dissection can achieve excellent results; such extensive surgery is accompanied by morbidities, especially more recurrent laryngeal nerve palsies, so its adoption should be selective balancing risks and benefits for individual patients.

3.3 Surgical Approaches for Resection

The esophagus extends anatomically from the cervical through the thoracic region into the abdominal region; there are several methods to carry out the esophageal cancer surgery (Fig. 2).

1. McKeown approach is a three-phase esophagectomy that consists of mobilization of the thoracic esophagus and lymphadenectomy followed by abdominal and neck incisions for the preparation of the esophageal substitute and its delivery to the neck for a cervical anastomosis.
2. Lewis-Tanner (or Ivor Lewis) procedure is a two-phase esophagectomy consisting of laparotomy for gastric mobilization

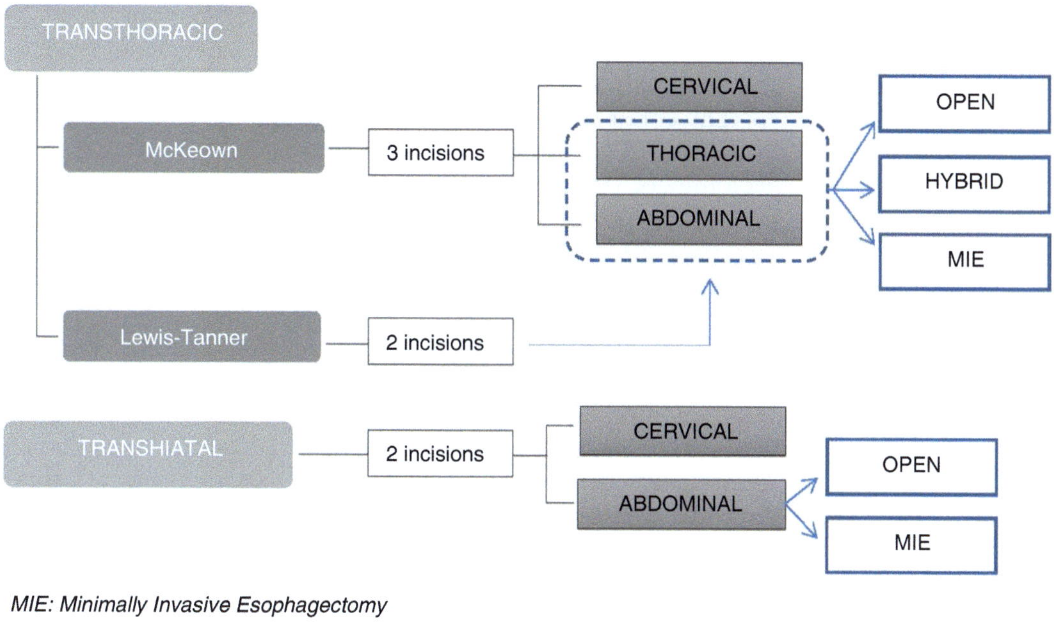

Fig. 2 Several surgical approaches in esophageal squamous cell carcinoma

and tubularization, followed by a right thoracotomy for esophageal resection and gastric pull-up for esophagogastrostomy.

3. Transhiatal approach is performed through laparotomy and left cervical incision; the esophagus is mobilized via the neck and through the diaphragmatic hiatus. The mobilization of the esophagus is partly a blind procedure, and adequate mediastinal lymphadenectomy cannot be carried out fully and safely. It is generally considered unsatisfactory for ESCC and will not be further discussed.
4. Minimally invasive techniques are gaining impetus in recent years. The same operation as open surgery can be carried out using a combination of video-assisted thoracoscopy (VATS) and laparoscopy (total minimally invasive esophagectomy MIE), or hybrid approaches whereby one phase is carried out with VATS or laparoscopy and the other phase by open approach. These techniques are becoming the preferred approach at many institutions because of reduced surgical trauma and lower respiratory complications, promoting earlier functional recovery and better quality of life [13, 14].

3.4 Reconstruction: Organ for Esophageal Substitution and Route of Reconstruction

Reconstruction of intestinal continuity is usually restored with a gastric conduit. The gastroplasty is easy to prepare, is reliable, and only one anastomosis is required. When the stomach is not available (such as previous gastrectomy) or when concomitant gastric resection is needed (such as synchronous stomach cancer), the colon (right ileo-colic, left, or transverse colon) can be used. This requires more extensive gastrointestinal mobilization and three anastomoses are required. Failing this, a long jejunal loop can be prepared. This can usually reach the tracheal bifurcation. If it is required to reach the neck, additional blood supply with "supercharge" and microvascular anastomosis is usually needed.

The conduit, usually the stomach, can be placed in the right thoracic cavity for intrathoracic anastomosis (Lewis-Tanner esophagectomy), or via the orthotopic route (posterior mediastinal) to the neck. The retrosternal (substernal) route is another option. The subcutaneous route to the neck is uncommonly used because of cosmesis.

3.5 Surgical Technique

3.5.1 Open Surgical Resection Method

Positioning and Anesthetic Technique

The patient is first placed in the supine position for the abdominal part of the surgery. To prepare for the subsequent right thoracotomy, a double-lumen endotracheal tube is usually positioned. At the author's institution, it is routine practice to place a single-lumen endotracheal tube, and during the thoracotomy phase, a right bronchial blocker is placed. This results in less airway trauma, and the more flexible tube allows better exposure of areas behind the trachea and around the left main bronchus. In the thoracic phase of surgery, the patient is placed in a full lateral decubitus position with the right arm approximately at a right angle at the shoulder.

Judicious use of intravenous fluid is important to avoid overhydration. Epidural analgesia for postoperative pain relief is standard practice. Other meaures to enhance postopearative outcome include avoidance of hypothermia, meticulous surgical technique.

As mentioned, esophagectomy can be carried out using different approaches. The following sections describe the different phases but can be combined in different ways and sequences depending on situation. For example, when a Lewis-Tanner operation is planned, the abdominal phase will precede the thoracic phase and an intrathoracic anastomosis is carried out. When a three-phase esophagectomy is selected, usually the thoracic phase will be first, followed by the abdominal and cervical phases. However, this operation can also be carried out with the abdominal and cervical phases first, with the conduit delivered to the neck for a cervical esophago-gastrostomy. This is then followed by the thoracic phase when the esophagus is taken out. The surgeon must be versatile in selecting the appropriate operation depending on clinical need.

Operating Technique: Abdominal Phase

Steps of Operation:

1. A midline or a bilateral subcostal incision is made. The author prefers the latter because it gives improved exposure to the upper abdomen, especially in obese patients.
2. The stomach is mobilized. The gastrocolic omentum is taken off the greater curvature of the stomach preserving the right gastroepiploic vessels and arcades (Fig. 3). Complete omentum resection is not necessary. The left crus is exposed when the

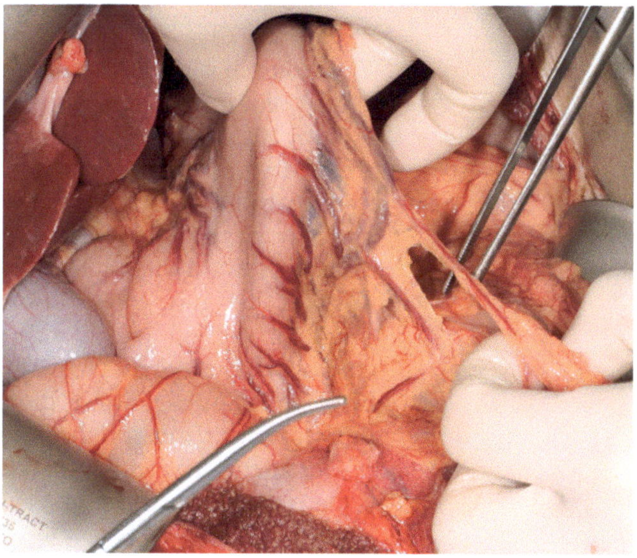

Fig. 3 Picture showing the gastro-colic ligament being divided. The right gastroepiploic vessels must be carefully preserved as this is the only reliable blood supply to the stomach tube

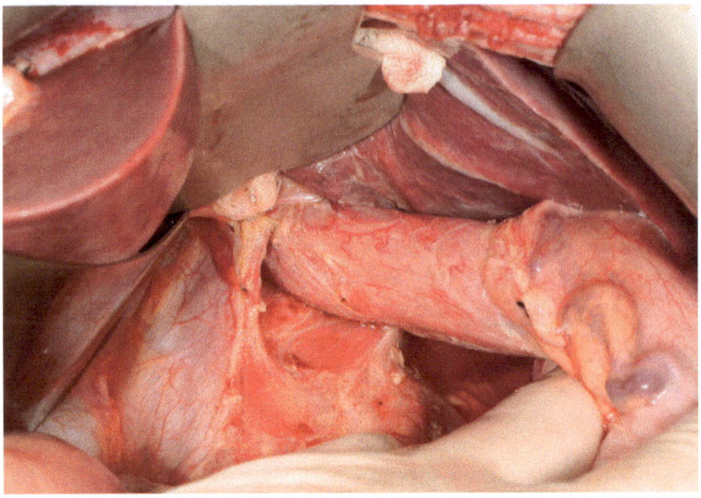

Fig. 4 The abdominal esophagus is mobilized from the esophageal hiatus. Both vagi have been divided

short gastric vessels are divided and the fundus mobilized medially. The phrenoesophageal membrane is detached and the abdominal esophagus and cardia can be freed on the left side.

3. The gastrohepatic ligament is then detached from the liver and from the portal structures. The anterior vagus nerve can be divided at this point. The esophagus is thus freed on both sides as well as anteriorly (Fig. 4). A sling placed around the lower esophagus, such as a Penrose or latex drain, may help later dissection by providing retraction.
4. The stomach is then reflected upward, and dissection is begun at the celiac trifurcation. Using fine electrocautery, dissection is performed along the anterior aspect of the common hepatic artery. Lymphadenectomy can then proceed laterally toward the hepatoduodenal ligament (Fig. 5). It is enough to remove nodes along the anterior surface of the common hepatic artery. Medially toward the origin of the left gastric artery at the celiac axis, the left gastric or coronary vein requires ligation. The origin of the left gastric artery is identified separately as it comes off the celiac axis, and it is doubly ligated and cut between ligatures. Further dissection toward the left will clear the lymphatic tissues on the proximal splenic artery. The areolar tissue superior to the common hepatic artery and splenic artery is therefore cleared en bloc with the abdominal esophagus toward the hiatus.
5. On the lesser curvature, the right gastric vessels are divided at the angular incisura (Fig. 6). One linear stapler is used to transect the stomach from this point upward toward the fundus. This is the first of a series of stapler used to transect the

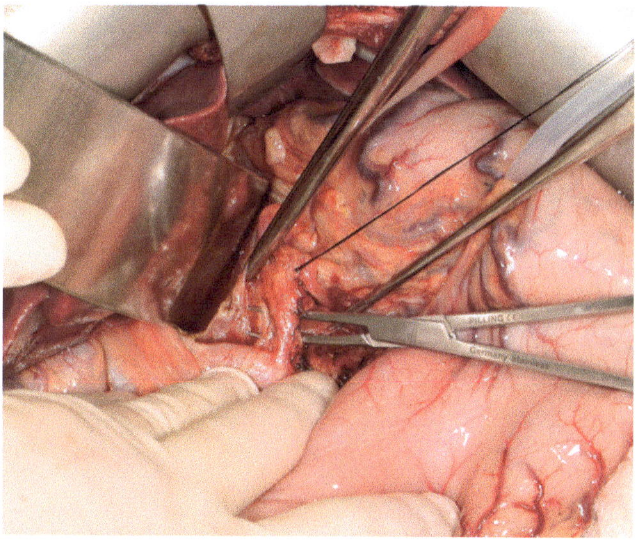

Fig. 5 Coeliac trifurcation lymphadenectomy. The left gastric artery is seen coming off the coeliac axis. The coronary vein has been ligated and divided (black stitch). The surface of the hepatic artery is clearly seen

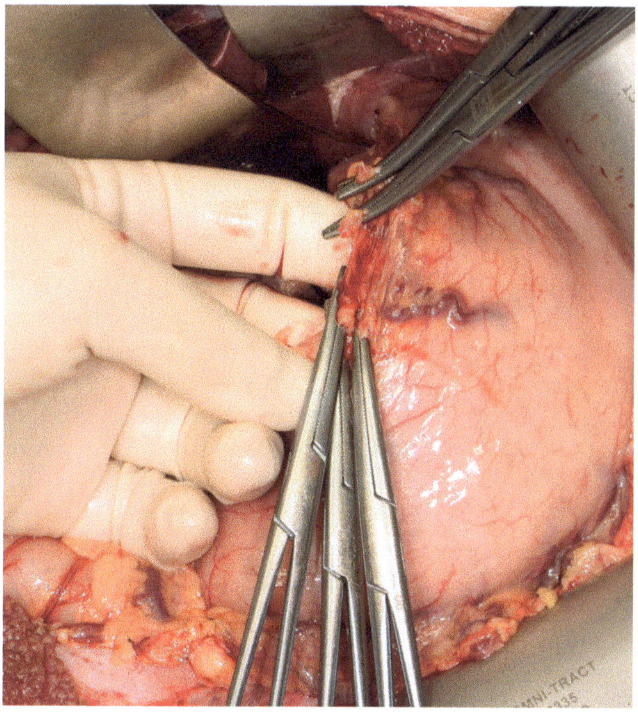

Fig. 6 The lesser curvature of the stomach is prepared; this point should be located at least distal to the third branch from the left gastric artery for an adequate lymphadenectomy. It can be more distally located if a narrower gastric tube is intended

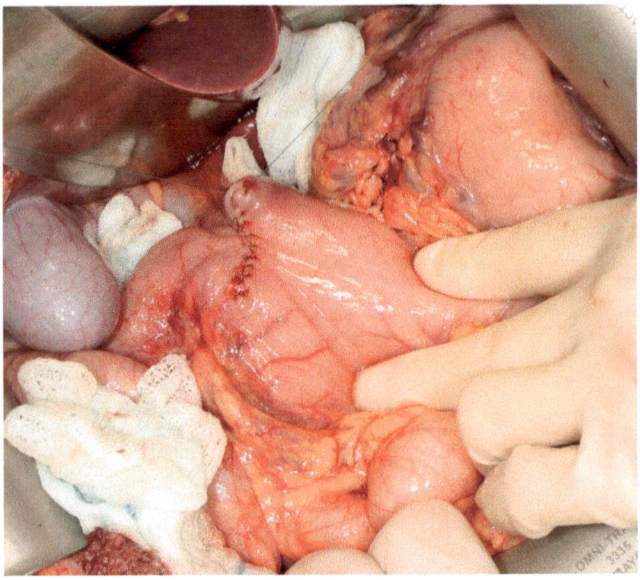

Fig. 7 A Heineke-Mikulicz pyloroplasty is performed

stomach to make a narrow gastric conduit. The application of one stapler at this stage of the operation will make the subsequent use of further staplers during the thoracic phase easier (*see* **Note 1**).

6. A Heineke-Mikulicz pyloroplasty is then performed although some surgeons would forgo his step (Fig. 7) (*see* **Note 2**). A Kocher maneuver is not mandatory provided the stomach is of enough length. However, this maneuver is easily performed and does have the advantage of straightening the "axis" of the pyloroduodenal region when the stomach is brought up to the right thoracic cavity. After careful hemostasis, the abdomen is closed. Abdominal drains are not required.

Operating Technique: Thoracic Phase

Steps of Operation:

1. A posterolateral thoracotomy through the fifth intercostal space is usually performed. Alternatively, an anterolateral thoracotomy can also be done with sparing of the latissimus dorsi. A controlled fracture of sixth rib posteriorly eases distraction of the rib space. Two rib spreaders placed at right angles to each other are used to open the rib space (Fig. 8).
2. The arch of the azygos vein as it crosses the esophagus is divided and transfixed. The right bronchial artery, which can be quite sizable, runs just beneath the vein. It can be preserved if desired. The superior mediastinal segment of the esophagus can be mobilized close to its wall. The mediastinal pleura is opened on the back of the trachea. The esophagus is freed from the back of the trachea anteriorly and posteriorly from the spine; it can be slung with a tape to ease later dissection. Dissection is carried out to near the apex.

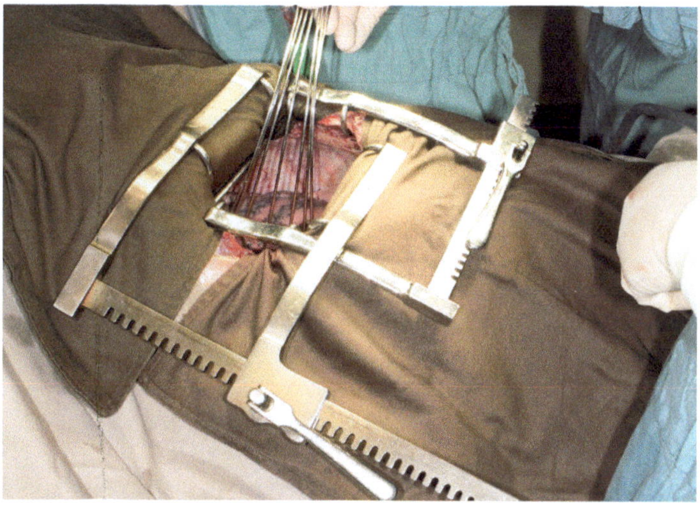

Fig. 8 Two rib spreaders placed at right angles to each other allow good exposure

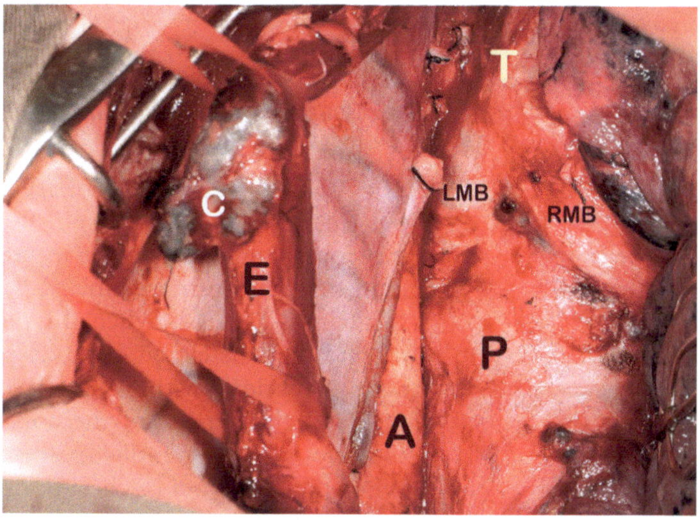

Fig. 9 Appearance after lower mediastinal dissection; the trachea (T), bronchi (LMB, RMB), pericardium (P), aorta (A) are clearly seen. The esophagus and carinal lymph nodes are resected en bloc (E and C)

3. The inferior pulmonary ligament is divided with electrocautery to the root of the inferior pulmonary vein. Dissection is then continued on the posterior surface of the pericardium. The right main bronchus is identified, and lymph nodes and connective tissue inferior to it are taken together with the esophagus. Further dissection will lead to the infracarinal lymph node package. The infracarinal dissection is followed toward the left to expose the left main bronchus and the lymph nodes and fatty tissues inferior to its edge (Fig. 9).

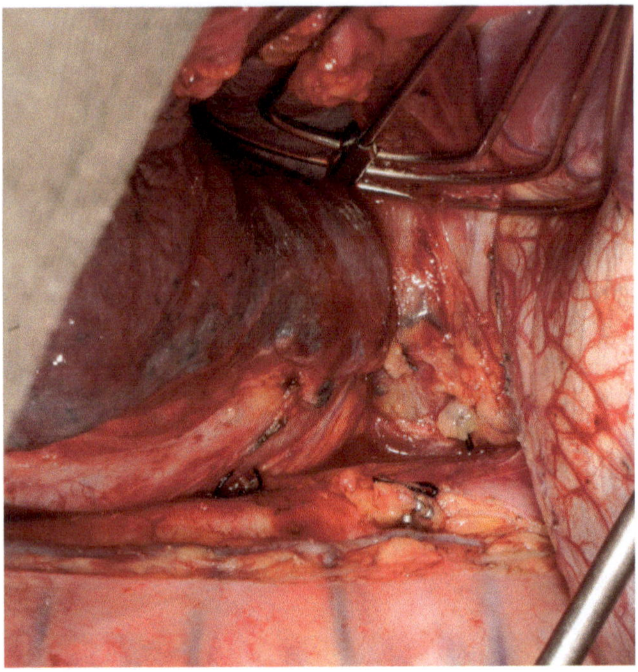

Fig. 10 The thoracic duct has been resected; the anal side was ligated on the surface of the aorta and marked with a metal clip

4. The mediastinal pleura is incised along the anterior aspect of the length of the azygos vein from above downward. Some surgeons remove the whole length of the azygos vein and its branches. The posterior limit of dissection can be defined using the vein as a guide. When the point just above the hiatus is reached, the dissection plane deepens onto the surface of the aorta. Anteriorly within the areola tissue between the azygos vein and the surface of the aorta is the thoracic duct. The thoracic duct is identified, isolated, and ligated (Fig. 10). When the dissection reaches the esophagus anteriorly, the thoracic duct, the areolar, and connective tissue on the aorta is removed en bloc with the esophagus (*see* **Note 3**). This resection continues from below upward, until the previous dissection plane from anteriorly on the left main bronchus is met. The limits of the lymph node dissection extend inferiorly to the crura of the diaphragm, anterior on the pericardium, right main bronchus, apically at the tracheal bifurcation, and posteriorly from the left main bronchus along the length of the descending aorta. Further dissection upward should meet the previously slung upper esophagus so that the whole intrathoracic esophagus is freed. The subaortic nodes could be removed at this point just above the left main bronchus, taking care not to damage the left recurrent laryngeal nerve medially, and the left pulmonary artery on the deep limit of dissection.

5. After esophageal mobilization and mediastinal nodal dissection, the gastric tube is delivered up through the diaphragmatic hiatus into the right chest. The gastric conduit can be tailored by starting transection at a chosen point of the fundus downward toward the already fired stapler from the distal lesser curvature during the abdominal phase of the operation. Usually two to three more linear staplers are necessary. A Satinsky clamp is then applied across the supra-aortic segment of the esophagus near the apex of the thoracic cavity. The esophagus is divided distal to the clamp. The esophagus with the cancer is removed. The gastric tube is placed in the mediastinum ready for anastomosis, which is performed either using a hand-sewn method or stapling (both circular and linear stapling work well, depending on the surgeon's preference) (Fig. 11).
6. After hemostasis, the thoracotomy is closed with a silicone chest drain (size 24 Fr) connected to underwater seal. Alternatively a simple closed suction drain can be used without the need for underwater seal, if no lung adhesions have required lysis [15]. This type of small drain is much more comfortable for the patient and encourages early mobilization as no underwater seal is needed.

The description above relates to a Lewis-Tanner esophagectomy, standard infracarinal lymphadenectomy, and intrathoracic anastomosis. For ESCC, most surgeons would perform extended or complete mediastinal dissection. Additional technique of superior mediastinal dissection is detailed below (Fig. 12).

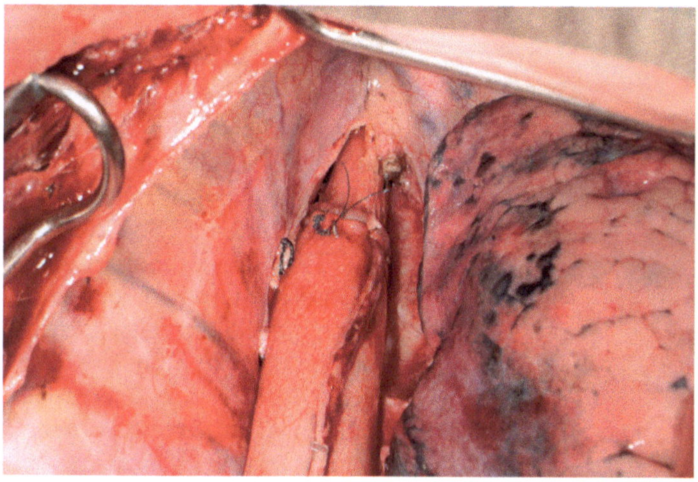

Fig. 11 The esophago-gastrostomy has been completed at the apex of the thoracic cavity using a hand-sewn technique

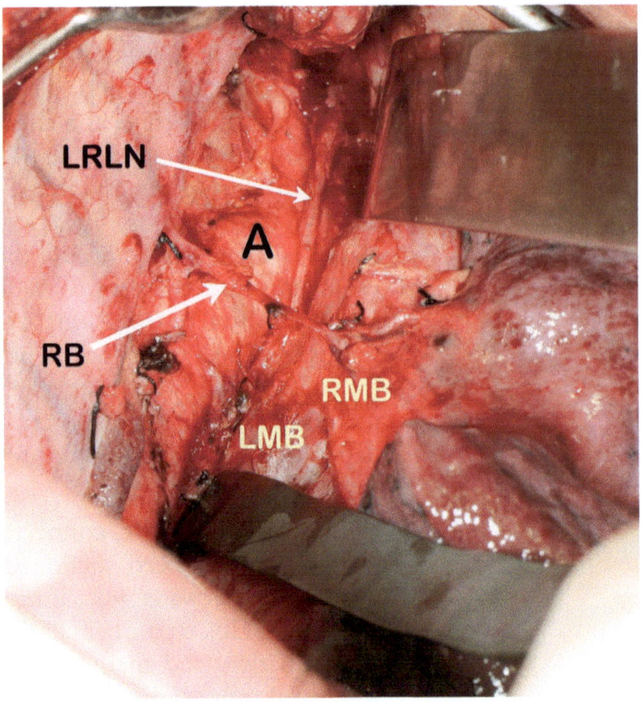

Fig. 12 Superior mediastinal lymphadenectomy. LRLN (left recurrent laryngeal nerve), A (aorta), RB (right bronchial artery), RMB (right main bronchus), LMB (left main bronchus). The right recurrent laryngeal nerve is at the apex outside the view in this figure

Superior Mediastinal Lymph Node Dissection (*See* **Note 4**)

1. After the arch of the azygos vein is divided, attention is turned to the right paratracheal area. The right vagus nerve is easily identified. The mediastinal pleura over it is opened and the nerve traced upward to the base of the subclavian artery. The right recurrent laryngeal nerve is found when the fatty tissue inferior to the subclavian artery and posterior to the vagus is dissected. The vagus from the neck and the recurrent laryngeal nerve together form the two prongs of a "fork" straddling the subclavian artery. Lymph nodes are removed with the fatty tissue. These nodes connect with the cervical paratracheal and paraesophageal nodes superior to the subclavian artery, which can be removed later in the cervical phase of the operation. One should be cautious in the use of electrocautery to avoid thermal injury to the recurrent laryngeal nerve. The use of a nerve stimulator as in thyroid surgery can aid identification of the nerve and its preservation.
2. The dissection of the left paratracheal area (left recurrent laryngeal nerve chain) is better commenced with the esophagus slung with a tape retracting it posteriorly but retaining the fibroareolar tissue attachment to the trachea (the mesentery). In this manner, the left recurrent laryngeal nerve is more easily

located within this "mesentery." If the esophagus has been isolated first, then the left recurrent laryngeal nerve tends to remain deeper in the left paratracheal area and therefore more difficult to dissect, especially the nodal tissues anterior to the nerve. A combination of blunt and sharp dissection longitudinally helps locate the left recurrent laryngeal nerve. Once the nerve is identified, lymph node tissue anterior to it in the paratracheal area is removed. This continues toward the apex of the thoracic cavity, reaching an area that can be dissected later from the neck. The thoracic duct, which has been isolated from below—its distal portion can be identified running upward—can be resected.

3. The recurrent laryngeal nerve is also traced downward on the aortic arch. The infra-aortic arch nodes can be removed by dissecting posteriorly toward the spine. In this area, the left bronchial artery arising from the arch of the aorta can be preserved. It is also very important not to injure the left pulmonary artery in the subaortic area.

Operating Technique: Cervical Phase

1. A left transverse supraclavicular incision is made extending from just beyond the sternocleidomastoid muscle to the right of the midline suffices. The left side is chosen because at this level the esophagus is more inclined to the left. Dissection is limited to medial to the carotid sheath. Once the middle thyroid vein is divided and the thyroid retracted to the right, the trachea and esophagus will come into view, especially when this follows the thoracic phase. Dissection of the esophagus should be easy if sufficient dissection has been performed from below. Next, attention is turned to isolating the esophagus from the trachea. Dissection should be made as close as possible to the esophageal wall. Traction and compression to the tracheoesophageal groove should be avoided to preserve the recurrent laryngeal nerve. A sling around the esophagus with a tape helps with retraction. If the thoracic phase precedes the cervical phase, a tape around the esophagus in the superior mediastinum, with the tails pushed up in the left paraesophageal area, will aid retrieval of the esophagus in the neck as the tape is readily located once the space medial to the carotid sheath is opened.
2. The conduit (usually stomach) can be delivered to the neck via the posterior mediastinal or retrosternal route for a cervical esophago-gastrotomy. If cervical lymphadenectomy is carried out, this is carried out in the standard fashion. Esophageal cancer rarely spreads above the level of the omohyoid muscle. So level IV, V, and VI nodal dissections are usually enough. The retrosternal route is easily created with blunt dissection from above (neck) and below (abdomen). It is usually avascular, and bleeding is uncommon.

Operating Technique: Minimally Invasive Esophagectomy

1. Video-Assisted Thoracoscopic Esophagectomy
   (a) A double-lumen endobronchial tube is introduced for single-lung ventilation, but a single-lumen endotracheal tube with a right bronchial blocker is preferred. The patient is placed in a left lateral decubitus position as for a posterolateral thoracotomy (Fig. 13). The right arm is raised to expose the armpit. This will allow more unimpeded use of thoracoscopic instruments. The surgeon stands at the back of the patient, and the first assistant stands on the opposite site. The second assistant using the videoscope stands next to the surgeon on his left side. His position will need to change to his right during the latter part of the operation when the videoscope changes direction. Two monitors are used: one opposite to the surgeon near the head end of the table and the other opposite to the first assistant.
   (b) Mobilization of the esophagus is begun by first incising the mediastinal pleura overlying the esophagus below the level of the inferior pulmonary vein. Once a short segment of esophagus is mobilized, a sling (a polydioxanone suture

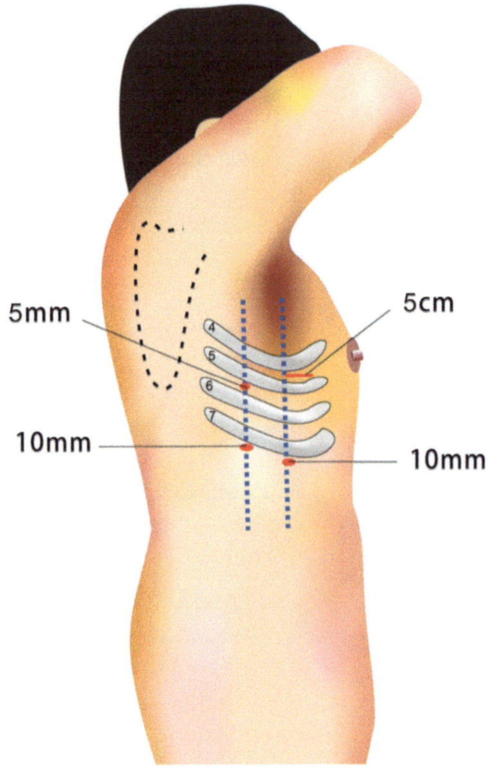

Fig. 13 Port sites used for video-assisted thoracoscopic surgery (VATS) esophagectomy. When superior mediastinal nodal dissection is carried out, an additional port at the third space posterior axillary line is often added

[PDS] 1 suture) is placed around the esophagus to ease retraction. Dissection essentially follows the same routine as in open surgery. The division of the azygos vein arch is eased using endovascular stapler. Once the posterior aspect of the esophageal dissection and periaortic tissue including the thoracic duct is dissected, the videoscope can switch to the seventh space port at the mid-axillary line. Anterior dissection along the right bronchus, carina, and left bronchus can proceed. Once infracarinal dissection is finished, the superior mediastinal lymphadenectomy can be performed just as that described in the section on open surgery. Dissection around the recurrent laryngeal nerves must be particularly meticulous; judicious use of energy source will lessen the chance of nerve injury. After the thoracoscopic phase is completed, the wounds can be closed with a small chest tube placed via the seventh spaceport pointing at the apex. The laparoscopic and cervical phase of the operation can then proceed.

2. Laparoscopic Gastric Mobilization
   (a) The patient is turned to the supine position with the legs apart (Fig. 14). The surgeon stands on the right side, the

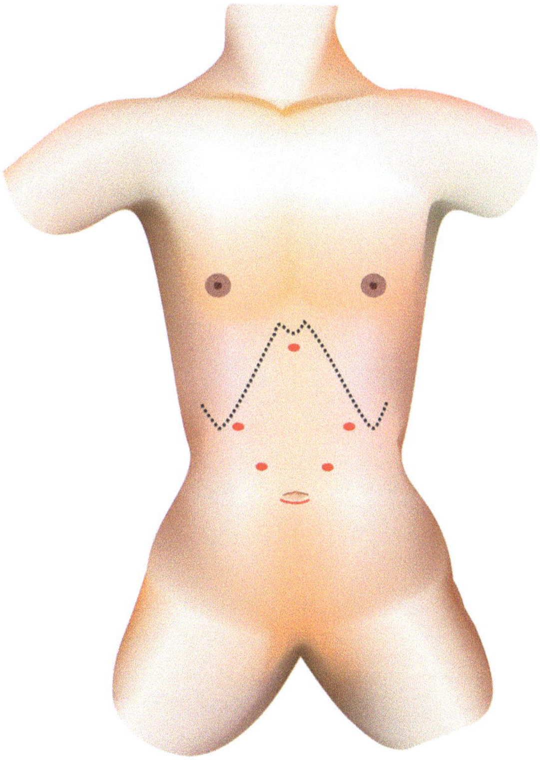

Fig. 14 Port sites used for laparoscopic gastric mobilization

first assistant on the left side, and the second assistant in between the legs holding the videoscope. The first port is placed with a sub-umbilical cut-down technique. Pneumoperitoneum is established. A 5-mm epigastric port is placed just below the xiphoid, and this is converted immediately into a Nathanson liver retractor. One 5-mm port is placed just below the right costal margin slightly medial to the anterior axillary line; another 10-mm port is placed in between this port and the umbilical port about one fist-length away. Two 5-mm ports are placed in the left side in similar positions. The gastric mobilization and lymphadenectomy are performed just like the open procedure as described.

(b) The abdominal esophagus is then divided using endostapler. The epigastric port is converted to a 5-cm midline mini-laparotomy. A silicone wound retractor is placed. The mobilized stomach is pulled outside the abdomen. The lesser curvature of the stomach is prepared just like in open surgery, and linear staplers are used to transect the stomach to make it into a gastric tube. The stomach can be delivered to the neck via the posterior mediastinal or retrosternal route for anastomosis.

3.6 Postoperative Management

The appropriate selection of surgical procedure, its meticulous execution, and perioperative care have causal relationship with morbidity and mortality. For most patients, a standardized clinical pathway is helpful, along the lines of enhanced recovery after surgery (ERAS) protocol (Table 1):

1. Most patients have endotracheal tube extubation in the recovery room, unless the surgery has been prolonged, complicated, or performed in high-risk patients.
2. Epidural analgesia is most important in postoperative pain relief. It is continued for the first 4–5 days after surgery and can be replaced by patient-controlled analgesia or oral medications. Recently, a propensity score-matched analysis revealed that postoperative scheduled intravenous acetaminophen decreased the rate of opioid use and may contribute to ERAS program for esophagectomy [16].
3. At the author's unit, the nasogastric tube is usually removed the day after surgery. Early removal of the tube results in more comfort and facilitates coughing. There is no need to replace the tube unless progressive dilatation of the gastroplasty is seen, but this is uncommon with a narrow gastric tube with a drainage procedure.
4. All patients have a bronchoscopic examination on the first postoperative day to check for recurrent laryngeal nerve injury,

although this is unusual in the absence of superior mediastinal or cervical lymphadenectomy. Judicious use of intravenous fluid is also important to avoid over-hydration and pulmonary edema.

5. Chest physiotherapy is instituted, and early ambulation encouraged.
6. Deep vein thrombosis prophylaxis is continued.
7. Chest drain is removed on day 4–5 post operation; the daily output should be less than 200–300 ml per day.
8. Liquid by mouth is started on day 1 post operation; usually, a carbohydrate drink can be taken as sips of fluid. Generally, by day 3–4 patients can take a liquid diet freely. A soft diet is started on day 5 post operation. The early oral intake does not increase the incidence of anastomotic leak and pneumonia (*see* **Note 5**) [17]. An oral contrast study is not routine unless leakage is suspected or if there is evidence of delayed gastric emptying. The author does not place feeding jejunostomy as a routine because early oral alimentation is successful in most patients, and most do not need supplementary nutritional support. Should oral intake be delayed, such as when anastomotic leak occurs, endoscopic placement of a naso-duodenal tube for feeding will suffice. A feeding jejunostomy is placed in high-risk patients who may be significantly malnourished preoperatively.

4 Notes

1. Conduit ischemia—Preparation of the gastric conduit requires care. The method of gastroplasty may affect vascular perfusion. The length of the right gastroepiploic arcade varies among individuals but the blood supply of the fundus of the stomach relies more on the intramural plexus. A narrower gastric tube may compromise the blood supply to the stomach (significant contribution comes from the lesser curvature side has been removed), but then the tube is longer and the suboptimally perfused top of the stomach can be resected. A wider gastric tube on the other hand tends to have a better blood supply but is shorter. Recent advances in indocyanine green fluorescence angiography allows for intraoperative assessment of gastric perfusion, with the potential to reduce the incidence of ischemia and anastomotic leak [18]. Other studies suggest that ischemic conditioning of the stomach as a staged procedure prior to esophagectomy improves perfusion of the gastric conduit but the results are inconclusive [19].

Gross ischemia of the conduit usually presents early, within the first 2–3 days after operation. Sepsis is obvious. However, in the early stage, signs may be subtle, which could simply be unexplained tachycardia, atrial arrhythmia, or poor arterial oxygenation [20]. It is important to treat this complication expeditiously so that further deterioration does not occur. A low threshold for endoscopic examination is recommended to examine the state of the conduit and anastomosis whenever there are signs of deterioration. Gross ischemia dictates taking down of the conduit, adequate drainage, and staged reconstruction later once sepsis is under control. In selected cases with ischemia limited to a small portion of the gastric conduit, when the patient is hemodynamically stable with minimal sepsis, and when an adequate length of stomach remains after resection of the ischemic portion, immediate re-anastomosis is an option.

2. Delayed gastric emptying—A routine pyloric drainage procedure is helpful but does not eliminate this complication because of other contributory factors. Mal-rotation of the gastric conduit is rare but is serious and should prompt immediate re-exploration. A larger gastric tube has more tendency of gastric retention, especially when an Ivor Lewis operation is performed; the redundant part of the stomach tends to form a pocket above the diagram, which turns anteriorly and medially before coming through the diaphragmatic hiatus into the abdomen. The stomach placed in the retrosternal route (when a cervical anastomosis is elected) also has less chance of delayed emptying.
3. Chylothorax—Routine mass ligation of areolar tissue on the aorta just above the hiatus should lessen the chance of chylous leak. Persistently high output from the chest tube, often more than a liter a day, should prompt the search for this complication. A milk challenge via a nasogastric tube or by mouth looking at the color change of the drain effluent into a milky fluid is diagnostic. Other biochemical parameters that could be looked at include triglyceride level and the presence of chylomicrons in the drain output after milk challenge. After the diagnosis is confirmed, low output chylothorax (less than 1 1L per day) could be treated by a short period of nil by mouth with total parenteral nutrition, or a diet with mid-chain triglyceride. Early surgical re-exploration however has a higher chance of success and prevents deterioration related to constant loss of lymphocytes and proteins from the effluent fluid. Preoperative lymphangiogram may help locate the site of chylous leak [21].
4. Recurrent laryngeal nerve injury—This should be uncommon unless bilateral recurrent laryngeal nerve lymphadenectomy is carried out. In these cases, it is most often due to careless and

forceful retraction. When it is unilateral, it would result in hoarseness of voice, poor cough effort, and increased chance of aspiration. When it is bilateral, airway patency could be compromised, and tracheostomy and delayed feeding may be required. Long-term quality of life is also affected.

5. Anastomotic leak—Conduit vascular perfusion plays a significant part in the etiology of this complication. The actual technique of anastomosis probably is less important than its proper application. Thus, hand-sewn or stapled methods should have similar leak rates [22, 23]. Cervical anastomosis tends to have a higher leak rate compared to intrathoracic leaks, though it is believed to be less lethal because drainage is more easily accomplished. Death from leaks should be uncommon with modern management. The location and magnitude of the leak can be visualized by a water-soluble contrast study. A carefully performed flexible endoscopic examination is also helpful. For small contained leaks, CT-guided drainage of pockets of collection may suffice. In septic patients with a sizable leak, exploration is warranted. Direct repair is seldom possible or effective; drainage is the key. Injection of fibrin glue or placement of intraluminal stents is increasingly used to treat leaks; sealing of the leak allows early control of sepsis and resumption of oral alimentation. The stent can be removed afterward, depending on the severity of the leak in the first place. Usually, 4–6 weeks will suffice for adequate healing.

References

1. Kitagawa Y, Uno T, Oyama T, Kato K, Kato H, Kawakubo H, Kawamura O, Kusano M, Kuwano H, Takeuchi H, Toh Y, Doki Y, Naomoto Y, Nemoto K, Booka E, Matsubara H, Miyazaki T, Muto M, Yanagisawa A, Yoshida M (2019) Esophageal cancer practice guidelines 2017 edited by the Japan esophageal society: part 1. Esophagus 16 (1):1–24. https://doi.org/10.1007/s10388-018-0641-9
2. Peyre CG, Hagen JA, DeMeester SR, Altorki NK, Ancona E, Griffin SM, Holscher A, Lerut T, Law S, Rice TW, Ruol A, van Lanschot JJ, Wong J, DeMeester TR (2008) The number of lymph nodes removed predicts survival in esophageal cancer: an international study on the impact of extent of surgical resection. Ann Surg 248(4):549–556
3. Tong D, Law S (2013) Extended lymphadenectomy in esophageal cancer is crucial. World J Surg 37(8):1751–1756. https://doi.org/10.1007/s00268-013-2068-8
4. Rizk NP, Ishwaran H, Rice TW, Chen LQ, Schipper PH, Kesler KA, Law S, Lerut TE, Reed CE, Salo JA, Scott WJ, Hofstetter WL, Watson TJ, Allen MS, Rusch VW, Blackstone EH (2010) Optimum lymphadenectomy for esophageal cancer. Ann Surg 251(1):46–50
5. Low DE, Kuppusamy MK, Alderson D, Cecconello I, Chang AC, Darling D, Davies A, D'Journo XB, Gisbertz SS, Griffin M, Harwick R, Hoelscher A, Hofstetter W, Jobe B, Kitagawa Y, Law S, Mariette C, Maynard N, Morse CR, Nafteux P, Pera M, Pramesh CS, Puig S, Reynolds JV, Schroeder W, Smithers M, Wijnhoven PL (2019) Benchmarking complications associated with esophagectomy. Ann Surg 269 (2):291–298
6. Audisio RA, Ramesh H, Longo WE, Zbar AP, Pope D (2005) Preoperative assessment of surgical risk in Oncogeriatric patients. Oncologist 10(4):262–268. https://doi.org/10.1634/theoncologist.10-4-262
7. Ferguson MK, Celauro AD, Prachand V (2011) Prediction of major pulmonary

complications after esophagectomy. Ann Thorac Surg 91(5):1494–1501. https://doi.org/10.1016/j.athoracsur.2010.12.036

8. Low DE, Allum W, De Manzoni G, Ferri L, Immanuel A, Kuppusamy M, Law S, Lindblad M, Maynard N, Neal J, Pramesh CS, Scott M, Mark Smithers B, Addor V, Ljungqvist O (2019) Guidelines for perioperative care in esophagectomy: enhanced recovery after surgery (ERAS((R))) society recommendations. World J Surg 43(2):299–330. https://doi.org/10.1007/s00268-018-4786-4
9. Markar SR, Karthikesalingam A, Low DE (2015) Enhanced recovery pathways lead to an improvement in postoperative outcomes following esophagectomy: systematic review and pooled analysis. Dis Esophagus 28 (5):468–475. https://doi.org/10.1111/dote.12214
10. Findlay MJ, Gillies SR, Millo KJ, Sgromo DB, Marshall DRE, Maynard DN (2014) Enhanced recovery for esophagectomy: a systematic review and evidence-based guidelines. Ann Surg 259(3):413–431. https://doi.org/10.1097/SLA.0000000000000349
11. Weimann A, Braga M, Carli F, Higashiguchi T, Hübner M, Klek S, Laviano A, Ljungqvist O, Lobo DN, Martindale R, Waitzberg DL, Bischoff SC, Singer P (2017) ESPEN guideline: clinical nutrition in surgery. Clin Nutr 36 (3):623–650. https://doi.org/10.1016/j.clnu.2017.02.013
12. Akiyama H, Tsurumaru M, Udagawa H, Kajiyama Y (1994) Radical lymph node dissection for cancer of the thoracic esophagus. Ann Surg 220(3):364–372; discussion 372–363
13. Biere S, van Henegouwen MI, Maas KW, Bonavina L, Rosman C, Garcia J, Gisbertz SS, Klinkenbijl JHG, Hollmann MW, de Lange E, Bonjer JH, van der Peet DL, Cuesta MA (2012) Minimally invasive versus open oesophagectomy for patients with oesophageal cancer: a multicentre, open-label, randomised controlled trial. Lancet 379 (9829):1887–1892. https://doi.org/10.1016/S0140-6736(12)60516-9
14. Mariette MMB, Pezet D, Dalban C, Collet D, Thomas PA, Brigand C, Perniceni T, Carrere N, Bonnetain F, Piessen G (2019) Hybrid minimally invasive versus open oesophagectomy for patients with oesophageal cancer: a multicenter, open- label randomized phase III controlled trial, the MIRO trial. N Engl J Med 380:2
15. Law S, Boey JP, Kwok KF, Wong KH, Chu KM, Wong J (2004) Pleural drainage after transthoracic esophagectomy: experience with a vacuum system. Dis Esophagus 17(1):81–86
16. Ohkura Y, Shindoh J, Ueno M, Iizuka T, Haruta S, Udagawa H (2018) A new postoperative pain management (intravenous acetaminophen: Acelio®) leads to enhanced recovery after esophagectomy: a propensity score-matched analysis. Surg Today 48(5):502–509. https://doi.org/10.1007/s00595-017-1616-5
17. Wong I, Law S (2018) Early oral intake through meticulous chewing after esophagectomy. J Thorac Dis 10(Suppl 17): S2070–S2073. https://doi.org/10.21037/jtd.2018.05.186
18. Zehetner J, DeMeester SR, Alicuben ET, Oh DS, Lipham JC, Hagen JA, DeMeester TR (2015) Intraoperative assessment of perfusion of the gastric graft and correlation with anastomotic leaks after esophagectomy. Ann Surg 262 (1):74–78. https://doi.org/10.1097/SLA.0000000000000811
19. Kechagias A, van Rossum PSN, Ruurda JP, van Hillegersberg R (2016) Ischemic conditioning of the stomach in the prevention of esophagogastric anastomotic leakage after esophagectomy. Ann Thorac Surg 101(4):1614–1623. https://doi.org/10.1016/j.athoracsur.2015.10.034
20. Murthy SC, Law S, Whooley BP, Alexandrou A, Chu KM, Wong J (2003) Atrial fibrillation after esophagectomy is a marker for postoperative morbidity and mortality. J Thorac Cardiovasc Surg 126(4):1162–1167
21. Lo OS, Law S, Chu KM, Wong J (2003) Chylothorax after esophagectomy. Surgery 133 (3):340–341
22. Law S, Fok M, Chu KM, Wong J (1997) Comparison of hand-sewn and stapled esophagogastric anastomosis after esophageal resection for cancer: a prospective randomized controlled trial. Ann Surg 226(2):169–173
23. Law S, Suen DT, Wong KH, Kwok KF, Wong J (2005) A single-layer, continuous, hand-sewn method for esophageal anastomosis: prospective evaluation in 218 patients. Arch Surg 140 (1):33–39

Chapter 26

Anesthetic Management for Squamous Cell Carcinoma of the Esophagus

Eva Y. F. Chan, Danny K. Y. Ip, and Michael G. Irwin

Abstract

While surgery plays a major role in the treatment and potential cure of esophageal cancers, esophagectomy remains a high-risk operation with significant perioperative morbidity and mortality compared to other oncosurgical procedures. Perioperative management for esophagectomy is complex, and close attention to detail in various areas of anesthetic and perioperative management is crucial to improve postoperative outcomes. Patients undergoing esophagectomy should be offered an evidence-based risk assessment for their postoperative outcomes to allow active participation and informed, shared-decision making. Novel perioperative risk scores have been developed to predict both short-term and long-term outcomes in patients with esophageal cancer, although independent validation of such scoring systems is still required. Apart from accurate preoperative risk assessment, further efforts to improve morbidity and mortality from esophagectomy is achieved through comprehensive Enhanced Recovery after Surgery (ERAS) protocols, which comprise an individualized bundle of care throughout the perioperative journey for each patient and should be implemented as a standard practice. Furthermore, anesthetic practice and perioperative anesthetic drug usage can potentially affect cancer progression and recurrence. This chapter reviews current evidence for various factors that contribute to the improvement of perioperative outcomes, including prehabilitation, preoperative optimization of anemia, thoracic epidural analgesia, intraoperative protective ventilatory strategies, goal-directed fluid therapy, as well as special attention to other perioperative issues that potentially reduce anastomotic and cardiopulmonary complications. In summary, it is difficult to show a measurable benefit from any one single intervention, and a multidisciplinary approach that encompasses multiple aspects of perioperative care is necessary to improve outcomes after esophagectomy.

Key words Esophagus, Complication, Anesthesia

1 Introduction

Esophageal cancer is one of the most fatal malignancies worldwide with a poor overall-5-year survival (10–40%) [1], and in many potentially curable solid tumors, surgical resection is the mainstay therapy [2]. However, despite advances in surgical techniques, the use of adjuvant chemoradiotherapy and improvements in anesthetic and perioperative management, tumor recurrence in patients who

Alfred K. Lam (ed.), *Esophageal Squamous Cell Carcinoma: Methods and Protocols*, Methods in Molecular Biology, vol. 2129, https://doi.org/10.1007/978-1-0716-0377-2_26,

were previously surgically treated still occurs and remains a condition that results in substantial morbidity and mortality.

There are two main subtypes of malignant esophageal carcinomas, namely, adenocarcinoma and squamous cell carcinoma (SCC). The latter is more prevalent in Southeast Asia and is notorious for its aggressiveness with a high recurrence rate, secondary to lymphatic and hematogenous spread [1, 3]. For instance, disease recurrence and/or distant metastases were found in approximately 50% of patients with SCC within 2–3 years despite primary tumur resection [4]. Apart from surgery itself, perioperative interventions as well as anesthetic techniques can play an important role in long-term outcomes via their effects on various malignant cell-signaling and immunomodulatory pathways [5–9].

Apart from the above, there is also a complex interplay between the immune system, tumor, surgery, and anesthesia (Fig. 1). An intact cellular immune system is the key host defence against tumor recurrence, and it has long been established that the immune system is able to recognize cancer cells as "non-self" and subsequently destroy them even before they are clinically detectable [8, 9]. Undoubtedly, complete tumor clearance is impossible from sole reliance on a competent immune system, and the process of cancer immunoediting, which is a dynamic and continuous process, will follow. It describes the process of immunosurveillance and the subsequent ability of tumor cells to undergo genomic

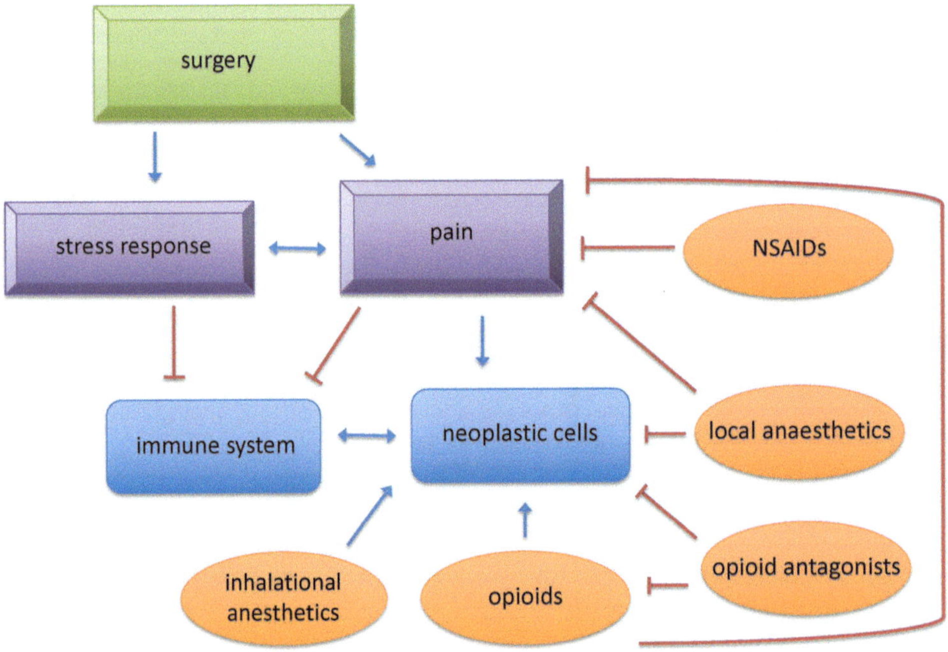

Fig. 1 The complex interplay between tumor cells and the immune system and how anesthesia may have a potential role in modulating the effects of cancer surgery

metamorphosis that can give rise to new tumor variants with increased mutations and enhanced resistance against host immune attack, whereby tumor cells finally evade the recognition system and eventually develop into clinically detectable malignancy [10, 11]. In particular, natural killer (NK) cells play an important role in this process. NK cell activity is suppressed after surgery [1–10, 12–14], and the degree of immunosuppression is directly proportional to the scale of surgery [7–9]. Surgical excision itself can also result in the dissemination of tumor cells into the systemic circulation, which further compounds the development of metastases and cancer recurrence [10, 15, 16]. Various anesthetic techniques and drugs have potential roles in altering immunosuppression and stress responses from surgery and, thus, play a promising role in surgical outcomes.

Patients with esophageal cancer are often cachexic and anemic. Their cardiopulmonary reserve is also frequently compromised, either due to the cancer itself or other co-existing diseases. Esophagectomy itself is an ultra-major surgery involving an extended period of procedural time, application of advanced anesthetic techniques such as thoracic epidural analgesia and one-lung ventilation, and potential major blood loss. It is, therefore, of utmost importance for every healthcare professional involved in managing this group of vulnerable patients to adopt best evidence practice contributing to better outcomes after surgery. This chapter will discuss various evidence-based anesthetic managements that are commonly adopted during esophagectomy for SCC. We will also describe how these techniques may contribute to the improvement of oncological outcomes after this ultra-major operation.

2 Materials

2.1 Patients

2.1.1 Risk Assessment and Stratification

1. Esophagectomy is an ultra-major surgery, and postoperative morbidity and mortality are some of the most important factors that determine prognoses in esophageal cancer.
2. Careful and detailed assessment of patients is required well before the procedure as their preoperative physiological status determines postoperative outcomes and well-being.
3. "Return to Intended Oncological Therapy" (RIOT) is one of the quality indicators specific to oncosurgical patients that describes the proportion of patients able to complete intended therapy after the initial cancer surgery, and the inability to RIOT is associated with poor outcome [17–19].
4. Efforts have been made to develop a composite risk score for predicting postoperative mortality specifically related to esophagectomy.

5. Several factors contribute to higher postoperative mortality in the "Bartels score," including compromised general condition and impaired cardiac, respiratory, and hepatic functions [20].
6. A comprehensive novel Preoperative Esophagectomy Risk (PER) Score assesses preoperative risks and predicts both short-term (morbidity and mortality) and long-term oncological outcomes for patients undergoing esophagectomy [21]. It is also an independent predictor of tumor recurrence.
7. The PER score is based on important organ functions, using diagnostic parameters such as pulmonary function tests, the revised cardiac risk index, and the model of end stage liver disease.
8. Points are allocated according to the severity of impairment of the corresponding organ systems, and summation of the above constitutes the final PER score.
9. Patients are then stratified into low-, intermediate-, and high-risk groups. Apart from predicting outcomes, proper risk stratification can also impact the decision of patient disposal immediately after surgery and allow clinicians to give a better informed consent during preoperative assessment.
10. Applicability of the above score is still subject to independent verification and validation through multicentered trials.
11. At present, no single risk scoring system is superior to others as risk prediction models, but they serve as a guide for anesthesiologists in terms of potential aspects to be aware of during preoperative assessment.

2.1.2 Preoperative Anemia

1. Preoperative anemia is common in the surgical population with a prevalence varying from 5% to 75% [22].
2. Common causes of anemia in patients with carcinoma of the esophagus include iron deficiency and anemia of chronic disease or inflammation [22, 23].
3. Uncorrected anemia before surgery will predispose patients to increased rates of perioperative allogenic blood transfusion, which has a negative impact on postoperative morbidity and survival [24–26].
4. Adverse outcomes associated with perioperative allogenic blood transfusion include disturbances in electrolyte balance, acid-base status, and body temperature. In addition, transfusion potentially causes immune-modulated injuries such as transfusion-related acute lung injury (TRALI), transfusion-associated immunomodulation (TRIM) and fluid overload, especially in patients with limited cardiovascular reserve [27–33].

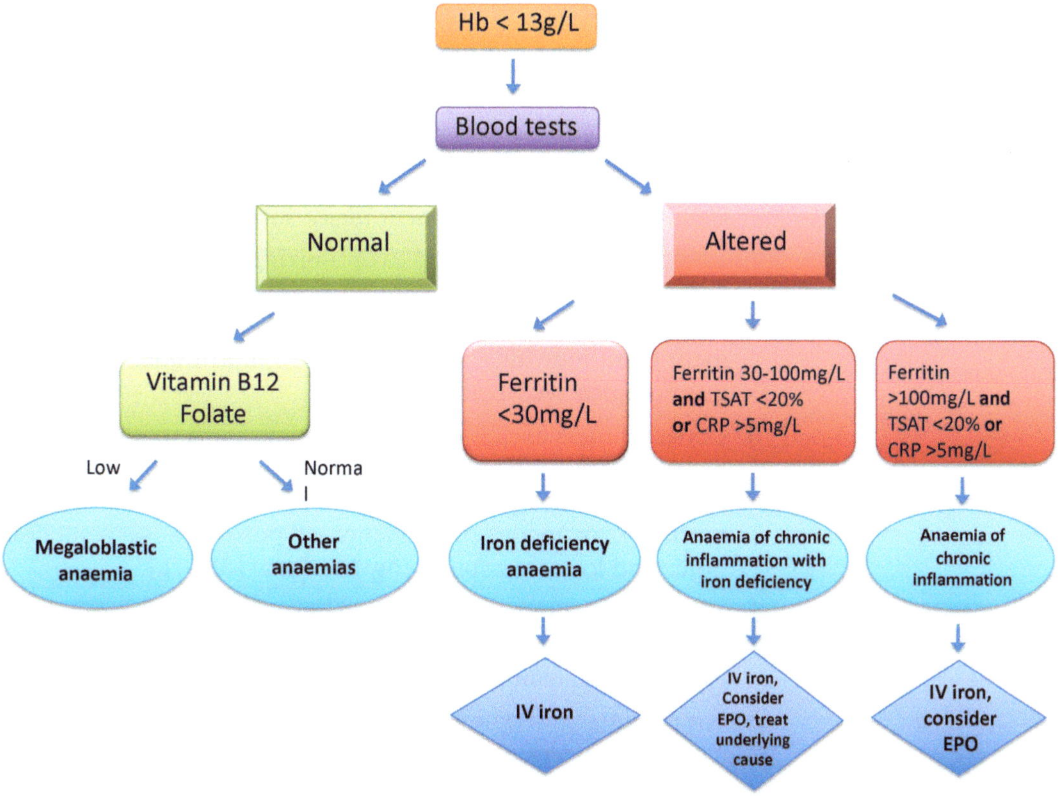

Fig. 2 The classification and management of preoperative anemia. *TSAT (transferrin saturation), CRP (C-reactive protein), EPO (recombinant erythropoietin)*

5. Recent evidence suggests that restrictive transfusion strategies after esophageal surgery are linked with improved outcomes [34]. Also, a recent large observational trial suggested inferior survival from thoracic resection of esophageal cancer with intraoperative red cell transfusion [28].
6. Figure 2 summarizes the classification and management of preoperative anemia.
7. Nowadays, with the development of newer intravenous iron preparations, for example, iron isomaltoside (Monofer™), anesthetists can safely prescribe the required iron dose to eligible patients during a single clinic visit. The newer generation also carries less allergic reactions compared to its older preparation.
8. A therapeutic response is seen as early as the fifth day after administration, with a maximal response in the elevation of hemoglobin level at 3 weeks [24–26].
9. According to the latest IVICA trial [35], preoperative treatment of iron deficiency anemia with intravenous iron can improve the quality of life in patients with colorectal surgery,

although whether this finding can be extrapolated to patients with esophageal cancer is yet to be confirmed by large-scale randomized trials.

2.1.3 Prehabilitation

1. Prehabilitation describes the process of strengthening the physiological reserve of patients in preparation for them to withstand the stress of subsequent major surgery [36, 37].
2. Its scope is not only limited to optimizing patients' pre-existing comorbidities. Rather, it comprises multidisciplinary, targeted interventions that also extend to include functional enhancement of an individual's physical fitness, nutritional status, and psychological well-being.
3. Physical fitness itself is an important determinant of postoperative outcomes, and evidence suggests that a suboptimal preoperative physical performance is associated with all-cause mortality, an increased incidence of postoperative complications, and longer hospital lengths of stay [38–41].
4. The main components of prehabilitation include preoperative exercise training, nutritional assessment and optimization, and psychological counseling [42, 43].
5. For patients undergoing surgery for thoracic and gastrointestinal cancer resection, multiple studies have confirmed a decrease in postoperative complications and, thus, a shorter length of stay with adequate presurgical exercise training and better physical fitness [41–46].
6. Apart from enhancing cardiopulmonary fitness, patients were more likely to return to their baseline fitness after surgical resection [44–46].
7. For exercise training to deliver a beneficial outcome, it must be conducted in the form of a structured program and prescribed at a "dose" that couples with the requirement of each individual patient.
8. Apart from muscle wasting, malnutrition is also a common phenomenon in patients with esophageal cancer, and the condition is further exacerbated before surgery as protein requirement is increased during stressed states.
9. According to guidelines from the European Society for Clinical Nutrition and Metabolism (ESPEN), patients who were malnourished will have a longer hospital stay and higher perioperative morbidity and/or mortality [47].
10. Patients at risk of malnutrition are recommended to receive dietary supplementation in combination with exercise training to maintain cardiorespiratory fitness and body composition, and resistance training has the potential to alleviate catabolic effects of cancer cachexia [48–50].

Table 1
Important nutritional interventions of patients before esophagectomy

• Assess nutritional status on confirmation of diagnosis and repeat the assessment after neoadjuvant chemoradiotherapy and before operation
• Initiate nutritional support in the early phase preoperatively
• Measure resting energy expenditure in patients with an altered body mass index
• Use fat free mass or skeletal muscle mass in calculating daily protein requirement
• Remind patients to take protein rich food or supplements
• Advise patients not to take alcoholic beverage at least before operation
• Advise against unnecessary and prolonged fasting before surgery
• Administer carbohydrate loading 2 h before operation unless contraindicated

11. A thorough nutritional pre-assessment followed by an individually tailored nutritional supplementation program designed by a specialist dietician is of paramount importance to maintain lean body mass and lower the subsequent risk of sarcopenia and frailty [51–57]. Table 1 is a summary of feasible nutritional interventions for this group of patients.
12. Anesthetists are important members of the multidisciplinary team for this group of patients during their perioperative journey, and they have an indispensable role to educate patients and provide support during anesthetic pre-assessments, as well as offering advice and maintaining motivation when patients encounter problems during their prehabilitation programs.

2.2 Equipment

2.2.1 Epidural Catheter and Thoracic Epidural Analgesia

1. Esophagectomy is a highly stressful and painful procedure, and proper pain management is crucial to enhance early recovery and to reduce postoperative complications [58].
2. The choice of analgesic technique thus plays an important role in influencing outcome from major surgery.
3. Neuraxial techniques such as thoracic epidural analgesia (TEA) have long been the preferred analgesic methods for major thoracic and upper abdominal surgeries with recognized benefits [59–64]. In particular, TEA is a well-established analgesic technique for postoperative pain relief [65–73], and the neuraxial catheter can be inserted during the immediate preoperative period or before the induction of general anesthesia in the operating room using aseptic techniques [60, 70, 71].
4. Figure 3 shows how TEA is inserted in the operating theater. TEA, when compared to intravenous patient-controlled analgesia, has a beneficial impact on outcome after cancer surgery, and was shown to improve postoperative pulmonary function, reduce pulmonary complications, and reduce postoperative pain, hence reducing ineffective cough [69, 71–73].

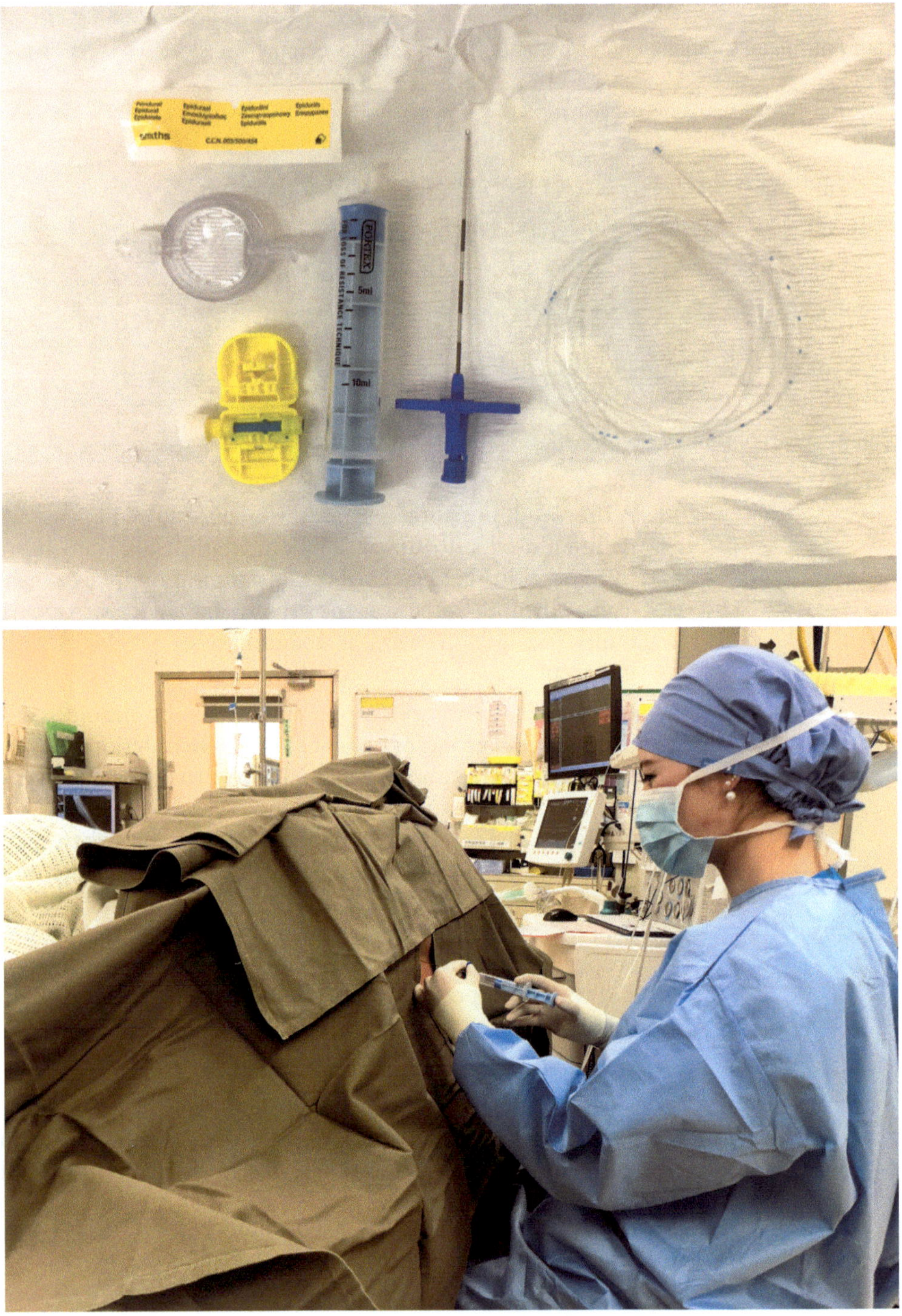

Fig. 3 Epidural catheter set (above) and insertion of epidural catheter inside the operating theater (below). The author (Chan) is performing the procedure (below)

5. Another advantage of TEA in esophagectomy is the associated sympathetic blockade that improves gastric conduit flow by differential effects on splanchnic perfusion and microcirculation [74, 75], thus promoting tissue healing in the anastomosis and reducing the duration of ileus, enabling early resumption of enteral feeding [63–67].
6. TEA also attenuates the stress response to surgery and reduces opioid requirements, thereby ameliorating perioperative immunosuppression [76–80].
7. There are some reports that regional anesthesia might protect against tumor recurrence and cancer progression, but its true effect on survival and recurrence in esophageal cancers is still largely unknown [9, 76, 80–93].

2.2.2 Special Endotracheal Tubes and Intraoperative Lung Isolation Techniques

1. Lung isolation techniques are frequently employed intraoperatively to facilitate surgical exposure [2, 94, 95]. Conventionally, a double-lumen tube or a single lumen endotracheal tube with subsequent placement of a bronchial blocker (Fig. 4) is used to achieve one-lung ventilation, and the final positioning of these airway devices is confirmed with fiberoptic bronchoscopic guidance.

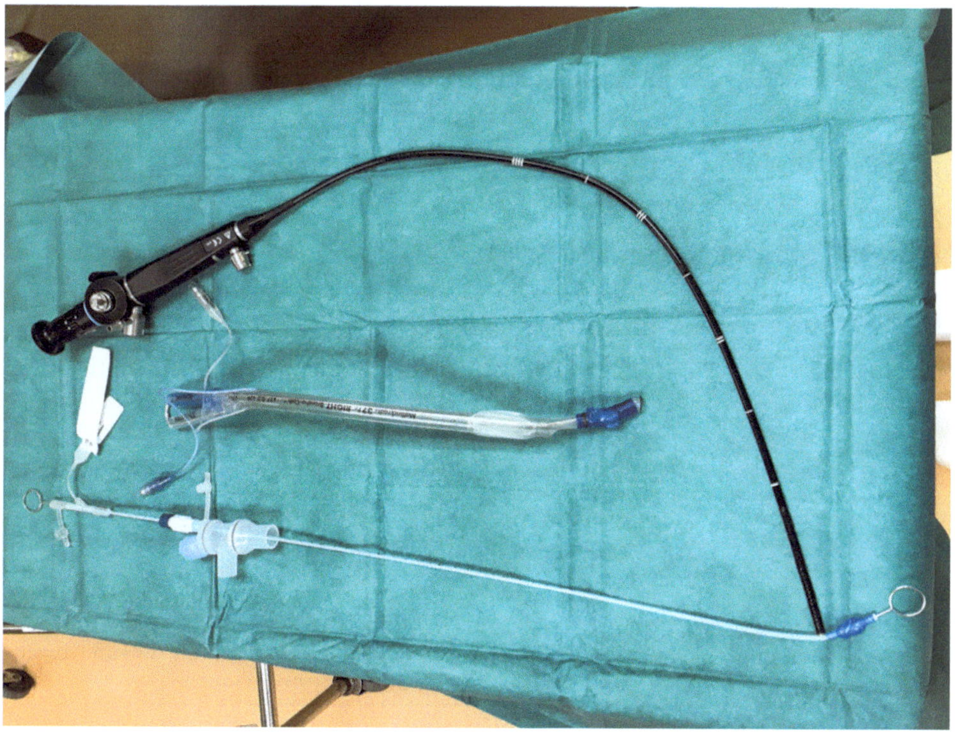

Fig. 4 Devices for achieving one-lung ventilation in theater. Bronchial blocker (left), double lumen tube (middle), fiberoptic bronchoscope (right)

2. The choice of airway device is largely a compromise between pre-existing conditions of the patient, surgical approach, as well as the attending anesthetist's preference.
3. Some centers employ commercially available endotracheal tubes with nerve monitoring devices that can detect intraoperative recurrent laryngeal nerve injury. However, the placement of these endotracheal tubes requires extra care and anesthetic expertise to ensure optimal electrical detection and minimal impedance during the operation, and they can be easily displaced during positional changes with different phases of surgery.
4. Protective lung ventilation strategies have been advocated by the ARDSNet trial [96] and, more recently, the Pulmonary Surgery with Protective Ventilation trial [97] during esophagectomy.
5. The goal of such strategies is to maintain adequate oxygenation and minimize pulmonary complications such as ventilator-induced lung trauma, inflammation, and lung injury [98–108]. The strategies are summarized in Table 2.
6. An individualized approach to ventilation strategies for each patient undergoing esophagectomy should be considered. Anesthetists should adjust ventilation parameters during one-lung ventilation to achieve a balance between adequate gas exchange and lung protection, facilitate surgical procedures, and minimize the incidence of postoperative pulmonary complications [109–113].

Table 2
Summary of lung protective ventilation strategies

Ventilation strategies	Recommendations
Low tidal volumes	• 4–6 ml/kg during one-lung ventilation [100–104, 114]
Optimization of positive end expiratory pressure (PEEP) [102, 105, 112]	• 5–10 cm H_2O • Add continuous positive airway pressure (5–10 cm H_2O) to non-ventilated lung [99] • Judicious use of PEEP in patients with chronic obstructive airway disease
Low inspiratory pressures	• Less than 30H_2O [106–108]
Adequate oxygenation with minimum fraction of inspired oxygen (FiO_2)	• Titrate FiO_2 as needed to maintain oxygen saturation > 90%

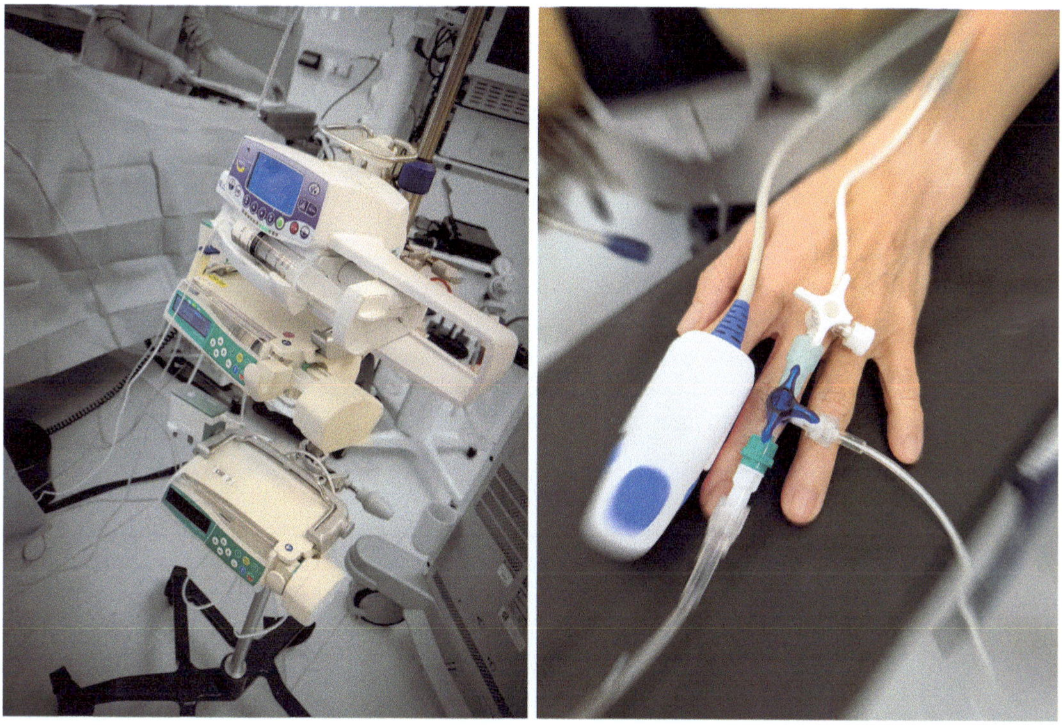

Fig. 5 The setup of TIVA in a patient during anesthesia

2.3 Drugs

2.3.1 Propofol-Based Total Intravenous Anesthesia

1. Anesthesia for esophagectomy can be achieved by inhalational agents or by propofol-based total intravenous anesthesia (TIVA) (Fig. 5).
2. Propofol is one of the most commonly used induction agents, and its use confers many additional advantages in anesthesia for cancer surgery. For example, a recent meta-analysis showed that propofol-based TIVA reduces the relative risk of postoperative nausea and vomiting by 39% [114].
3. Propofol is also believed to play a role in pain signaling by inhibiting the phosphorylation of a subunit of the *N*-methyl-D-aspartate receptor leading to reduced glutamatergic transmission [115] and inhibiting HCN1 channels. A meta-analysis, composed of randomized controlled trials only, also showed that it was associated with reduced pain scores at 24 h when compared with anesthesia maintained by inhalational agents [116, 117].
4. Apart from the anesthetic and analgesic characteristics, propofol also contains other beneficial properties, such as free radical scavenging and organ protection. It also appears to demonstrate a protective effect on the immune system.
5. Unlike inhalational agents, propofol does not inhibit the hypoxic vasoconstrictor response that reduces shunt during one lung ventilation.

6. Propofol-based TIVA appears to be associated with an enhanced recurrence-free survival and overall survival in patients undergoing cancer surgery, as demonstrated in a meta-analysis conducted in 2019 [118].
7. Therefore, based on current available evidence, TIVA is the preferred anesthetic technique in patients receiving major cancer surgery.

2.3.2 Nonsteroidal Anti-Inflammatory Drugs (NSAIDs)

1. NSAIDs are widely prescribed for postoperative pain relief, as they contain analgesic, antipyretic, and anti-inflammatory properties [119–126]. They are also potentially opioid-sparing and lack the respiratory depressive effects of the other stronger analgesics used perioperatively.
2. Despite their widespread use in surgery, there may be associated renal, cardiovascular, and gastrointestinal side effects, especially in susceptible patients. Several studies have even shown an association between NSAIDs and postoperative leakage of anastomosis in colorectal and gastroesophageal junction cancers, although the results are conflicting [127–134].
3. A recently available new intravenous preparation of cyclooxygenase (COX)-2 inhibitor is incorporated as a component of the multi-modal analgesia regimen in a wide range of surgeries. COX-2 selective NSAIDs have been shown to exhibit protective effects against cancer [135–140], and specifically, celecoxib caused substantial tumor regression in rat mammary tumor models [141, 142]. Being a selective COX-2 inhibitor, it has less gastrointestinal side effects and no platelet inhibition.
4. Therefore, its administration as a part of a balanced analgesia regimen can be considered in esophagectomy unless contraindicated by renal impairment [143–148].

2.3.3 Perioperative Beta-Blockers

1. Perioperative levels of catecholamines are elevated because of surgical stress and pain, and these neurotransmitters are believed to play a role in cancer progression [149–161].
2. Also, resultant overt and persistent intraoperative tachycardia will increase myocardial oxygen demand, which is undesirable especially in patients at risk of cardiac complications.
3. While abrupt initiation of high dose beta-blockers preoperatively may result in more deaths according to the POISE trial [162], careful and stepwise administration intraoperatively is usually well-tolerated in indicated cases, especially when full physiological monitoring is in place. Also, $beta_1$- selective agents such as propranolol have been shown to reduce the risk of cancers of the head and neck, esophagus, stomach, colon, and prostate [163–168], and the protective effect was most substantial with an increased duration of exposure.

3 Methods

3.1 Preoperative Anesthetic Management

1. Patients with a confirmed diagnosis of esophageal cancer will consult anesthetists for the assessment of fitness for potential surgery. Meanwhile, surgeons will perform a complete workup of the disease, such as arranging appropriate imaging for detailed staging and discussing the case in multidisciplinary rounds for the exact surgical plan, as well as deciding the plausibility of neoadjuvant chemoradiotherapy.
2. A detailed preoperative assessment is conducted with special focus on the cardiopulmonary status of the patients, to prepare for the intended ultra-major surgery. Baseline investigations to be included and reviewed include complete blood count, liver and renal function tests, and coagulation profile. Pulmonary function tests will also be arranged as they will predict potential difficulties during one-lung ventilation intraoperatively, and the test itself is an important element for risk stratification for esophagectomy.
3. Individualized prehabilitation programs are carried out by paramedical staff simultaneously, which include supervised exercise training conducted by physiotherapists and nutritional assessment followed by necessary nutritional supplementation recommended by dietitians.
4. For a holistic approach, medical conditions will be optimized before surgery. For instance, preoperative anemia will be investigated and treated where appropriate. For patients with multiple comorbidities which are not under control, referral to physicians will be made for advice and optimization.

3.2 Intraoperative Anesthetic Assessment

1. Unless contraindications exist, such as clinical coagulopathy, documented back pathology or patient refusal, a thoracic epidural catheter will be placed by the anesthetist before induction of anesthesia.
2. The preferred mode of anesthesia will be propofol-based TIVA, with the depth of anesthesia monitored by processed electroencephalography. Invasive blood pressure monitoring will be implemented to enable beat-to-beat monitoring of hemodynamic parameters throughout the operation and permit periodic blood-taking to check and correct changes in hemoglobin levels, electrolyte balance, and acid-base status intraoperatively. Cardiac output and changes in cardiopulmonary status can also be monitored with an arterial line [169–173]. External warming devices will be applied to maintain normothermia.
3. One-lung ventilation will be achieved by either placing a double lumen catheter or a bronchial blocker during thoracic resection of the tumor. Protective ventilation strategies will be carried out with close monitoring of oxygen saturation.

4. Pain control will be multimodal. In patients who are contraindicated for TEA, wound infiltration by local anesthetics will be performed by surgeons at the conclusion of the surgery. Anesthetists will also prescribe morphine-based patient-controlled analgesia for immediate postoperative pain control.
5. Goal-directed fluid therapy (*see* **Note 1**) will be employed throughout the operation to avoid unnecessary over-administration of intravenous fluids throughout the operation.
6. After the surgery, patients will be extubated awake and sent to recovery area for observation of any immediate surgical or anesthetic-related complications. Pain control must be satisfactory before they are discharged from the theater area.

3.3 Postoperative Anesthetic Management

1. Patients will usually be monitored in the intensive care unit or high dependency unit after the operation.
2. All the patients will be enrolled in the ERAS program. It is mainly a protocol-driven program, which consists of a bundle of care aiming at helping patients to return to their preoperative functional status as early as possible (*see* **Note 2**).
3. Anesthetists play an important role in this phase, especially in managing problems arising from the thoracic epidural catheters and to ensure that patients have adequate pain control, so that they can participate in chest physiotherapy as early as possible and can also be mobilized as much as tolerated. Table 3 summarizes the important elements of anesthetic management during esophagectomy.

Table 3
Anesthetic management of patients presented for esophagectomy

Preoperative phase
• Risk assessment and stratification
• Investigation and management of preoperative anemia
• Prehabilitation
Intraoperative phase
• Thoracic epidural anesthesia and multimodal analgesia
• Maintenance of anesthesia by Total intravenous Anesthesia (TIVA)
• Goal-directed fluid therapy (GDFT)
• Lung isolation techniques and lung protective ventilation strategy
Postoperative phase
• Special care unit (immediate postoperative period)
• Enhanced recovery after surgery (ERAS)

4 Notes

1. Goal-directed fluid therapy
   (a) Perioperative fluid balance is associated with the incidence of postoperative complications after esophagectomy; therefore, it is of paramount importance for anesthetists to optimize fluid administration as a strategy to mitigate morbidity in these patients [5, 174].
   (b) The main goal of fluid management in this group of patients is to optimize organ perfusion pressures, tissue blood flow, and oxygen delivery to vital organs and the gut mucosa [174, 175].
   (c) Many studies advocate restrictive fluid regimens over liberal fluid administration in both gastrointestinal and pulmonary surgeries, and in general, a greater cumulative fluid balance in the perioperative period is associated with increased morbidities [175–181].
   (d) However, there is a lack of standardization of such regimens, and a large heterogeneity in fluid administration exists across centers.
   (e) Recently, goal-directed therapy has been introduced as an attempt to achieve objective hemodynamic goals with rational fluid administration, and the approach has been linked with decreased use of vasopressors, reduced postoperative anastomotic/cardiopulmonary complications, and shorter length of stay in intensive care unit [182–188].
   (f) In summary, perioperative fluid optimization should be individualized, which includes optimization of intraoperative stroke volume during the abdominal and thoracic phases, and the avoidance of aggressive fluid loading to counteract hypotensive episodes [189–192].
2. Enhanced Recovery after Surgery (ERAS)
   (a) Although the term ERAS is frequently mistaken as a bundle of care that is to be implemented only after surgery, it is instead a holistic approach involving multidisciplinary care throughout the preoperative, intraoperative, and postoperative phases for patients undergoing major surgery, and these programs have been shown to predictably improve short-term outcomes associated with different surgical procedures [64–66].
   (b) A summary of the current recommendations with components relevant to anesthetists is highlighted in Table 4.

Table 4
Current recommendations for ERAS in esophagectomy relevant to the anesthetist

Preoperative phase	*General considerations* • Preoperative counseling should be provided with an emphasis on perioperative and postoperative targets and goals • Smoking cessation and alcohol abstinence should be considered 4 weeks before surgery • Postoperative nausea and vomiting (PONV) prophylaxis should be considered in high-risk patients *Nutrition* • Nutritional assessment by dieticians to delineate and optimize preoperative nutritional status • For high-risk cases, enteral support is indicated • However, routine use of pharmaco-nutrition for esophageal cancer surgery is not currently supported *Fasting* • Prolonged fasting should be avoided • Clear liquids allowed until 2 h before surgery • Caution is warranted in patients with significant dysphagia or other obstructive symptoms *Anemia* • Detection and optimization of preoperative anemia with iron supplements • Possible reduction in the need for transfusion and related adverse events *Prehabilitation* • Multimodal prehabilitation programs can reduce sarcopenia and improve cardiorespiratory functions • Limited evidence supports the use of exercise-derived parameters in risk stratification of patients undergoing esophagectomy
Intraoperative phase	*Conduct of anesthesia* • Inhalational or intravenous anesthetics are equally effective for maintenance of anesthesia, although propofol-based TIVA has considerable advantages • Intermediate-acting neuromuscular blockers, bispectral index monitoring, avoidance of volume overload, and the use of lung-protective strategies facilitate early extubation and reduce postoperative complications • Goal-directed fluid therapy, preferably with balanced crystalloids, is recommended [193–195] • Measures to maintain normothermia intraoperatively are recommended *Analgesia* • Thoracic epidural analgesia (TEA) should be considered as the first-line approach to postoperative analgesia • Paravertebral blocks are a good alternative • Regular acetaminophen dosing should be considered [196]. • Nonsteroidal anti-inflammatory drugs (NSAIDs) may be initiated on an individualized basis • Current evidence is limited for gabapentinoids, ketamine, magnesium, and lidocaine
Postoperative phase	*DVT prophylaxis and early mobilization* • Antithrombotic prophylaxis with low-molecular-weight heparin (LMWH), together with mechanical measures, should be started preoperatively and continued in the postoperative phase • Early postoperative mobilization should be encouraged as soon as possible

(continued)

Table 4 (continued)

• Early (≤48 h) removal of urinary catheters may be considered to facilitate mobilization
Feeding
• Early removal of NG tube and introduction of early enteral feeding may be considered when clinically appropriate
• Bowel stimulation with oral laxatives given postoperatively are safe and can accelerate gastrointestinal transit
Fluid management
• Optimal fluid balance should be sought. A positive fluid balance resulting in weight gain >2 kg/day should be avoided

References

1. Jun IJ, Jo JY, Kim JI (2017) Impact of anaesthetic agents on overall and recurrence-free survival in patients undergoing esophageal cancer surgery: a retrospective observational study. Sci Rep 7(1):14020
2. Carney A, Dickinson M (2015) Anaesthesia for esophagectomy. Anaesthesiol Clin 33 (1):143
3. Hirahara N, Tajima Y, Fujii Y (2018) A novel prognostic scoring system using inflammatory response biomarkers for esophageal squamous cell carcinoma. World J Surg 42:172–184
4. Su XD, Zhang DK, Zhang X (2014) Prognostic factors in patients with recurrence after complete resection of esophageal squamous cell carcinoma. J Thorac Dis 6(7):949–957
5. Durkin C, Schisler T, Lohser J (2017) Current trends in anaesthesia for esophagectomy. Curr Opin Anaesthesiol 30(1):30–35
6. Bartels K, Fiegel M, Stevens Q, Ahlgren B, Qeitzel N (2015) Approaches to perioperative care for esophagectomy. J Cardiothorac Vasc Anesth 29(2):472–480
7. Kim R (2017) Anaesthetic technique and cancer recurrence in oncologic surgery: unraveling the puzzle. Cancer Metastasis Rev 36:159–177
8. Snyder GL, Greenberg S (2010) Effect of anaesthetic technique and other perioperative factors on cancer recurrence. Br J Anaesth 105(2):106–115
9. Cassinello F, Prieto I, del Olmo M (2015) Cancer surgery: how may anesthesia influence outcome? J Clin Anesth 27(3):262–272
10. Dunn GP, Old LJ, Schreiber RD (2004) The immunobiology of cancer immunosurveillance and immunoediting. Immunity 21:137–148
11. Smyth MJ, Dunn GP, Schreiber RD (2006) Cancer immunosurveillance and immunoediting: the roles of immunity in suppressing tumor development and shaping tumor immunogenicity. Adv Immunol 90:1–50
12. Brittenden J, Heys SD, Ross J, Eremin O (1996) Natural killer cells and cancer. Cancer 77:1226–1243
13. Tai LH, de Souza CT, Belanger S (2012) Preventing postoperative metastatic disease by inhibiting surgery-induced dysfunction in natural killer cells. Cancer Res 73(1):97–107
14. Kurosawa S, Kato M (2008) Anaesthetics, immune cells, and immune responses. J Anesth 22:263–277
15. Reiche EM, Nunes SO, Morimoto HK (2004) Stress, depression, the immune system, and cancer. Lancet Oncol 5:617–625
16. Balkwill F, Mantovani A (2001) Inflammation and cancer: back to Virchow? Lancet 357:539–545
17. Aloia TA, Zimmitti G, Conrad C, Gottumukalla V, Kopetz S, Vauthey JN (2014) Return to intended oncologic treatment (RIOT): a novel metric for evaluating the quality of oncosurgical therapy for malignancy. J Surg Oncol 110(2):107–114
18. Merkow RP, Bilimoria KY, Tomlinson JS (2014) Postoperative complications reduce adjuvant chemotherapy use in resectable pancreatic cancer. Ann Surg 260(2):372–377
19. Slankamenac K, Slankamenac M, Schlegel A (2017) Impact of postoperative complications on readmission and long-term survival in patients following surgery for colorectal cancer. Int J Color Dis 32(6):805–811
20. Bartels H, Stein HJ, Siewert JR (2000) Risk analysis in Esophageal surgery. Recent Results Cancer Res 155:89–96
21. Reeh M, Metze J, Uzunoglu FG (2016) The PER (preoperative esophagectomy risk) score:

a simple risk score to predict short-term and long-term outcome in patients with surgically treated esophageal cancer. Medicine (Baltimore) 95(7):e2724

22. Shander A, Knight K, Thurer R, Adamson J, Spence R (2004) Prevalence and outcomes of anemia in surgery: a systematic review of the literature. Am J Med 116:58S–69S
23. Cappell MS, Goldberg ES (1992) The relationship between the clinical presentation and spread of colon cancer in 315 consecutive patients. A significant trend of earlier cancer detection from 1982 through 1988 at a university hospital. J Clin Gastroenterol 14:227–235
24. Munting KE, Klein AA (2019) Optimisation of pre-operative anaemia in patients before elective major surgery—why, who, when and how? Anaesthesia 74(Suppl 1):49–57
25. Muñoz M, Acheson AG, Auerbach M (2017) International consensus statement on the peri-operative management of anaemia and iron deficiency. Anaesthesia 72:233–247
26. Leichtle SW, Mouawad NJ, Lampman R, Singal B, Cleary RK (2011) Does preoperative anemia adversely affect colon and rectal surgery outcomes? J Am Coll Surg 212:187–194
27. Fields RC, Meyers BF (2006) The effects of perioperative blood transfusion on morbidity and mortality after esophagectomy. Thorac Surg Clin 16(1):75–86
28. Boshier PR, Ziff C, Adam ME (2018) Effect of perioperative blood transfusion on the long-term survival of patients undergoing esophagectomy for esophageal cancer: a systematic review and meta-analysis. Dis Esophagus 31(4)
29. Schneider C, Boddy AP, Fukuta J, Groom WD, Streets CG (2014) Predicting blood transfusion in patients undergoing minimally invasive oesophagectomy. Int J Surg 12 (12):1342–1347
30. Reeh M, Ghadban T, Dedow J (2017) Allogenic blood transfusion is associated with poor perioperative and long-term outcome in esophageal cancer. World J Surg 41 (1):208–215
31. Gottschalk A, Sharma S, Ford J, Durieux ME, Tiouririne M (2010) The role of the perioperative period in recurrence after cancer surgery. Anaesth Analg 110(6):1636–1643
32. Liu J, Chen S, Chen Y (2018) Perioperative blood transfusion has no effect on overall survival after esophageal resection for esophageal squamous cell carcinoma: a retrospective cohort study. Int J Surg 55:24–30
33. Ling FC, Hoelscher AH, Vallbohmer D (2009) Leukocyte depletion in allogeneic blood transfusion does not change the negative influence on survival following transthoracic resection for esophageal cancer. J Gastrointest Surg 13(4):581–586
34. Towe CW, Gulack BC, Kim S (2018) Restrictive transfusion practices after esophagectomy are associated with improved outcome: a review of the society of thoracic surgeons general thoracic database. Ann Surg 267 (5):886–891
35. Keeler BD, Dickson EA, Simpson JA (2019) The impact of preoperative intravenous iron on quality of life after colorectal cancer surgery: outcomes from the intravenous iron in colorectal cancer-associated anaemia (IVICA) trial. Anaesthesia 74:696–699
36. Doganay E, Moorthy K (2019) Prehabilitation for esophagectomy. J Thorac Dis 11(5): S632–S638
37. Steenhagen E (2019) Preoperative nutritional optimisation of esophageal cancer patients. J Thorac Dis 11(5):S645–S653
38. Hughes MJ, Hackney RJ, Lamb PJ, Wigmore SJ, Christopher Deans DA, Skipworth RJE (2019) Prehabilitation before major abdominal surgery: a systematic review and meta-analysis. World J Surg 43(7):1661–1668
39. Barberan-Garcia A, Ubre M, Roca J (2018) Personalised prehabilitation in high-risk patients undergoing elective major abdominal surgery - a randomised controlled trial. Ann Surg 267(1):50–56
40. Carli F, Gillis C, Scheede-Bergdahl C (2017) Promoting a culture of prehabilitation for the surgical cancer patient. Acta Oncol 56 (2):128–133
41. Valkenet K, van de Port IG, Dronkers JJ (2011) The effects of preoperative exercise therapy on postoperative outcome: a systematic review. Clin Rehabil 25(2):99–111
42. Wyner-Blyth V, Moorthy K (2017) Prehabilitation: preparing patients for surgery. BMJ 358:j3702
43. Huang DD, Ji YB, Zhou DL (2017) Effect of surgery-induced acute muscle wasting on postoperative outcomes and quality of life. J Surg Res 218:58–96
44. Vermillion SA, James A, Dorrell RD (2018) Preoperative exercise therapy for gastrointestinal cancer patients: a systematic review. Syst Rev 7(1):103
45. Moran J, Guinan E, McCormick (2016) The ability of prehabilitation to influence postoperative outcome after intra-abdominal

operation: a systematic review and meta-analysis. Surgery 160:1189–1201
46. West MA, Loughney L, Lythgoe D (2015) Effect of prehabilitation on objectively measured physical fitness after neoadjuvant treatment in preoperative rectal cancer patients: a blinded interventional pilot study. Br J Anaesth 114(2):244–251
47. Arends J, Bachmann P, Baracos V (2017) ESPEN guidelines on nutrition in cancer patients. Clin Nutr 36(1):11–48
48. Minnella EM, Awasthi R, Loiselle SE (2018) Effect of exercise and nutrition prehabilitation on functional capacity in esophagogastric cancer surgery. JAMA Surg 153(12):1081–2089
49. Santa Mina D, Clarke H, Ritvo P, Leung YW, Matthew AG, Katz J (2014) Effect of total-body prehabilitation on postoperative outcomes: a systematic review and meta-analysis. Physiotherapy 100(3):196–207
50. Dewberry LC, Wingrove LJ, Marsh MD, Glode AE (2019) Pilot prehabilitation program for patients with esophageal cancer during neoadjuvant therapy and surgery. J Surg Res 235:66–72
51. Cruz-Jentoft AJ, Bahat G, Bauer J (2019) Sarcopenia: revised European consensus on definition and diagnosis. Age Ageing 48 (1):16–31
52. Fearon K, Strasser F, Anker SD (2011) Definition and classification of cancer cachexia: an international consensus. Lancet Oncol 12 (5):489–495
53. Elliott JA, Doyle SL, Murphy CF (2017) Sarcopenia: prevalence, and impact on operative and oncologic outcomes in the multimodal management of locally advanced esophageal cancer. Ann Surg 266:822–830
54. Jack S, West MA, Raw D (2014) The effect of neoadjuvant chemotherapy on physical fitness and survival in patients undergoing oesophagogastric cancer surgery. Eur J Surg Oncol 40 (10):1313–1320
55. Makiura D, Ono R, Inoue J, Kashiwa M (2016) Preoperative sarcopenia is a predictor of postoperative pulmonary complications in esophageal cancer following esophagectomy: a retrospective cohort study. J Geriatr Oncol 7 (6):430–436
56. Awad S, Tan BH, Cui H (2012) Marked changes in body composition following neoadjuvant chemotherapy for oesophagogastric cancer. Clin Nutr 31(1):74–77
57. Paireder M, Asari R, Kristo I (2017) Impact of sarcopenia on outcome in patients with esophageal resection following neoadjuvant chemotherapy for esophageal cancer. Eur J Surg Oncol 43(2):478–484
58. Templeton R, Greenhalgh D (2019) Preoperative rehabilitation for thoracic surgery. Curr Opin Anaesthesiol 32(1):23–28
59. Li Y, Dong H, Tan S (2019) Effects of thoracic epidural anaesthesia/analgesia on the stress response, pain relief, hospital stay and treatment costs of patients with esophageal carcinoma undergoing thoracic surgery: a single-center, randomized controlled trial. Medicine (Baltimore) 98(7):e14362
60. Feltracco P, Bortolato A, Barbieri S (2018) Perioperative benefit and outcome of thoracic epidural in esophageal surgery: a clinical review. Dis Esophagus 1(31):5
61. Ng JM (2011) Update on anesthetic management for esophagectomy. Curr Opin Anaesthesiol 24(1):37–43
62. Li W, Li Y, Huang Q (2016) Short and long-term outcomes of epidural or intravenous analgesia after esophagectomy: a propensity-matched cohort study. PLoS One 11(4): e0154380
63. Findlay JM, Gillies RS, Millo J (2014) Enhanced recovery for esophagectomy: a systematic review and evidence-based guidelines. Ann Surg 259(3):413–431
64. Liu F, Wang W, Wang C (2018) Enhanced recovery after surgery (ERAS) programs for esophagectomy protocol for a systematic review and meta-analysis. Medicine (Baltimore) 97(8):e0016
65. Low DE, Allum W, De Manzoni G (2019) Guidelines for perioperative care in esophagectomy: enhanced recovery after surgery (ERAS®) society recommendations. World J Surg 43(2):299–330
66. Steinthorsdottir KJ, Wildgaard L, Hansen HJ (2014) Regional analgesia for video-assisted thoracic surgery: a systematic review. Eur J Cardiothorac Surg 45(6):959–966
67. Jaeger JM, Collins SR, Blank RS (2012) Anesthetic management for esophageal resection. Anesthesiol Clin 30(4):731–747
68. Manion SC, Brennan TJ (2011) Thoracic epidural analgesia and acute pain management. Anesthesiology 115(1):181–188
69. Pöpping DM, Elia N, Marret E (2008) Protective effects of epidural analgesia on pulmonary complications after abdominal and thoracic surgery: a meta-analysis. Arch Surg 143(10):990–999
70. Flisberg P, Tornebrandt K, Walther B (2001) Pain relief after esophagectomy: thoracic epidural analgesia is better than parental opioids. J Cardiothorac Vasc Anesth 15(3):282–287

71. Tsui SL, Law S, Fok M (1997) Postoperative analgesia reduces mortality and morbidity after esophagectomy. Am J Surg 173 (6):472–478
72. Brodner G, Pogatzki E, Van Aken H et al (1998) A multimodal approach to control postoperative pathophysiology and rehabilitation in patients undergoing abdominothoracic esophagectomy. Anesth Analg 86 (2):228–234
73. Smedstad KG, Beattie WS, Blair WS, Buckley DN (1992) Postoperative pain relief and hospital stay after total esophagectomy. Clin J Pain 8(2):149–153
74. Michelet P, D'Journo XB, Roch A (2005) Perioperative risk factors for anastomotic leakage after esophagectomy: influence of thoracic epidural analgesia. Chest 128(5):3461–3466
75. Al-Rawi OY, Pennefather SH, Page RD (2008) The effect of thoracic epidural bupivacaine and an intravenous adrenaline infusion on gastric tube blood flow during esophagectomy. Anesth Analg 106 (3):884–887
76. Zura M, Kozmar A, Sakic K (2012) Effect of spinal and general anesthesia on serum concentration of pro-inflammatory and anti-inflammatory cytokines. Immunobiology 217(6):622–627
77. Beilin B, Shavit Y, Trabekin E (2003) The effects of postoperative pain management on immune response to surgery. Anesth Analg 97 (3):822–827
78. Beilin B, Bessler H, Mayburd E (2003) Effects of preemptive analgesia on pain and cytokine production in the postoperative period. Anesthesiology 98(1):151–155
79. Yokoyama M, Itano Y, Katayama H (2005) The effects of continuous epidural anesthesia and analgesia on stress response and immune function in patients undergoing radical esophagectomy. Anaesth Analg 101 (5):1532–1527
80. Fares KM, Mohamed SA, Hamza HM (2014) Effect of thoracic epidural analgesia on pro-inflammatory cytokines in patients subjected to protective lung ventilation during Ivor Lewis esophagectomy. Pain Physician 17 (5):305–315
81. Rudin A, Flisberg P, Johansson J (2005) Thoracic epidural analgesia or intravenous morphine analgesia after thoracoabdominal esophagectomy: a prospective follow-up of 201 patients. J Cardiothorac Vasc Anesth 19 (3):350–357
82. Werawatganon T, Charuluxanun S (2005) Patient controlled intravenous opioid analgesia versus continuous epidural analgesia for pain after intra-abdominal surgery. Cochrane Database Syst Rev 1:CD004088
83. Guay J, Kopp S (2016) Epidural pain relief versus systemic opioid-based pain relief for abdominal aortic surgery. Cochrane Database Syst Rev 5(1):CD005059
84. Kahn L, Baxter FJ, Dauphin A (1999) A comparison of thoracic and lumbar epidural techniques for post-thoracoabdominal esophagectomy analgesia. Can J Anaesth 46 (5):415–422
85. Davies RG, Myles PS, Graham JM (2006) A comparison of the analgesic efficacy and side-effects of paravertebral vs epidural blockade for thoracotomy--a systematic review and meta-analysis of randomized trials. Br J Anaesth 96(4):418–426
86. Ding X, Jin S, Niu X (2014) A comparison of the analgesia efficacy and side effects of paravertebral compared with epidural blockade for thoracotomy: an updated meta-analysis. PLoS One 9(5):e96233
87. Yeung JH, Gates S, Naidu BV (2016) Paravertebral block versus thoracic epidural for patients undergoing thoracotomy. Cochrane Database Syst Rev 2:CD009121
88. Kehlet H, Wilkinson RC, Fischer HB (2007) PROSPECT: evidence-based, procedure-specific postoperative pain management. Best Pract Res Clin Anaesthesiol 21(1):149–159
89. Shanthanna H, Moisuik P, O'Hare T (2018) Survey of postoperative regional analgesia for Thoracoscopic surgeries in Canada. J Cardiothorac Vasc Anesth 32(4):1750–1755
90. Cummings KC 3rd, Xu F, Cummings LC, Cooper GS (2012) A comparison of epidural analgesia and traditional pain management effects on cancer recurrence after colectomy: a population based study. Anesthesiology 116 (4):797–806
91. Weng M, Chen W, Hou W, Li L, Ding M, Miao C (2016) The effect of neuraxial anesthesia on cancer recurrence and survival after cancer surgery: an updated meta-analysis. Oncotarget 7(12):15262–15273
92. Pöpping DM, Elia N, Van Aken HK, Marret E, Schug SA, Kranke P (2014) Impact of epidural analgesia on mortality and morbidity after surgery: systematic review and meta-analysis of randomized controlled trials. Ann Surg 259(6):1056–1067
93. Cummings KC III, Kou TD, Chak A (2019) Surgical approach and the impact of epidural analgesia on survival after esophagectomy for cancer: a population based retrospective cohort study. PLoS One 14(1):e0211125

94. Law S, Wong KH, Kwok KF (2004) Predictive factors for postoperative pulmonary complications and mortality after esophagectomy for cancer. Ann Surg 240(5):791–800
95. Ferguson MK, Durkin AE (2002) Preoperative prediction of the risk of pulmonary complications after esophagectomy for cancer. J Thorac Cardiovasc Surg 123(4):661–669
96. Brower RG, Matthay MA, Morris A (2000) Ventilation with lower tidal volumes as compared with traditional tidal volumes for acute lung injury and the acute respiratory distress syndrome. The acute respiratory distress syndrome network. N Engl J Med 342 (18):1301–1308
97. Marret E, Cinotti R, Berard L (2018) Protective ventilation during anaesthesia reduces major postoperative complications after lung cancer surgery: a double-blind randomised controlled trial. Eur J Anaesthesiol 35:727–735
98. Verhage RJ, Boone J, Rijkers GT (2014) Reduced local immune response with continuous positive airway pressure during one-lung ventilation for oesophagectomy. Br J Anaesth 112(5):920–928
99. Gajic O, Dara SI, Mendez JL (2004) Ventilator-associated lung injury in patients without acute lung injury at the onset of mechanical ventilation. Crit Care Med 32 (9):1817–1824
100. Determann RM, Royakkers A, Wolthuis EK (2010) Ventilation with lower tidal volumes as compared with convential tidal volumes for patients without acute lung injury: a preventive randomised controlled trial. Crit Care 14 (1):R1
101. Michelet P, D'Journo XB, Roch A, Doddoli C (2006) Protective ventilation influences systemic inflammation after esophagectomy: a randomised controlled study. Anaesthesiology 105(5):911–919
102. Wrigge H, Uhlig U, Zinserling J (2004) The effects of different ventilatory settings on pulmonary and systemic inflammatory responses during major surgery. Anesth Analg 98 (3):775–781
103. Schiling T, Kozian A, Huth C (2005) The pulmonary immune effects of mechanical ventilation in patients undergoing thoracic surgery. Anesth Analg 101(4):957–965
104. Yang M, Ahn HJ, Kim K (2011) Does a protective ventilation strategy reduce the risk of pulmonary complications after lung cancer surgery? A randomised controlled trial. Chest 139(3):530–537
105. Tugrul M, Camci E, Karadeniz H, Senturk M, Pembeci K, Akpir K (1997) Comparison of volume controlled with pressure controlled ventilation during one lung anaesthesia. Br J Anaesth 79(3):306–310
106. Senturk NM, Dilek A, Camci E, Senturk E (2005) Effects of positive end-expiratory pressure on ventilatory and oxygenation parameters during pressure-controlled one-lung ventilation. J Cardiothorac Vasc Anesth 19 (1):71–75
107. Nichols D, Haranath S (2007) Pressure control ventilation. Crit Care Clin 23(2):183–199
108. Choi H, Cho JH, Kim HK (2019) Prevalence and clinical course of postoperative acute lung injury after esophagectomy for esophageal cancer. J Thorac Dis 11(1):200–205
109. Weijs TJ, Ruurda JP, Luyer MDP (2013) Strategies to reduce pulmonary complications after esophagectomy. World J Gastroenterol 19(39):6509–6514
110. Hu XY, Du B (2019) Lung-protective ventilation during one-lung ventilation: known knowns, and known unknowns. J Thorac Dis 11(3):S237–S240
111. Hemmes SN, Gama de Abreu M, Pelosi P (2014) High versus low positive end-expiratory pressure during general anaesthesia for open abdominal surgery (PROVHILO trial): a multicentre randomised controlled trial. Lancet 384 (9942):495–503
112. Serpa NA, Hemmes SN, Barbas CS (2015) Protective versus conventional ventilation for surgery: a systematic review and individual patient data meta-analysis. Anesthesiology 123(1):66–78
113. Blank RS, Colquhoun DA, Duriex ME (2016) Management of one-lung ventilation: impact of tidal volume on complications after thoracic surgery. Anesthesiology 124 (6):1286–1295
114. Schraag S, Pradelli L, Alsaleh AJO (2018) Propofol vs. inhalational agents to maintain general anaesthesia in ambulatory and in-patient surgery: a systematic review and meta-analysis. BMC Anesthesiol 18(1):162
115. Kingston S, Mao L, Yang L, Arora A, Fibuch EE, Wang JQ (2006) Propofol inhibits phosphorylation of N-methyl-D-aspartate NR1 subunits in neurons. Anaesthesiology 104 (4):763–769
116. Qiu Q, Choi SW, Wong SS, Irwin MG, Cheung CW (2016) Effects of intraoperative maintenance of general anaesthesia with Propofol on postoperative pain outcomes – a systematic review and meta-analysis. Anaesthesia 71(10):1222–1233
117. Song JG, Shin JW, Lee EH, Choi DK (2012) Incidence of post-thoracotomy pain: a

comparison between total intravenous anaesthesia and inhalation anaesthesia. Eur J Cardiothorac Surg 41(5):1078–1082

118. Yap A, Lopez-Olivo MA, Duboiwitz J, Hiller J, Ruedel B (2019) Anesthetic technique and cancer outcomes: a meta-analysis of total intravenous versus volatile anesthesia. Can J Anaesth 66(5):546–561

119. Dierssen-Sotos T, Gómez-Acebo I, de Pedro M (2016) Use of non-steroidal anti-inflammatory drugs and risk of breast cancer: the Spanish multi-case-control (MCC) study. BMC Cancer 16(1):660

120. Vidal AC, Howard LE, Moreira DM (2015) Aspirin, NSAIDs, and risk of prostate cancer: results from the REDUCE study. Clin Cancer Res 21(4):756–762

121. Friis S, Riis AH, Erichsen R, Baron JA (2015) Low-dose aspirin or nonsteroidal anti-inflammatory drug use and colorectal cancer risk. Ann Intern Med 163(5):347–355

122. Shi J, Leng W, Zhao L, Xu C (2017) Nonsteroidal anti-inflammatory drugs using and risk of head and neck cancer: a dose–response meta-analysis of prospective cohort studies. Oncotarget 8(58):99066–99074

123. Thun MJ, Henley SJ, Patrono C (2002) Nonsteroidal anti-inflammatory drugs as anticancer agents: mechanistic, pharmacologic, and clinical issues. J Natl Cancer Inst 94 (4):252–266

124. Zamarron BF, Chen W (2011) Dual roles of immune cells and their factors in cancer development and progression. Int J Biol Sci 7 (5):651–658

125. Landskron G, De la Fuente M, Thuwajit P, Thuwajit C, Hermoso MA (2014) Chronic inflammation and cytokines in the tumor microenvironment. J Immunol Res 2014:149185

126. Wong RSY (2019) Role of Nonsteroidal Anti-Inflammatory Drugs (NSAIDs) in Cancer Prevention and Cancer Promotion. Adv Pharmacol Sci 2019:3418975

127. Rushfeldt CF, Agledahl UC, Sveinbjornsson B (2016) Effect of perioperative dexamethasone and different NSAIDs on anastomotic leak risk: a propensity score analysis. World J Surg 40(11):2782–2789

128. Fjederholt KT, Okholm C, Svendsen LB (2018) Ketorolac and other NSAIDs increase the risk of anastomotic leakage after surgery for GEJ cancers: a cohort study of 557 patients. J Gastrointest Surg 22 (4):587–594

129. McDermott FD, Heeney A, Kelly ME, Steele RJ, Carlson GL, Winter DC (2015) Systematic review of preoperative, intraoperative and postoperative risk factors for colorectal anastomic leaks. Br J Surg 102(5):462–479

130. Paulasir S, Kaoutzanis C, Welch KB (2015) Nonsteroidal anti-inflammatory drugs: do they increase the risk of anastomotic leaks following colorectal operations? Dis Colon Rectum 58(9):870–877

131. Rutegard M, Westermark S, Kverneng Hultberg D (2016) Nonsteroidal anti-inflammatory drug use and risk of anastomotic leakage after anterior resection: a protocol-based study. Dig Surg 33 (2):129–135

132. Hakkarainen TW, Steele SR, Bastaworous A (2015) Nonsteroidal anti-inflammatory drugs and the risk for anastomotic failure: a report from Washington State's surgical care and outcomes assessment program (SCOAP). JAMA Surg 150(3):223–228

133. Hassan I (2014) NSAID use and colorectal anastomotic leaks. Caution and further investigation. J Gastrointest Surg 18 (8):1405–1406

134. Bhangu A, Singh P, Fitzgeral JE (2014) Postoperative nonsteroidal anti-inflammatory drugs and risk of anastomotic leak: meta-analysis of clinical and experimental studies. World J Surg 38(9):2247–2257

135. Hao WM, Shen YX, Feng MX (2018) Aspirin acts in esophageal cancer: a brief review. J Thorac Dis 10(4):2490–2497

136. Sun L, Yu S (2011) Meta-analysis: non-steroidal anti-inflammatory drug use and the risk of esophageal squamous cell carcinoma. Dis Esophagus 24(8):544–549

137. Husain SS, Szabo IL, Tamawski AS (2002) NSAID inhibition of GI cancer growth: clinical implications and molecular mechanisms of action. Am J Gastroenterol 97(3):542–553

138. Li M, Lotan R, Levin B, Tahara E, Lippman SM, Xu SC (2000) Aspirin induction of apoptosis in esophageal cancer: a potential for chemoprevention. Cancer Epidemiol Biomark Prev 9(6):545–549

139. Krishnan K, Ruffin MT, Brenner DE (1997) Colon cancer chemoprevention: clinical development of aspirin as a chemopreventive agent. J Cell Biochem 28-29:148–158

140. Gupta RA, DuBois RN (1998) Aspirin, NSAIDs, and colon cancer prevention: mechanisms? Gastoenterology 114 (5):1095–1098

141. Alshafie GA, Abou-Issa HM, Seibert K, Harris RE (2000) Chemotherapeutic evaluation of celecoxib, a cyclooxygenase-2 inhibitor, in a rat mammary tumour model. Oncol Rep 7:1377–1381

142. Yao M, Zhou W, Sangha S, Albert A (2005) Effects of nonselective cyclooxygenase inhibition with low-dose ibuprofen on tumor growth, angiogenesis, metastasis, and survival in a mouse model of colorectal cancer. Clin Cancer Res 11(4):1618–1628
143. Liu X, Li P, Zhang ST, You H, Jia JD, Yu ZL (2008) COX-2 mRNA expression in esophageal squamous cell carcinoma (ESCC) and effect by NSAID. Dis Esophagus 21(1):9–14
144. Liu JF, Jamieson GG, Drew PA, Zhu GJ (2005) Aspirin induces apoptosis in esophageal cancer cells by inhibiting the pathway of NF-kappaB downstream regulation of cyclooxygenase-2. ANZ J Surg 75 (11):1011–1016
145. Kase S, Osaki M, Honjo S (2004) A selective cyclooxygenase-2 inhibitor, NS 398, inhibits cell growth and induces cell cycle arrest in the G2/M phase in human esophageal squamous cell carcinoma cells. Cancer Res 23 (2):301–307
146. Masferrer J (2001) Approach to angiogenesis inhibition based on cyclooxygenase-2. Cancer J 7:144–150
147. Bolieva LZ, Dzhioev FK, Kakabadze SA (2007) Effects of acetylsalicyclic acid and celecoxib on the N-nitrosodiethylamine induced carcinogenesis in rat liver and esophagus. Bull Exp Biol Med 143:87–90
148. Deasy BM, O'Sullivan-Coyne G, O'Donovan TR (2007) Cyclooxygenase-2 inhibitors demonstrate anti-proliferative effects in esophageal cancer cells by prostaglandin E-2 independent mechanisms. Cancer Lett 256:246–258
149. Ji Y, Chen SY, Xiao X (2012) B-blockers: a novel class of antitumor agents. Onco Targets Ther 5:391–401
150. Cole SW (2012) Sood AK (2012) molecular pathways: beta-adrenergic signaling in cancer. Clin Cancer Res 18(5):1201–1206
151. Lutgendorf SK, Cole S, Costanzo E (2003) Stress-related mediators stimulate vascular endothelial growth factor secretion by two ovarian cancer cell lines. Clin Cancer Res 9 (12):4514–4521
152. Palm D, Lang K, Niggemann B (2006) The norepinephrine-driven metastasis development of PC-3 human prostate cancer cells in BALB/c nude mice is inhibited by beta-blockers. Int J Cancer 118 (11):2744–2749
153. Benish M, Bartal I, Goldfarb Y (2008) Perioperative use of beta-blockers and COX-2 inhibitors may improve immune competence and reduce the risk of tumor metastasis. Ann Surg Oncol 15(7):2042–2052
154. Akbar S, Alsharidah MS (2014) Are beta blockers new potential anticancer agents? Asian Pac J Cancer Prev 15(22):9567–9574
155. Melhem-Bertrandt A, Chavez-Macgregor M, Lei X (2011) Beta-blocker use is associated with improved relapse-free survival in patients with triple-negative breast cancer. J Clin Oncol 29(19):2645–2652
156. Grytli HH, Fagerland MW, Fosså SD (2014) Association between use of β-blockers and prostate cancer-specific survival: a cohort study of 3561 prostate cancer patients with high-risk or metastatic disease. Eur Urol 65 (3):635–641
157. Diaz ES, Karlan BY, Li AJ (2012) Impact of beta blockers on epithelial ovarian cancer survival. Gynecol Oncol 127(3):375–378
158. Johannesdottir SA, Schmidt M, Phillips G (2013) Use of β-blockers and mortality following ovarian cancer diagnosis: a population-based cohort study. BMC Cancer 13:85
159. McCourt C, Coleman HG, Murray LJ (2014) Beta-blocker usage after malignant melanoma diagnosis and survival: a population-based nested case-control study. Br J Dermatol 170(4):930–938
160. Shah SM, Carey IM, Owen CG (2011) Does β-adrenoceptor blocker therapy improve cancer survival? Findings from a population-based retrospective cohort study. Br J Clin Pharmacol 72(1):157–161
161. Coleman CI, Baker WL, Kluger J (2008) Antihypertensive medication and their impact on cancer incidence: a mixed treatment comparison meta-analysis of randomized controlled trials. J Hypertens 26(4):622–629
162. Fleisher LA, Fleischmann KE, Auerbach AD (2014) 2014 ACC/AHA guideline on perioperative cardiovascular evaluation and management of patients undergoing noncardiac surgery: a report of the American College of Cardiology/American Heart Association task force on practice guidelines. Circulation 130 (24):2215–2245
163. Chang PY, Huang WY, Lin CL (2015) Propanolol reduces cancer risk: a population-based cohort study. Medicine (Baltimore) 94 (27):e1097
164. Monami M, Filippi L, Ungar A (2013) Further data on beta-blockers and cancer risk: observational study and meta-analysis of randomised clinical trials. Curr Med Res Opin 29 (4):369–378

165. Zhang D, Ma Q, Shen S (2009) Inhibition of pancreatic cancer cell proliferation by propranolol occurs through apoptosis induction: the study of beta-adrenoceptor antagonist's anticancer effect in pancreatic cancer cell. Pancreas 38(1):94–100
166. Guo K, Ma Q, Wang L (2009) Norepinephrine-induced invasion by pancreatic cancer cells is inhibited by propranolol. Oncol Rep 22(4):825–830
167. Pantziarka P, Bouche G, Sukhatme V (2016) Repurposing drugs in oncology (ReDO)—propanolol as an anti-cancer agent. Ecancermedicalscience 10:680
168. Liao X, Che X, Zhao W (2010) The β-adrenoceptor antagonist, propranolol, induces human gastric cancer cell apoptosis and cell cycle arrest via inhibiting nuclear factor κB signaling. Oncol Rep 24(6):1669–1676
169. Ito K, Ito M, Ando A (2017) Simplified intraoperative goal-directed therapy using the FloTrac/Vigileo system: an analysis of its usefulness and safety. Open J Anesthesiol 7 (1):1–14
170. Cannesson M, Musard H, Desebbe O, Boucau C, Simon R, Henaine R (2009) The ability of stroke volume variations obtained with Vigileo/Frotrac system to monitor fluid responsiveness in mechanically ventilated patients. Anesth Analg 108(2):513–517
171. Ramsingh DS, Sanghvi C, Gamboa J, Cannesson M, Applegate RL 2nd (2013) Outcome impact of goal directed fluid therapy during high risk abdominal surgery in Low to moderate risk patients: a randomized controlled trial. J Clin Monit Comput 27 (3):249–257
172. Scheeren TW, Wiesenack C, Gerlach H, Marx G (2013) Goal-directed intraoperative fluid therapy guided by stroke volume and its variation in high-risk surgical patients: a prospective randomized multicentre study. J Clin Monit Comput 27(3):225–233
173. Cannesson M, Le Manach Y, Hofer CK, Goarin JP, Lehot J, Vallet B (2011) Assessing the diagnostic accuracy of pulse pressure variations for the prediction of fluid responsiveness: a "Gray zone" approach. Anesthesiology 115(2):231–241
174. Eng OS, Arlow RL, Moore D (2016) Fluid administration and morbidity in transhiatal esophagectomy. J Surg Res 200(1):91–97
175. Xing X, Gao Y, Wang H (2015) Correlation of fluid balance and postoperative pulmonary complications in patients after esophagectomy for cancer. J Thorac Dis 7 (11):1986–1993
176. Chau EH, Slinger P (2014) Perioperative fluid management for pulmonary resection surgery and esophagectomy. Semin Cardiothorac Vasc Anesth 18(1):36–44
177. Brandstrup B, Tonnesen H, Beier-Holgersen R (2003) Effects of intravenous fluid restriction on postoperative complications: comparisons of two perioperative fluid regimens: a randomized assessor-blinded multicenter trial. Ann Surg 238(5):641–648
178. Nisanevich V, Felsentein I, Almogy G (2005) Effect of intraoperative fluid management on outcome after intraabdominal surgery. Anesthesiology 103(1):25–32
179. Wei S, Tian J, Song X (2008) Association of perioperative fluid balance and adverse surgical outcomes in esophageal cancer and esophagogastric junction cancer. Ann Thorac Surg 86(1):266–272
180. Kita T, Mammoto T, Kishi Y (2002) Fluid management and postoperative respiratory disturbances in patients with transthoracic esophagectomy for carcinoma. J Clin Anesth 14(4):252–256
181. Casado D, Lopez F, Marti R (2010) Perioperative fluid management and major respiratory complications in patients undergoing esophagectomy. Dis Esophagus 23:523–528
182. Goepfert MS, Reuter DA, Akyol D (2007) Goal-directed fluid management reduces vasopressor and catecholamine use in cardiac surgery patients. Intensive Care Med 33 (1):96–103
183. Gan TJ, Soppitt A, Maroof M (2002) Goal-directed intraoperative fluid administration reduces length of hospital stay after major surgery. Anesthesiology 97(4):820–826
184. Pearse R, Dawson D, Fawcett J (2005) Early goal-directed therapy after major surgery reduces complications and duration of hospital stay: a randomized, controlled trial. Crit Care 9(6):R687–R693
185. Donati A, Loggi S, Preiser JC (2007) Goal-directed intraoperative therapy reduces morbidity and length of hospital stay in high-risk surgical patients. Chest 132(6):1817–1824
186. Neal JM, Wilcox RT, Allen HW (2003) Near-total esophagectomy: the influence of standardized multimodal management and intraoperative fluid restriction. Reg Anesth Pain Med 28(4):328–334
187. Pearse RM, Harrison DA, MacDonald N (2014) OPTIMISE study group. Effect of a perioperative, cardiac output-guided

hemodynamic therapy algorithm on outcomes following major gastrointestinal surgery: a randomized clinical trial and systematic review. JAMA 311(21):2181–2190

188. Veelo DP, van Berge Henegouwen MI, Ouwehand KS (2017) Effect of goal-directed therapy on outcome after esophageal surgery: a quality improvement study. PLoS One 12 (3):e0172806
189. Assaad S, Popescu W, Perrino A (2013) Fluid management in thoracic surgery. Curr Opin Anaesthesiol 26(1):31–39
190. Jin J, Min S, Liu D (2018) Clinical and economic impact of goal-directed fluid therapy during elective gastrointestinal surgery. Periop Med 7(22):1–8
191. Hamilton MA, Cecconi M, Rhodes A (2011) A systematic review and meta-analysis on the use of Preemptive hemodynamic intervention to improve postoperative outcomes in moderate and high-risk surgical patients. Anesth Analg 112(6):1392–1402
192. Secher NH (2013) When is enough? Individualized goal-directed fluid therapy for surgery. J Clin Monit Comput 27(3):223–224
193. Kotake Y, Fukuda M, Yamagata A, Iwasaki R, Toyoda D, Sato N (2014) Low molecular weight pentastarch is more effective than crystalloid solution in goal-directed fluid management in patients undergoing major gastrointestinal surgery. J Anesth 28 (2):180–188
194. Yates DR, Davies SJ, Milner HE, Wilson RJ (2014) Crystalloid or colloid for goal-directed fluid therapy in colorectal surgery. Br J Anaesth 112(2):281–289
195. Feldheiser A, Pavlova V, Bonomo T, Jones A, Fotopoulou C, Sehouli J (2013) Balanced crystalloid compared with balanced colloid solution using a goal-directed haemodynamic algorithm. Br J Anaesth 110(2):231–240
196. Ogata T, Nakajima T, Kano K (2016) Multimodal analgesia combined with intravenous administration of acetaminophen in perioperative management of esophagectomy using modified ERAS protocol. J Clin Oncol 34 (4):94

INDEX

Alfred K. Lam (ed.), *Esophageal Squamous Cell Carcinoma: Methods and Protocols*, Methods in Molecular Biology, vol. 2129, https://doi.org/10.1007/978-1-0716-0377-2, © Springer Science+Business Media, LLC, part of Springer Nature 2020

MIX
Papier aus verantwortungsvollen Quellen
Paper from responsible sources
FSC® C105338

If you have any concerns about our products,
you can contact us on
ProductSafety@springernature.com

In case Publisher is established outside the EU,
the EU authorized representative is:
Springer Nature Customer Service Center GmbH
Europaplatz 3, 69115 Heidelberg, Germany

Printed by Libri Plureos GmbH
in Hamburg, Germany